To Jack and Eva
For being so wonderful and sleeping when it really mattered

Commissioning Editor: *Rita Demetriou-Swanwick*
Development Editor: *Veronika Watkins*
Project Manager: *Frances Affleck*
Design Direction: *George Ajayi*
Illustrator: *Graeme Chambers*
Illustration Manager: *Bruce Hogarth*

The Physiotherapist's Pocket Book

ESSENTIAL FACTS AT YOUR FINGERTIPS

Karen Kenyon BSc (Hons), BA (Hons), MCSP

Department of Physiotherapy, East Sussex Hospitals NHS Trust

Jonathan Kenyon BSc (Hons), MCSP

Department of Physiotherapy, Brighton and Sussex University Hospitals NHS Trust

CHURCHILL LIVINGSTONE

ELSEVIER

EDINBURGH LONDON NEW YORK OXFORD PHILADELPHIA ST LOUIS SYDNEY TORONTO 2009

CHURCHILL
LIVINGSTONE
ELSEVIER

An imprint of Elsevier Ltd

1st edition © 2004 Churchill Livingstone

ISBN: 978-0-08-044984-5
Reprinted 2009, 2010, 2011 (twice)

British Library Cataloguing in Publication Data
A catalogue record for this book is available from the British Library

Library of Congress Cataloging in Publication Data
A catalog record for this book is available from the Library of Congress

Notice
Knowledge and best practice in this field are constantly changing. As new research and experience broaden our knowledge, changes in practice, treatment and drug therapy may become necessary or appropriate. Readers are advised to check the most current information provided (i) on procedures featured or (ii) by the manufacturer of each product to be administered, to verify the recommended dose or formula, the method and duration of administration, and contraindications. It is the responsibility of the practitioner, relying on their own experience and knowledge of the patient, to make diagnoses, to determine dosages and the best treatment for each individual patient, and to take all appropriate safety precautions. To the fullest extent of the law, neither the Publisher nor the Authors assume any liability for any injury and/or damage to persons or property arising out or related to any use of the material contained in this book.

The Publisher

The Publisher's policy is to use **paper manufactured from sustainable forests**

Printed in China

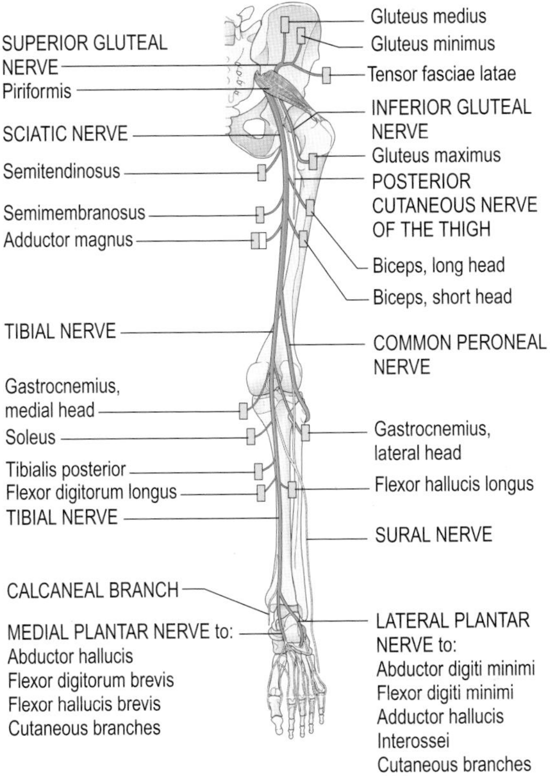
SUPERIOR GLUTEAL NERVE
Piriformis
SCIATIC NERVE
Semitendinosus
Semimembranosus
Adductor magnus
TIBIAL NERVE
Gastrocnemius, medial head
Soleus
Tibialis posterior
Flexor digitorum longus
TIBIAL NERVE
CALCANEAL BRANCH
MEDIAL PLANTAR NERVE to:
Abductor hallucis
Flexor digitorum brevis
Flexor hallucis brevis
Cutaneous branches
Gluteus medius
Gluteus minimus
Tensor fasciae latae
INFERIOR GLUTEAL NERVE
Gluteus maximus
POSTERIOR CUTANEOUS NERVE OF THE THIGH
Biceps, long head
Biceps, short head
COMMON PERONEAL NERVE
Gastrocnemius, lateral head
Flexor hallucis longus
SURAL NERVE
LATERAL PLANTAR NERVE to:
Abductor digiti minimi
Flexor digiti minimi
Adductor hallucis
Interossei
Cutaneous branches

Figure 1.36 Posterior aspect of lower limb.

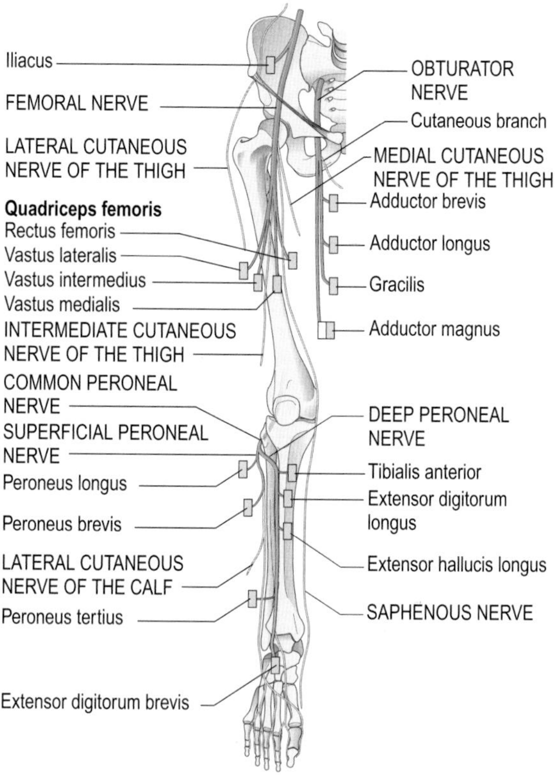
Iliacus
FEMORAL NERVE
LATERAL CUTANEOUS NERVE OF THE THIGH
Quadriceps femoris
Rectus femoris
Vastus lateralis
Vastus intermedius
Vastus medialis
INTERMEDIATE CUTANEOUS NERVE OF THE THIGH
COMMON PERONEAL NERVE
SUPERFICIAL PERONEAL NERVE
Peroneus longus
Peroneus brevis
LATERAL CUTANEOUS NERVE OF THE CALF
Peroneus tertius
Extensor digitorum brevis
OBTURATOR NERVE
Cutaneous branch
MEDIAL CUTANEOUS NERVE OF THE THIGH
Adductor brevis
Adductor longus
Gracilis
Adductor magnus
DEEP PERONEAL NERVE
Tibialis anterior
Extensor digitorum longus
Extensor hallucis longus
SAPHENOUS NERVE

Figure 1.35 Anterior aspect of lower limb.

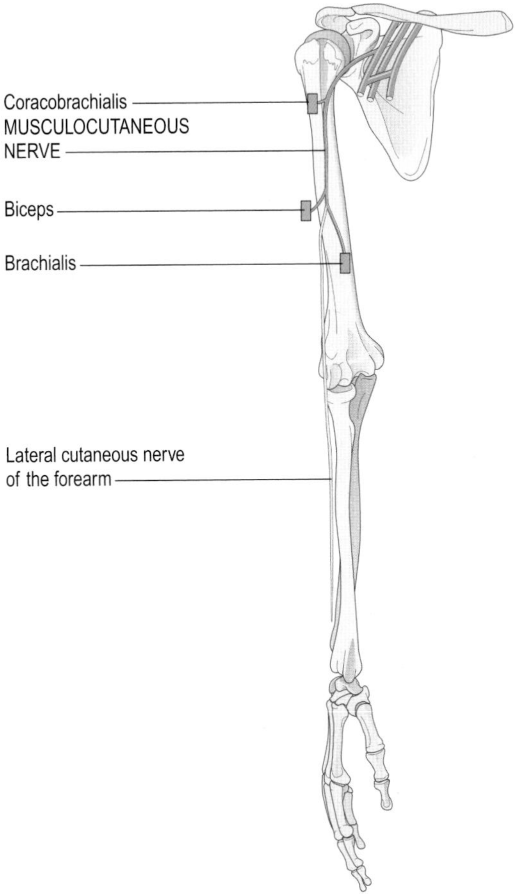
Coracobrachialis
MUSCULOCUTANEOUS
NERVE
Biceps
Brachialis
Lateral cutaneous nerve
of the forearm

Figure 1.34 Musculocutaneous nerve.

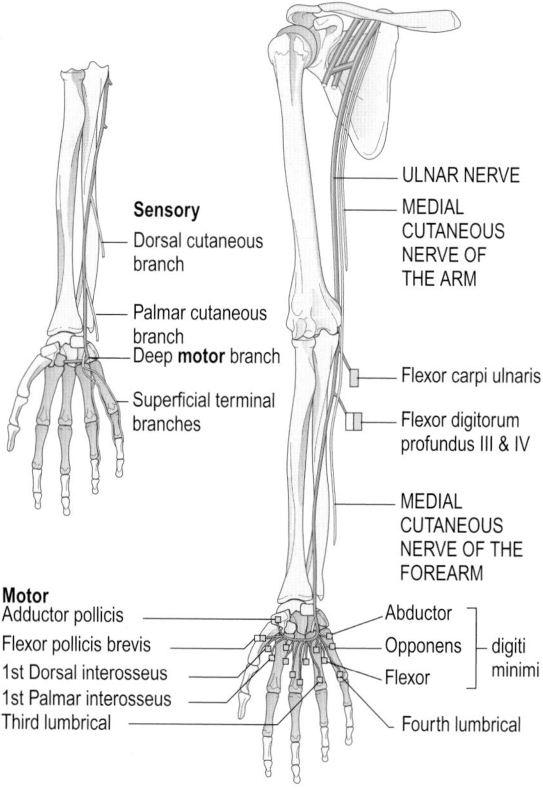
Sensory
Dorsal cutaneous branch
Palmar cutaneous branch
Deep motor branch
Superficial terminal branches
ULNAR NERVE
MEDIAL CUTANEOUS NERVE OF THE ARM
Flexor carpi ulnaris
Flexor digitorum profundus III & IV
MEDIAL CUTANEOUS NERVE OF THE FOREARM
Motor
Adductor pollicis
Flexor pollicis brevis
1st Dorsal interosseus
1st Palmar interosseus
Third lumbrical
Abductor
Opponens
Flexor
digiti minimi
Fourth lumbrical

Figure 1.33 Ulnar nerve.

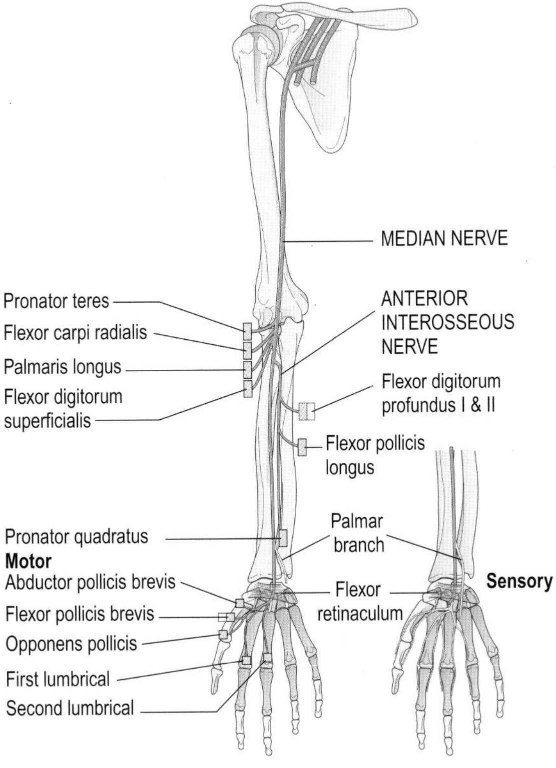
MEDIAN NERVE
Pronator teres
Flexor carpi radialis
Palmaris longus
Flexor digitorum superficialis
ANTERIOR INTEROSSEOUS NERVE
Flexor digitorum profundus I & II
Flexor pollicis longus
Pronator quadratus
Motor
Abductor pollicis brevis
Flexor pollicis brevis
Opponens pollicis
First lumbrical
Second lumbrical
Palmar branch
Flexor retinaculum
Sensory

Figure 1.32 Median nerve.

Peripheral nerve motor innervation (from O'Brien 2000, with permission)

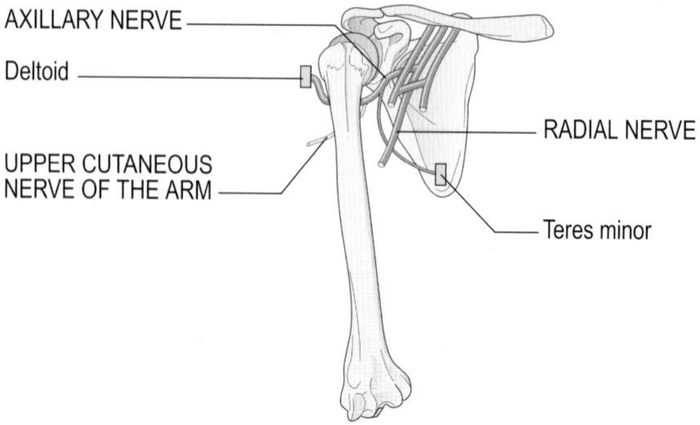

AXILLARY NERVE
Deltoid
UPPER CUTANEOUS
NERVE OF THE ARM
RADIAL NERVE
Teres minor

Figure 1.30 Upper cutaneous nerve of the arm.

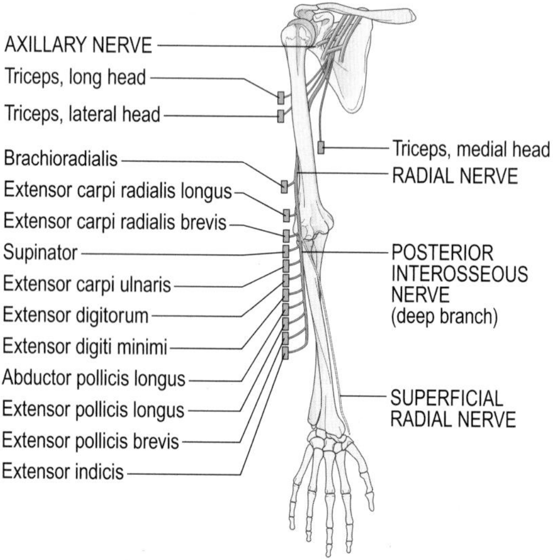

AXILLARY NERVE
Triceps, long head
Triceps, lateral head
Brachioradialis
Extensor carpi radialis longus
Extensor carpi radialis brevis
Supinator
Extensor carpi ulnaris
Extensor digitorum
Extensor digiti minimi
Abductor pollicis longus
Extensor pollicis longus
Extensor pollicis brevis
Extensor indicis
Triceps, medial head
RADIAL NERVE
POSTERIOR
INTEROSSEOUS
NERVE
(deep branch)
SUPERFICIAL
RADIAL NERVE

Figure 1.31 Axillary and radial nerve.

Dermatomes (from O'Brien 2000, with permission)

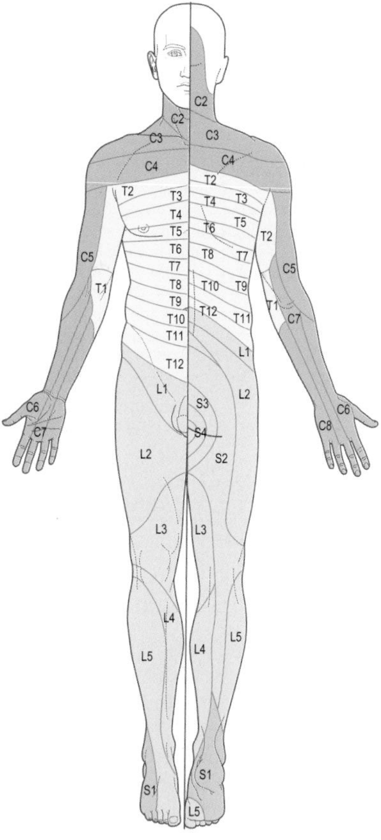
C2
C2
C3
C3
C4
C4
T2
T2
T3
T4
T3
T4
T5
T6
T5
T6
T8
T7
T2
T7
T8
T10
T9
T9
T12
T11
T10
T11
T12
C5
C5
T1
T1
C7
L1
L1
L2
S3
C6
C6
C7
C8
S4
L2
S2
L3
L3
L4
L4
L5
L5
S1
S1
L5

Figure 1.39 Dermatomes of the whole body.

The above illustration is used extensively in clinical practice to define the body's dermatonal patterns. It represents the dermatones as lying between clearly defined boundaries with no overlap between areas. However, it is worth noting that studies have shown that there is significant variability in the pattern of segmental innervation and that the above dermatones do not always describe the patterns found in a large number of patients.

Myotomes

Root	Joint action	Root	Joint action
C1–C2	Cervical flexion	T1	Finger abduction/ adduction
C3	Cervical lateral flexion	T1–L1	No muscle test
C4	Shoulder girdle elevation	L2	Hip flexion
C5	Shoulder abduction	L3	Knee extension
C6	Elbow flexion	L4	Ankle dorsiflexion
C7	Elbow extension	L5	Great toe extension
C8	Thumb extension	S1	Ankle eversion/hip extension/ankle plantarflexion/ knee flexion
		S2	Knee flexion

Reflexes

When testing reflexes, the patient must be relaxed and the muscle placed on a slight stretch. Look for symmetry of response between reflexes on both sides and ensure that both limbs are positioned identically. When a reflex is difficult to elicit, a reinforcement manoeuvre can be used to facilitate a stronger response. This is performed while the reflex is being tested. Usually upper limb reinforcement manoeuvres are used for lower limb reflexes and vice versa. Examples of reinforcement manoeuvres include clenching the teeth or the fists, hooking the hands together by the flexed fingers and pulling one hand against the other (Jendrassik's manoeuvre), crossing the legs at the ankle and pulling one ankle against the other.

Reflexes may be recorded as follows, noting any asymmetry (Petty 2006):

0 or −	absent
1 or −	diminished
2 or +	average/normal
3 or + +	exaggerated
4 or + + +	clonus

An abnormal reflex response may or may not be indicative of a neurological lesion. Findings need to concur with other neurological observations in order to be considered as significant evidence of an abnormality.

An exaggerated response (excessively brisk or prolonged) may simply be caused by anxiety. However, it may also indicate an upper motor neurone lesion, i.e. central damage. Clonus is associated with exaggerated reflexes and also indicates an upper motor neurone lesion. A diminished or absent response may indicate a lower motor neurone lesion, i.e. loss of ankle jerk with lumbosacral disc prolapse.

Deep tendon reflex	Root	Nerve
Biceps jerk	C5–C6	Musculocutaneous
Brachioradialis jerk	C5–C6	Radial
Triceps jerk	C7–C8	Radial
Knee jerk	L3–L4	Femoral
Ankle jerk	S1–S2	Tibial

Other reflexes	Method	Normal response	Abnormal response (indicating possible upper motor neurone lesion)
Plantar (superficial reflex)	Run a blunt object over lateral border of sole of foot from the heel up towards the little toe and across the foot pad	Flexion of toes	Extension of big toe and fanning of other toes (Babinski response)
Clonus (tone)	Apply sudden and sustained dorsiflexion to the ankle	Oscillatory beats may occur but they are not rhythmic or sustained	More than three rhythmic contractions of the plantarflexors
Hoffman reflex	Flick distal phalanx of third or fourth finger downwards	No movement of thumb	Reflex flexion of distal phalanx of thumb

Common locations for palpation of pulses

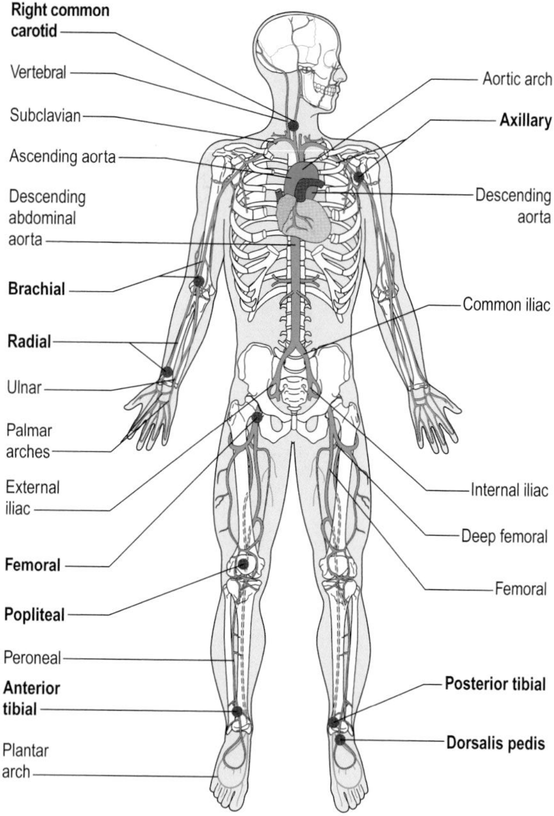
Right common carotid
Vertebral
Subclavian
Ascending aorta
Descending abdominal aorta
Brachial
Radial
Ulnar
Palmar arches
External iliac
Femoral
Popliteal
Peroneal
Anterior tibial
Plantar arch
Aortic arch
Axillary
Descending aorta
Common iliac
Internal iliac
Deep femoral
Femoral
Posterior tibial
Dorsalis pedis

Figure 1.40 Pulse points.

Common carotid	Between the trachea and the sternocleidomastoid muscle
Axillary	Lateral wall of axilla in the groove behind coracobrachialis
Brachial	(a) Between the humerus and biceps on the medial aspect of arm (b) Cubital fossa
Radial	Lateral to flexor carpi radialis tendon
Femoral	In femoral triangle (sartorius, adductor longus and inguinal ligament)
Popliteal	In popliteal fossa. Palpated more easily in prone with the knee flexed about 45°
Anterior tibial	Above level of ankle joint, between tibialis anterior and extensor hallucis longus tendons
Posterior tibial	Posterior aspect of medial malleolus
Dorsalis pedis	Dorsum of foot, between first and second metatarsal bones

References and further reading

Drake R L, Vogl W, Mitchell A W M 2005 Gray's anatomy for students. Churchill Livingstone, Philadelphia

Middleditch A, Oliver J 2005 Functional anatomy of the spine, 2nd edn. Butterworth Heinemann, Edinburgh

O'Brien M D 2000 Guarantors of 'Brain' 1999–2000 (prepared by O'Brien M D). Aids to the examination of the peripheral nervous system, 4th edn. W B Saunders, Edinburgh

Palastanga N, Field D, Soames R 2006 Anatomy and human movement: structure and function, 5th edn. Butterworth-Heinemann, Oxford

Petty N J 2006 Neuromusculoskeletal examination and assessment: a handbook for therapists, 2nd edn. Churchill Livingstone, Edinburgh

Standring S 2004 Gray's anatomy, 39th edn. Churchill Livingstone, Edinburgh

Stone R J, Stone J A 2005 Atlas of skeletal muscles, 5th edn. McGraw-Hill, Boston

Thompson J C 2002 Netter's concise atlas of orthopaedic anatomy. Icon Learning Systems, Teterboro, NJ

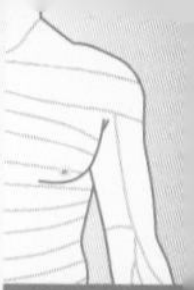

SECTION 2

Musculoskeletal

Muscle innervation chart **49**

Muscles listed by function **54**

Alphabetical listing of muscles **57**

The Medical Research Council scale for muscle power **84**

Trigger points **85**

Normal joint range of movement **97**

Average range of segmental movement **99**

Close packed positions and capsular patterns for selected joints **101**

Common postures **103**

Beighton hypermobility score **108**

Beighton criteria: diagnostic criteria for benign joint hypermobility syndrome **109**

Common classifications of fractures **110**

Classification of ligament and muscle sprains **114**

Common musculoskeletal tests **114**

Neurodynamic tests **130**

Precautions with physical neural examination and management **138**

Nerve pathways **139**

Diagnostic triage for back pain (including red flags) **154**

Psychosocial yellow flags **156**

Musculoskeletal assessment **160**

References and further reading **162**

Muscle innervation chart (data from Standring 2004, with permission)

Upper limb

C1	C2	C3	C4	C5	C6	C7	C8	T1
Inferior and superior oblique								
Rectus capitis posterior major and minor								
Rectus capitis anterior and lateralis								
Longus capitis								
	Longissimus cervicis							
	Longus colli							
		Levator scapulae						
		Trapezius						
		Diaphragm						
		Splenius capitis						
		Scalenus medius						
			Rhomboid major					
			Rhomboid minor					
			Scalenus anterior					
			Longissimus capitis					
				Biceps brachii				
				Brachioradialis				
				Deltoid				
				Infraspinatus				

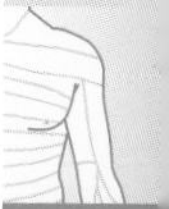

<table>
<tr><th>C1</th><th>C2</th><th>C3</th><th>C4</th><th>C5</th><th>C6</th><th>C7</th><th>C8</th><th>T1</th></tr>
<tr><td></td><td></td><td></td><td></td><td colspan="2">Subscapularis</td><td></td><td></td><td></td></tr>
<tr><td></td><td></td><td></td><td></td><td colspan="2">Supraspinatus</td><td></td><td></td><td></td></tr>
<tr><td></td><td></td><td></td><td></td><td colspan="2">Teres minor</td><td></td><td></td><td></td></tr>
<tr><td></td><td></td><td></td><td></td><td colspan="3">Brachialis</td><td></td><td></td></tr>
<tr><td></td><td></td><td></td><td></td><td colspan="3">Coracobrachialis</td><td></td><td></td></tr>
<tr><td></td><td></td><td></td><td></td><td colspan="3">Serratus anterior</td><td></td><td></td></tr>
<tr><td></td><td></td><td></td><td></td><td colspan="3">Splenius cervicis</td><td></td><td></td></tr>
<tr><td></td><td></td><td></td><td></td><td colspan="3">Teres major</td><td></td><td></td></tr>
<tr><td></td><td></td><td></td><td></td><td colspan="5">Pectoralis major</td></tr>
<tr><td></td><td></td><td></td><td></td><td colspan="5">Pectoralis minor</td></tr>
<tr><td></td><td></td><td></td><td></td><td></td><td colspan="2">Extensor carpi radialis longus</td><td></td><td></td></tr>
<tr><td></td><td></td><td></td><td></td><td></td><td colspan="2">Flexor carpi radialis</td><td></td><td></td></tr>
<tr><td></td><td></td><td></td><td></td><td></td><td colspan="2">Pronator teres</td><td></td><td></td></tr>
<tr><td></td><td></td><td></td><td></td><td></td><td colspan="2">Supinator</td><td></td><td></td></tr>
<tr><td></td><td></td><td></td><td></td><td></td><td colspan="3">Anconeus</td><td></td></tr>
<tr><td></td><td></td><td></td><td></td><td></td><td colspan="3">Latissimus dorsi</td><td></td></tr>
<tr><td></td><td></td><td></td><td></td><td></td><td colspan="3">Scalenus posterior</td><td></td></tr>
<tr><td></td><td></td><td></td><td></td><td></td><td colspan="3">Triceps brachii</td><td></td></tr>
<tr><td></td><td></td><td></td><td></td><td></td><td></td><td colspan="2">Abductor pollicis longus</td><td></td></tr>
<tr><td></td><td></td><td></td><td></td><td></td><td></td><td colspan="2">Extensor carpi radialis brevis</td><td></td></tr>
<tr><td></td><td></td><td></td><td></td><td></td><td></td><td colspan="2">Extensor carpi ulnaris</td><td></td></tr>
<tr><td></td><td></td><td></td><td></td><td></td><td></td><td colspan="2">Extensor digiti minimi</td><td></td></tr>
<tr><td></td><td></td><td></td><td></td><td></td><td></td><td colspan="2">Extensor digitorum</td><td></td></tr>
<tr><td></td><td></td><td></td><td></td><td></td><td></td><td colspan="2">Extensor indicis</td><td></td></tr>
</table>

C1	C2	C3	C4	C5	C6	C7	C8	T1
						Extensor pollicis brevis		
						Extensor pollicis longus		
						Flexor pollicis longus		
						Palmaris longus		
						Pronator quadratus		
						Flexor carpi ulnaris		
							Abductor digiti minimi	
							Abductor pollicis brevis	
							Adductor pollicis	
							Dorsal interossei	
							Flexor digiti minimi brevis	
							Flexor digitorum profundus	
							Flexor digitorum superficialis	
							Flexor pollicis brevis	
							Lumbricals	
							Opponens digiti minimi	
							Opponens pollicis	
							Palmar interossei	

SECTION 2 MUSCULOSKELETAL

Lower limb

<table>
<tr><th>T12</th><th>L1</th><th>L2</th><th>L3</th><th>L4</th><th>L5</th><th>S1</th><th>S2</th><th>S3</th></tr>
<tr><td colspan="5">Quadratus lumborum</td><td></td><td></td><td></td><td></td></tr>
<tr><td></td><td>Psoas minor</td><td></td><td></td><td></td><td></td><td></td><td></td><td></td></tr>
<tr><td></td><td colspan="3">Psoas major</td><td></td><td></td><td></td><td></td><td></td></tr>
<tr><td></td><td></td><td colspan="2">Adductor brevis</td><td></td><td></td><td></td><td></td><td></td></tr>
<tr><td></td><td></td><td colspan="2">Gracilis</td><td></td><td></td><td></td><td></td><td></td></tr>
<tr><td></td><td></td><td colspan="2">Iliacus</td><td></td><td></td><td></td><td></td><td></td></tr>
<tr><td></td><td></td><td colspan="2">Pectineus</td><td></td><td></td><td></td><td></td><td></td></tr>
<tr><td></td><td></td><td colspan="2">Sartorius</td><td></td><td></td><td></td><td></td><td></td></tr>
<tr><td></td><td></td><td colspan="2">Adductor longus</td><td></td><td></td><td></td><td></td><td></td></tr>
<tr><td></td><td></td><td colspan="2">Adductor magnus</td><td></td><td></td><td></td><td></td><td></td></tr>
<tr><td></td><td></td><td colspan="2">Rectus femoris</td><td></td><td></td><td></td><td></td><td></td></tr>
<tr><td></td><td></td><td colspan="2">Vastus intermedius</td><td></td><td></td><td></td><td></td><td></td></tr>
<tr><td></td><td></td><td colspan="2">Vastus lateralis</td><td></td><td></td><td></td><td></td><td></td></tr>
<tr><td></td><td></td><td colspan="2">Vastus medialis</td><td></td><td></td><td></td><td></td><td></td></tr>
<tr><td></td><td></td><td></td><td colspan="2">Obturator externus</td><td></td><td></td><td></td><td></td></tr>
<tr><td></td><td></td><td></td><td colspan="3">Gluteus medius</td><td></td><td></td><td></td></tr>
<tr><td></td><td></td><td></td><td colspan="3">Gluteus minimus</td><td></td><td></td><td></td></tr>
<tr><td></td><td></td><td></td><td colspan="3">Popliteus</td><td></td><td></td><td></td></tr>
<tr><td></td><td></td><td></td><td></td><td colspan="2">Tibialis anterior</td><td></td><td></td><td></td></tr>
<tr><td></td><td></td><td></td><td></td><td colspan="2">Tibialis posterior</td><td></td><td></td><td></td></tr>
<tr><td></td><td></td><td></td><td></td><td colspan="3">Tensor fascia lata</td><td></td><td></td></tr>
<tr><td></td><td></td><td></td><td></td><td></td><td>Extensor hallucis longus</td><td></td><td></td><td></td></tr>
<tr><td></td><td></td><td></td><td></td><td></td><td colspan="2">Extensor digitorum brevis</td><td></td><td></td></tr>
<tr><td></td><td></td><td></td><td></td><td></td><td colspan="2">Extensor digitorum longus</td><td></td><td></td></tr>
</table>

T12	L1	L2	L3	L4	L5	S1	S2	S3
					Gemellus inferior			
					Gemellus superior			
					Obturator internus			
					Peroneus brevis			
					Peroneus longus			
					Peroneus tertius			
					Quadratus femoris			
					Biceps femoris			
					Flexor digitorum longus			
					Flexor hallucis longus			
					Gluteus maximus			
					Piriformis			
					Semimembranosus			
					Semitendinosus			
						Abductor hallucis		
						Flexor digitorum brevis		
						Flexor hallucis brevis		
						Gastrocnemius		
						Plantaris		
						Soleus		
						Abductor digiti minimi		
						Flexor digitorum accessorius		
							Adductor hallucis	
							Dorsal interossei	
							Flexor digiti minimi brevis	
							Lumbricals	
							Plantar interossei	

Muscles listed by function

Head and neck

Flexors: longus colli, longus capitis, rectus capitis anterior, sternocleidomastoid, scalenus anterior
Lateral flexors: erector spinae, rectus capitis lateralis, scalenes (anterior, medius and posterior), splenius cervicis, splenius capitis, trapezius, levator scapulae, sternocleidomastoid
Extensors: levator scapulae, splenius cervicis, trapezius, splenius capitis, semispinalis, superior oblique, sternocleidomastoid, erector spinae, rectus capitis posterior major, rectus capitis posterior minor
Rotators: semispinalis, multifidus, scalenus anterior, splenius cervicis, sternocleidomastoid, splenius capitis, rectus capitis posterior major, inferior oblique

Trunk

Flexors: rectus abdominis, external oblique, internal oblique, psoas minor, psoas major, iliacus
Rotators: multifidus, rotatores, semispinalis, internal oblique, external oblique
Lateral flexors: quadratus lumborum, intertransversarii, external oblique, internal oblique, erector spinae, multifidus
Extensors: quadratus lumborum, multifidus, semispinalis, erector spinae, interspinales, rotatores

Scapula

Retractors: rhomboid minor, rhomboid major, trapezius, levator scapulae
Protractors: serratus anterior, pectoralis minor
Elevators: trapezius, levator scapulae
Depressors: trapezius
Lateral rotators: trapezius, serratus anterior
Medial rotators: rhomboid major, rhomboid minor, pectoralis minor, levator scapulae

Shoulder

Flexors: pectoralis major, deltoid (anterior fibres), biceps brachii (long head), coracobrachialis

Lumbosacral plexus

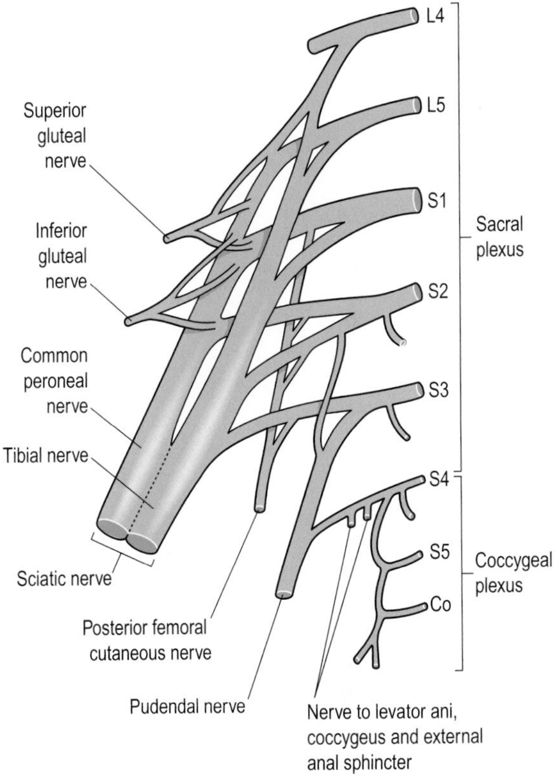

L4
L5
S1
S2
S3
S4
S5
Co
Sacral plexus
Coccygeal plexus
Superior gluteal nerve
Inferior gluteal nerve
Common peroneal nerve
Tibial nerve
Sciatic nerve
Posterior femoral cutaneous nerve
Pudendal nerve
Nerve to levator ani, coccygeus and external anal sphincter

Figure 1.29 Schematic of lumbosacral plexus.

Brachial plexus

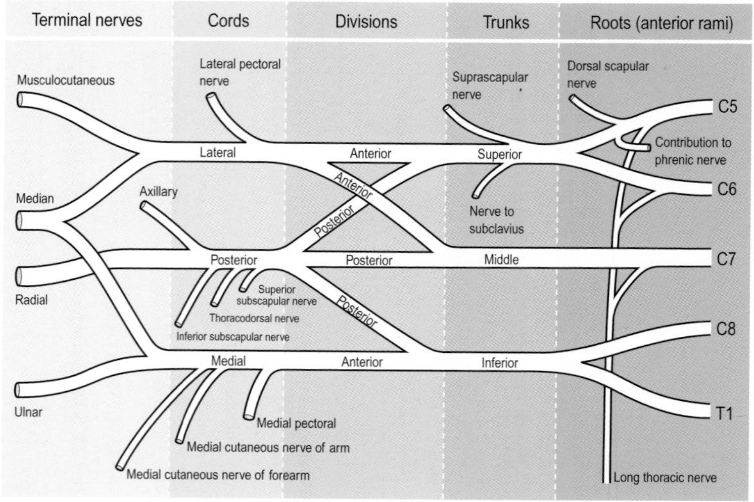

Terminal nerves
Cords
Divisions
Trunks
Roots (anterior rami)
Musculocutaneous
Lateral pectoral nerve
Suprascapular nerve
Dorsal scapular nerve
C5
Lateral
Anterior
Superior
Contribution to phrenic nerve
C6
Median
Axillary
Anterior
Posterior
Nerve to subclavius
Posterior
Posterior
Middle
C7
Radial
Superior subscapular nerve
Thoracodorsal nerve
Inferior subscapular nerve
Posterior
C8
Medial
Anterior
Inferior
Ulnar
T1
Medial pectoral
Medial cutaneous nerve of arm
Medial cutaneous nerve of forearm
Long thoracic nerve

Figure 1.28 Schematic of brachial plexus.

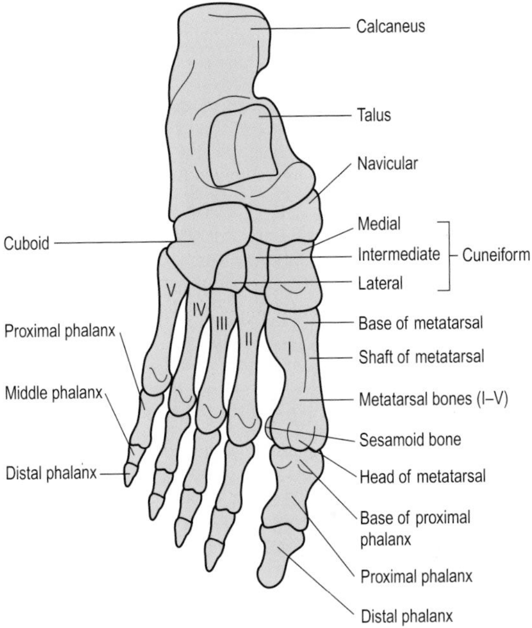
Calcaneus
Talus
Navicular
Medial
Intermediate
Lateral
Cuneiform
Cuboid
V
IV
III
II
I
Base of metatarsal
Shaft of metatarsal
Metatarsal bones (I–V)
Sesamoid bone
Head of metatarsal
Base of proximal phalanx
Proximal phalanx
Distal phalanx
Proximal phalanx
Middle phalanx
Distal phalanx

Figure 1.27 Bones of the right foot.

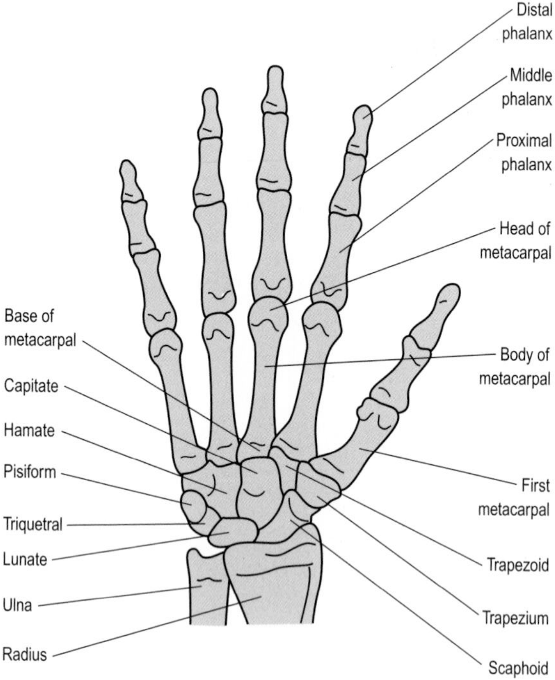
Distal phalanx
Middle phalanx
Proximal phalanx
Head of metacarpal
Base of metacarpal
Body of metacarpal
Capitate
Hamate
Pisiform
Triquetral
Lunate
Ulna
Radius
First metacarpal
Trapezoid
Trapezium
Scaphoid

Figure 1.26 Bones of the right hand.

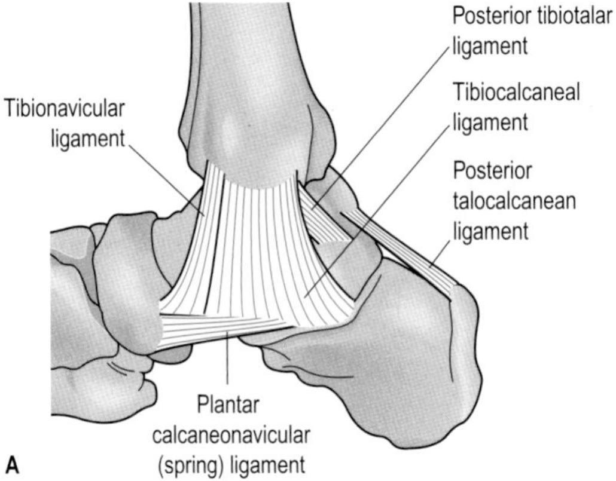
Tibionavicular ligament
Posterior tibiotalar ligament
Tibiocalcaneal ligament
Posterior talocalcanean ligament
Plantar calcaneonavicular (spring) ligament
A

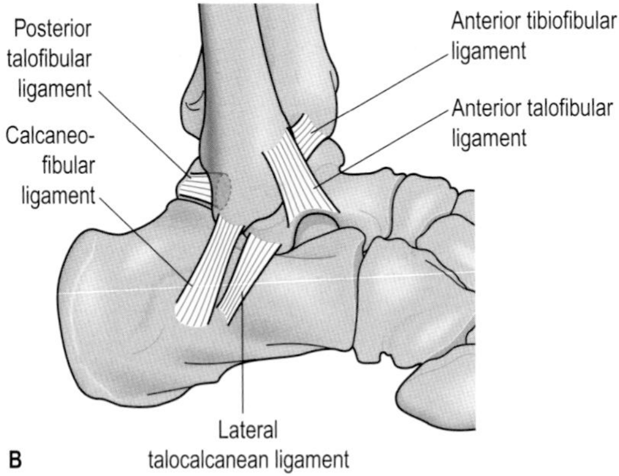
Posterior talofibular ligament
Calcaneo-fibular ligament
Anterior tibiofibular ligament
Anterior talofibular ligament
Lateral talocalcanean ligament
B

Figure 1.25 Ligaments of the ankle joint. **A** Medial. **B** Lateral.

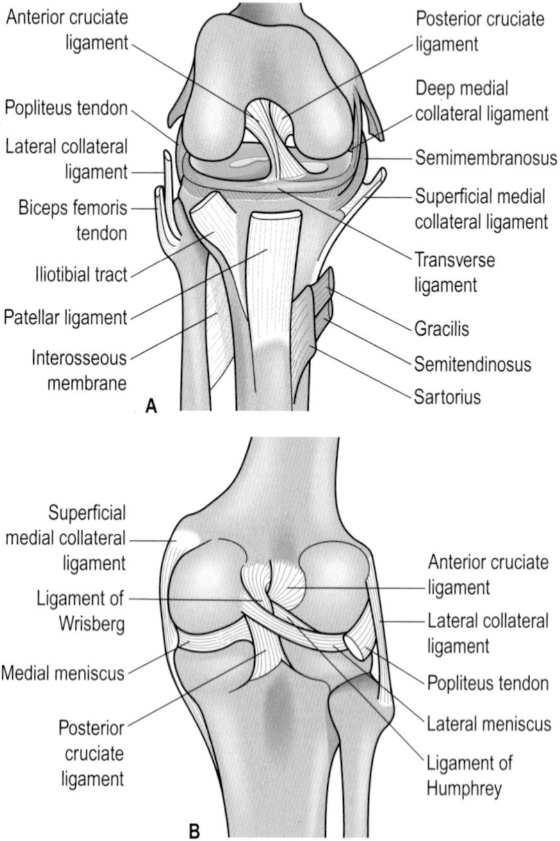

Anterior cruciate ligament
Popliteus tendon
Lateral collateral ligament
Biceps femoris tendon
Iliotibial tract
Patellar ligament
Interosseous membrane
A
Posterior cruciate ligament
Deep medial collateral ligament
Semimembranosus
Superficial medial collateral ligament
Transverse ligament
Gracilis
Semitendinosus
Sartorius
Superficial medial collateral ligament
Ligament of Wrisberg
Medial meniscus
Posterior cruciate ligament
B
Anterior cruciate ligament
Lateral collateral ligament
Popliteus tendon
Lateral meniscus
Ligament of Humphrey

Figure 1.24 Ligaments of the knee joint. **A** Anterior. **B** Posterior.

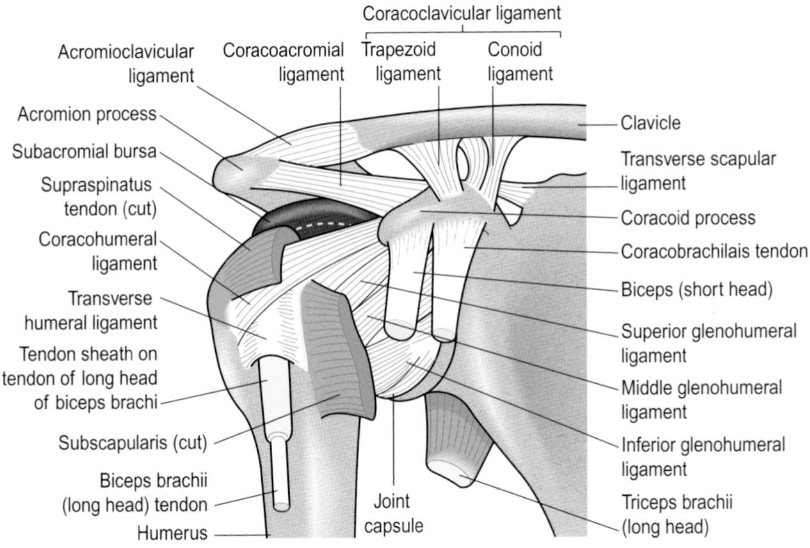
Coracoclavicular ligament
Acromioclavicular ligament
Coracoacromial ligament
Trapezoid ligament
Conoid ligament
Acromion process
Subacromial bursa
Supraspinatus tendon (cut)
Coracohumeral ligament
Transverse humeral ligament
Tendon sheath on tendon of long head of biceps brachi
Subscapularis (cut)
Biceps brachii (long head) tendon
Humerus
Joint capsule
Clavicle
Transverse scapular ligament
Coracoid process
Coracobrachilais tendon
Biceps (short head)
Superior glenohumeral ligament
Middle glenohumeral ligament
Inferior glenohumeral ligament
Triceps brachii (long head)

Figure 1.19 Ligaments of the glenohumeral joint.

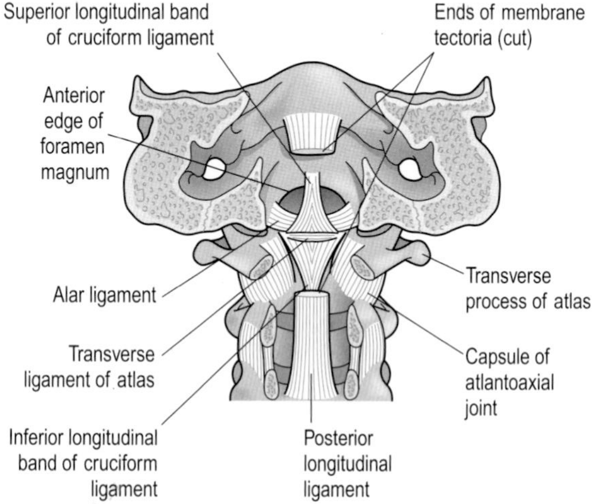
Superior longitudinal band of cruciform ligament
Ends of membrane tectoria (cut)
Anterior edge of foramen magnum
Alar ligament
Transverse process of atlas
Transverse ligament of atlas
Capsule of atlantoaxial joint
Inferior longitudinal band of cruciform ligament
Posterior longitudinal ligament

Figure 1.18 Ligaments of the atlanto-axial and atlanto-occipital joints.

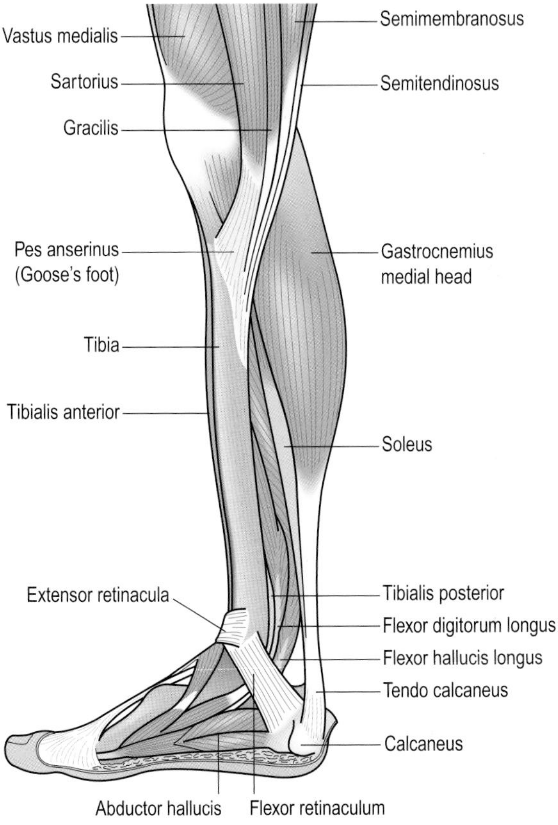
Vastus medialis
Sartorius
Gracilis
Pes anserinus
(Goose's foot)
Tibia
Tibialis anterior
Extensor retinacula
Semimembranosus
Semitendinosus
Gastrocnemius
medial head
Soleus
Tibialis posterior
Flexor digitorum longus
Flexor hallucis longus
Tendo calcaneus
Calcaneus
Abductor hallucis
Flexor retinaculum

Figure 1.17 Muscles of the medial right leg.

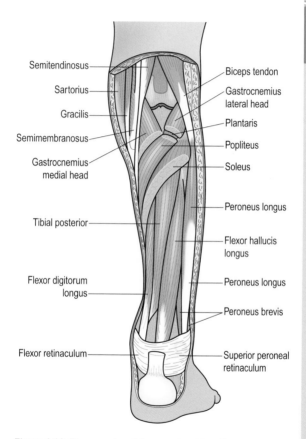

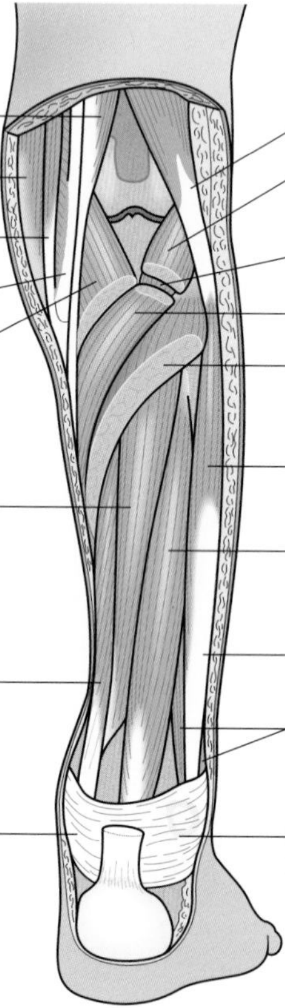
Semitendinosus
Sartorius
Gracilis
Semimembranosus
Gastrocnemius medial head
Tibial posterior
Flexor digitorum longus
Flexor retinaculum
Biceps tendon
Gastrocnemius lateral head
Plantaris
Popliteus
Soleus
Peroneus longus
Flexor hallucis longus
Peroneus longus
Peroneus brevis
Superior peroneal retinaculum

Figure 1.16 Deep muscles of the posterior right calf.

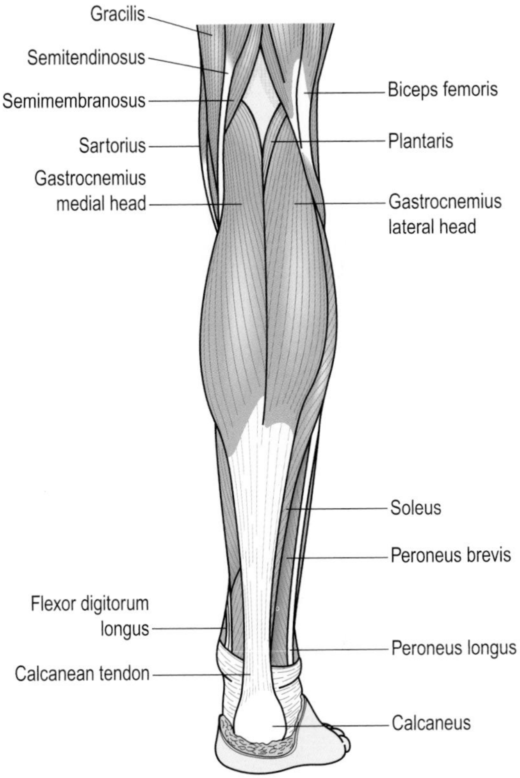
Gracilis
Semitendinosus
Semimembranosus
Sartorius
Gastrocnemius medial head
Biceps femoris
Plantaris
Gastrocnemius lateral head
Soleus
Peroneus brevis
Flexor digitorum longus
Calcanean tendon
Peroneus longus
Calcaneus

Figure 1.15 Superficial muscles of the posterior right calf.

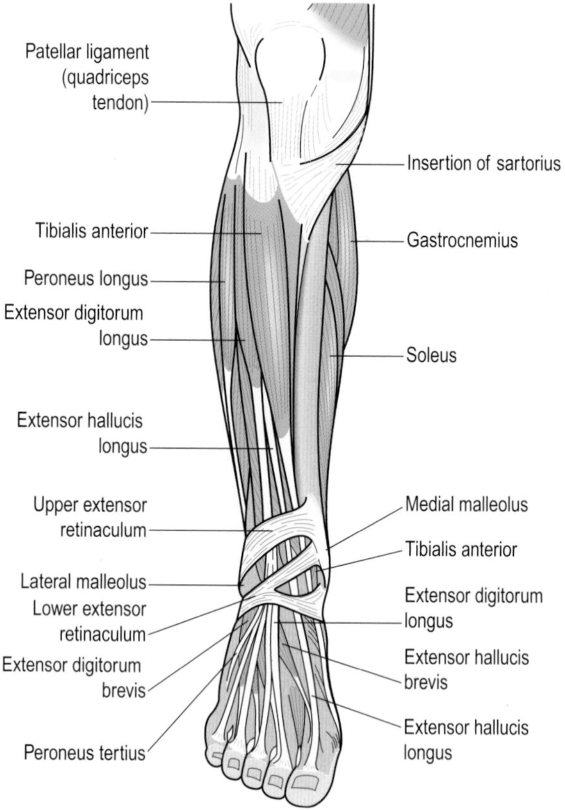
Patellar ligament
(quadriceps
tendon)
Insertion of sartorius
Tibialis anterior
Gastrocnemius
Peroneus longus
Extensor digitorum
longus
Soleus
Extensor hallucis
longus
Upper extensor
retinaculum
Medial malleolus
Tibialis anterior
Lateral malleolus
Lower extensor
retinaculum
Extensor digitorum
longus
Extensor digitorum
brevis
Extensor hallucis
brevis
Extensor hallucis
longus
Peroneus tertius

Figure 1.14 Muscles of the anterior right leg.

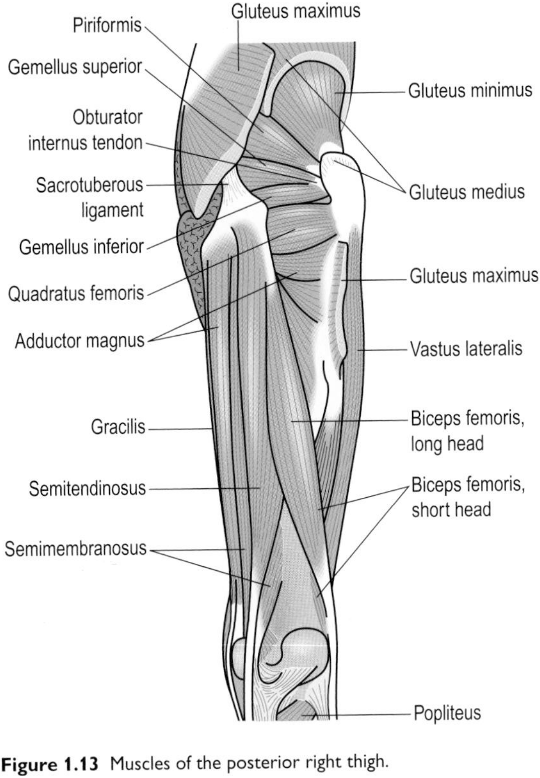
Gluteus maximus
Piriformis
Gemellus superior
Obturator internus tendon
Sacrotuberous ligament
Gemellus inferior
Quadratus femoris
Adductor magnus
Gracilis
Semitendinosus
Semimembranosus
Gluteus minimus
Gluteus medius
Gluteus maximus
Vastus lateralis
Biceps femoris, long head
Biceps femoris, short head
Popliteus

Figure 1.13 Muscles of the posterior right thigh.

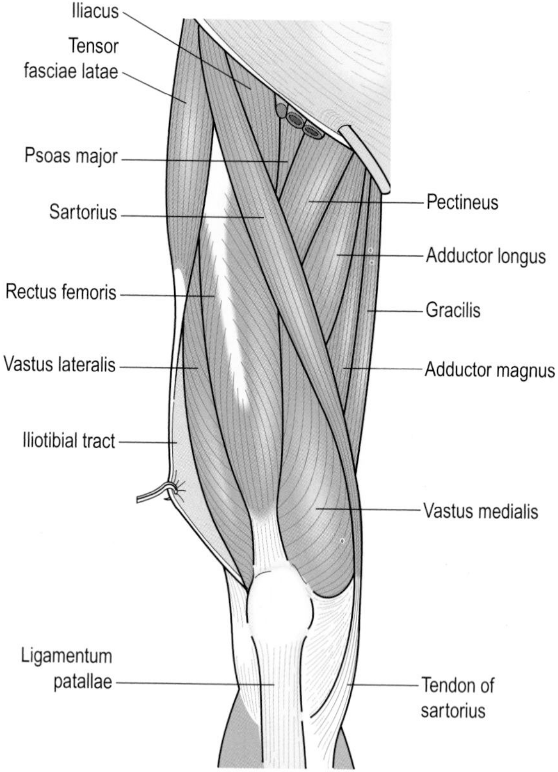
Iliacus
Tensor fasciae latae
Psoas major
Sartorius
Rectus femoris
Vastus lateralis
Iliotibial tract
Ligamentum patallae
Pectineus
Adductor longus
Gracilis
Adductor magnus
Vastus medialis
Tendon of sartorius

Figure 1.12 Superficial muscles of the anterior right thigh.

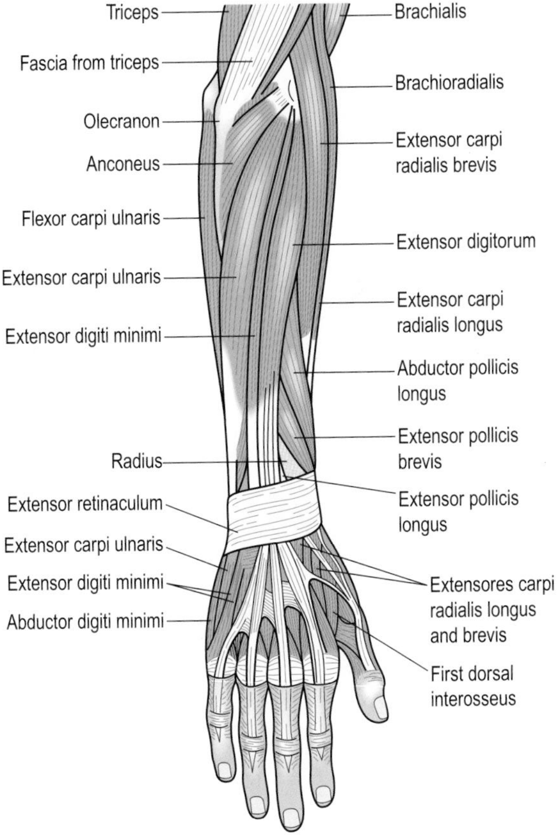
Triceps
Fascia from triceps
Olecranon
Anconeus
Flexor carpi ulnaris
Extensor carpi ulnaris
Extensor digiti minimi
Radius
Extensor retinaculum
Extensor carpi ulnaris
Extensor digiti minimi
Abductor digiti minimi
Brachialis
Brachioradialis
Extensor carpi radialis brevis
Extensor digitorum
Extensor carpi radialis longus
Abductor pollicis longus
Extensor pollicis brevis
Extensor pollicis longus
Extensores carpi radialis longus and brevis
First dorsal interosseus

Figure 1.11 Superficial extensors of the right forearm.

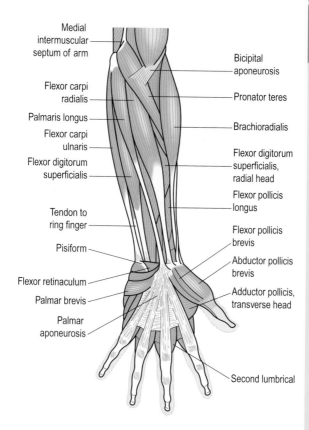

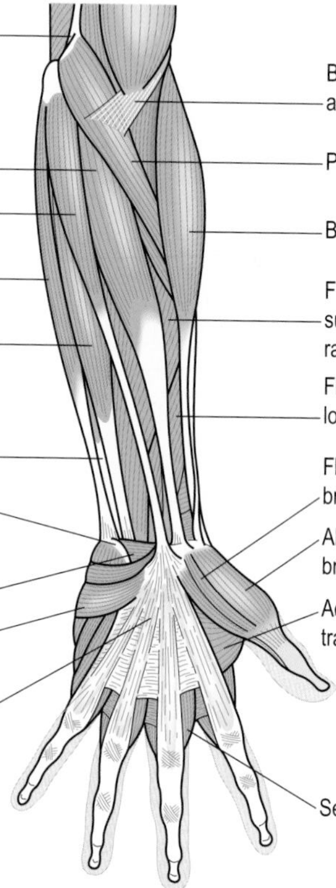
Medial
intermuscular
septum of arm
Flexor carpi
radialis
Palmaris longus
Flexor carpi
ulnaris
Flexor digitorum
superficialis
Tendon to
ring finger
Pisiform
Flexor retinaculum
Palmar brevis
Palmar
aponeurosis
Bicipital
aponeurosis
Pronator teres
Brachioradialis
Flexor digitorum
superficialis,
radial head
Flexor pollicis
longus
Flexor pollicis
brevis
Abductor pollicis
brevis
Adductor pollicis,
transverse head
Second lumbrical

Figure 1.10 Superficial flexors of the left forearm.

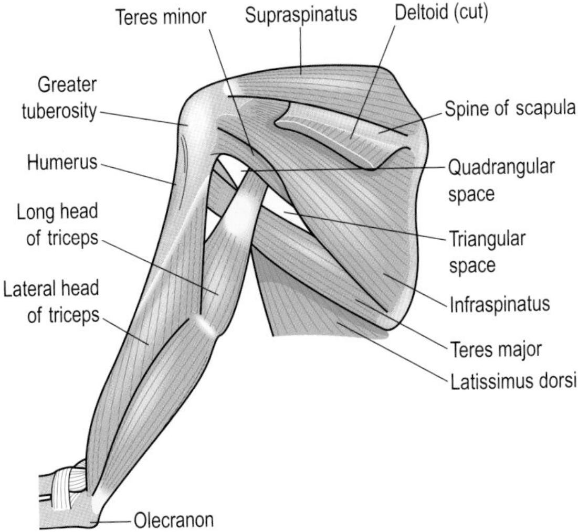
Teres minor
Supraspinatus
Deltoid (cut)
Greater tuberosity
Spine of scapula
Humerus
Quadrangular space
Long head of triceps
Triangular space
Lateral head of triceps
Infraspinatus
Teres major
Latissimus dorsi
Olecranon

Figure 1.9 Muscles of the posterior scapula and upper arm. Left side.

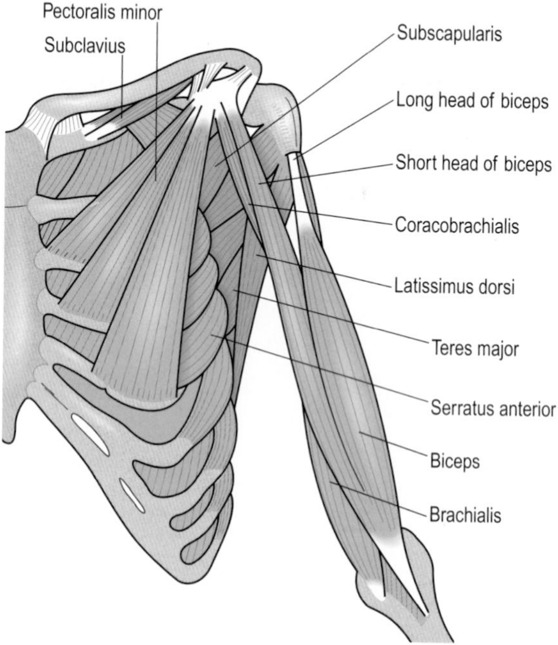
Pectoralis minor
Subclavius
Subscapularis
Long head of biceps
Short head of biceps
Coracobrachialis
Latissimus dorsi
Teres major
Serratus anterior
Biceps
Brachialis

Figure 1.8 Deep muscles of the anterior chest and upper arm. Left side.

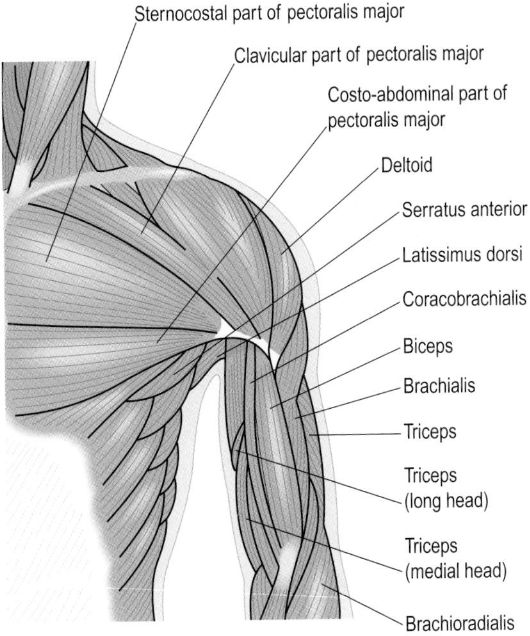
Sternocostal part of pectoralis major
Clavicular part of pectoralis major
Costo-abdominal part of pectoralis major
Deltoid
Serratus anterior
Latissimus dorsi
Coracobrachialis
Biceps
Brachialis
Triceps
Triceps (long head)
Triceps (medial head)
Brachioradialis

Figure 1.7 Superficial muscles of the anterior chest and arm. Left side.

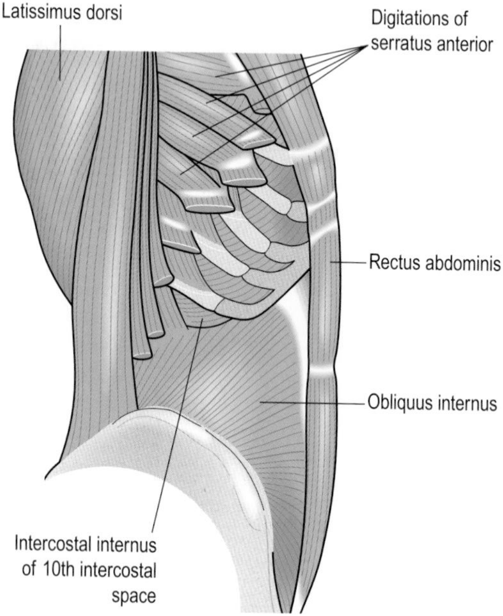
Latissimus dorsi
Digitations of serratus anterior
Rectus abdominis
Obliquus internus
Intercostal internus of 10th intercostal space

Figure 1.6 Muscles of the right side of the trunk.

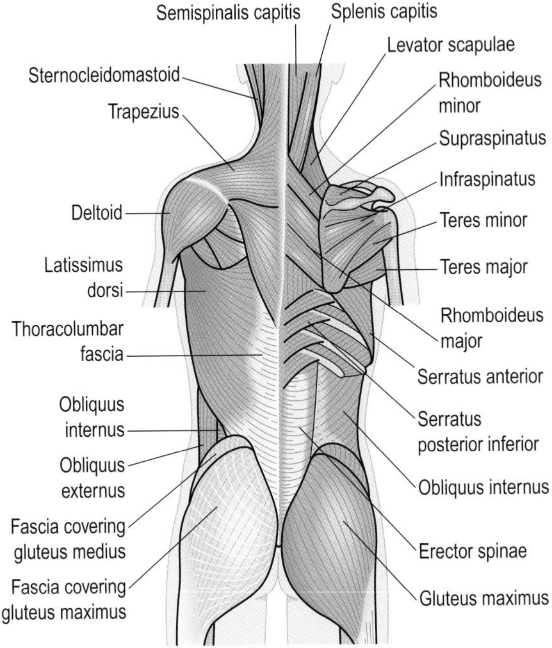
Semispinalis capitis
Splenis capitis
Levator scapulae
Sternocleidomastoid
Rhomboideus minor
Trapezius
Supraspinatus
Infraspinatus
Deltoid
Teres minor
Latissimus dorsi
Teres major
Rhomboideus major
Thoracolumbar fascia
Serratus anterior
Obliquus internus
Serratus posterior inferior
Obliquus externus
Obliquus internus
Fascia covering gluteus medius
Erector spinae
Fascia covering gluteus maximus
Gluteus maximus

Figure 1.5 Superficial muscles of the back, neck and trunk.

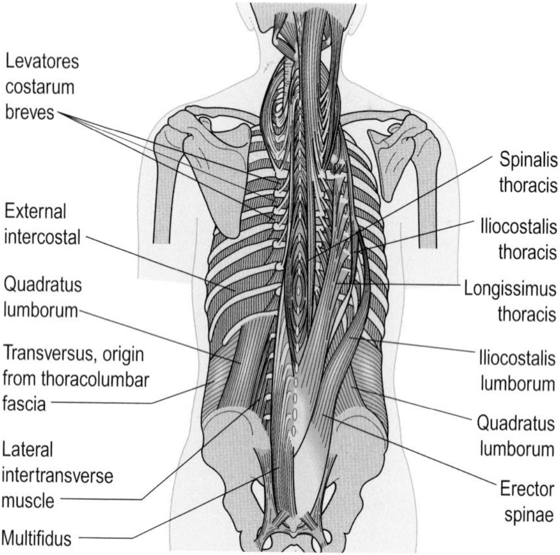
Levatores costarum breves
External intercostal
Quadratus lumborum
Transversus, origin from thoracolumbar fascia
Lateral intertransverse muscle
Multifidus
Spinalis thoracis
Iliocostalis thoracis
Longissimus thoracis
Iliocostalis lumborum
Quadratus lumborum
Erector spinae

Figure 1.4 Deep muscles of the back.

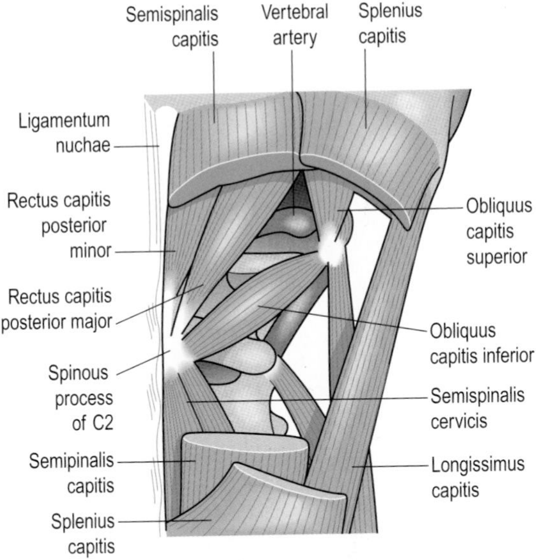
Semispinalis capitis
Vertebral artery
Splenius capitis
Ligamentum nuchae
Rectus capitis posterior minor
Rectus capitis posterior major
Spinous process of C2
Semipinalis capitis
Splenius capitis
Obliquus capitis superior
Obliquus capitis inferior
Semispinalis cervicis
Longissimus capitis

Figure 1.3 Posterior and lateral muscles of the neck.

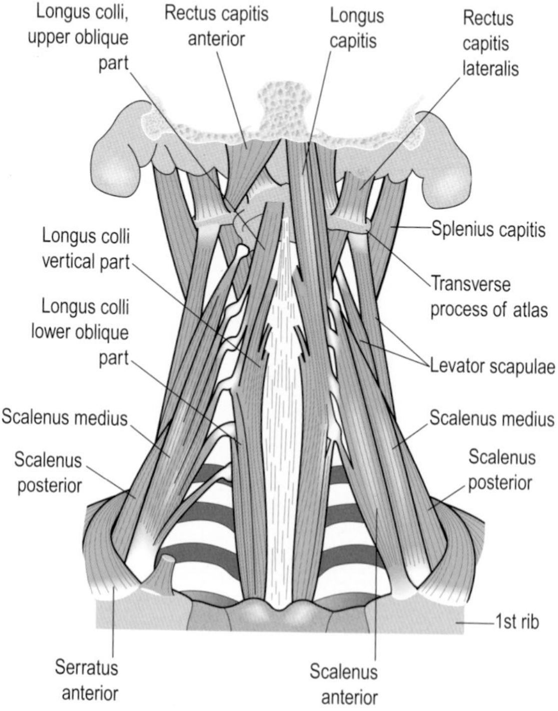
Longus colli, upper oblique part
Rectus capitis anterior
Longus capitis
Rectus capitis lateralis
Splenius capitis
Longus colli vertical part
Transverse process of atlas
Longus colli lower oblique part
Levator scapulae
Scalenus medius
Scalenus medius
Scalenus posterior
Scalenus posterior
1st rib
Serratus anterior
Scalenus anterior

Figure 1.2 Anterior and lateral muscles of the neck.

Musculoskeletal anatomy illustrations

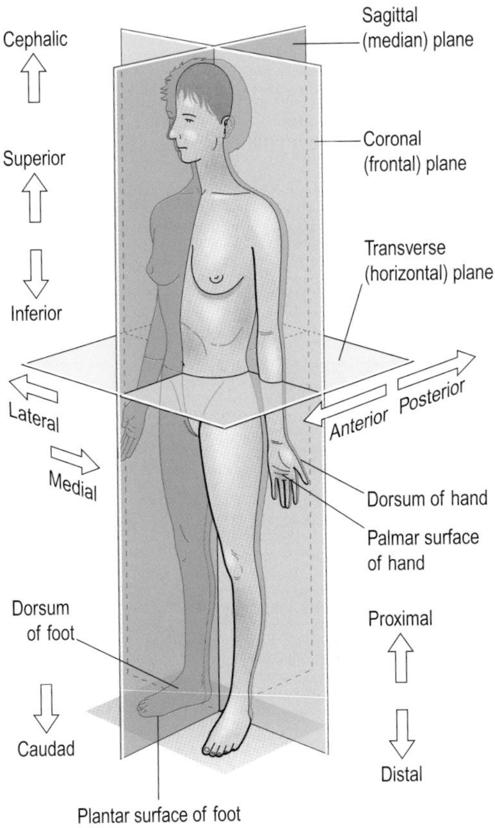
Cephalic
Superior
Inferior
Lateral
Medial
Dorsum of foot
Caudad
Plantar surface of foot
Sagittal (median) plane
Coronal (frontal) plane
Transverse (horizontal) plane
Anterior
Posterior
Dorsum of hand
Palmar surface of hand
Proximal
Distal

Figure 1.1 Anatomical position showing cardinal planes and directional terminology.

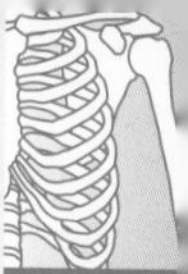

SECTION 1

Neuromusculoskeletal anatomy

Musculoskeletal anatomy illustrations **2**

Brachial plexus **29**

Lumbosacral plexus **30**

Peripheral nerve motor innervation **31**

Peripheral nerve sensory innervation **37**

Dermatomes **39**

Myotomes **40**

Reflexes **40**

Common locations for palpation of pulses **43**

References and further reading **44**

Acknowledgements

Once again we are indebted to all our colleagues, friends and students for the feedback, advice and encouragement they have offered over the past few years. If we could name them all this would definitely not be a pocket-sized book. Hopefully, they know who they are and appreciate how grateful we are for all their help.

We would like to say a special thanks to the Association of Chartered Physiotherapists in Respiratory Care (ACPRC) for working so hard to meet our deadline, Janet Deane for her contribution to the pathology section and Domenico Spina for reviewing the pharmacology section. We would also like to give our heartfelt thanks to the team at Elsevier – Rita, Veronika, Siobhan and Heidi – for all their support and understanding.

Preface

This edition of *The Physiotherapist's Pocket Book* was written with all physiotherapists in mind. We were overwhelmed by the favourable response to the first edition and, thanks to all the invaluable feedback we have had from colleagues, students and academics, have endeavoured to make this edition as comprehensive and as useful as possible to all clinicians.

We have tried to ensure that the contents reflect the dynamic and ever-changing profession we work in. We felt that the book could be expanded without compromising its portability and so have included more definitions of common pathologies, drugs, musculoskeletal special tests and assessment tools, as well as additional anatomical illustrations. The content has also been reorganized and new sections have been created to make it easier to find the relevant information.

We hope that this book continues to fulfil its main purpose – to provide quick and easy access to essential clinical information during everyday practice.

Karen and Jonathan Kenyon
East Sussex, 2009

Modes of mechanical ventilation 212
Cardiorespiratory monitoring 215
ECGs 218
Biochemical and haematological studies 225
Treatment techniques 232
Tracheostomies 237
Respiratory assessment 240
References and further reading 242

Section 5 Pathology 245

Alphabetical listing of pathologies 246
Diagnostic imaging 281
Electrodiagnostic tests 283

Section 6 Pharmacology 285

Drug classes 286
A–Z of drugs 289
Prescription abbreviations 316
Further reading 316

Section 7 Appendices 317

Maitland symbols 318
Grades of mobilization/manipulation 319
Abbreviations 319
Prefixes and suffixes 331
Adult basic life support 336
Paediatric basic life support 337
Conversions and units 338
Laboratory values 339
Physiotherapy management of the spontaneously breathing, acutely breathless patient 342

Index 345

Inside back cover
Normal values
The Glasgow Coma Scale

Common classifications of fractures 110
Classification of ligament and muscle sprains 114
Common musculoskeletal tests 114
Neurodynamic tests 130
Precautions with physical neural examination and management 138
Nerve pathways 139
Diagnostic triage for back pain (including red flags) 154
Psychosocial yellow flags 156
Musculoskeletal assessment 160
References and further reading 162

Section 3 Neurology 165

Neuroanatomy illustrations 166
Signs and symptoms of cerebrovascular lesions 171
Signs and symptoms of injury to the lobes of the brain 175
Signs and symptoms of haemorrhage to other areas of the brain 178
Cranial nerves 179
Key features of upper and lower motor neurone lesions 183
Functional implications of spinal cord injury 184
Glossary of neurological terms 187
Neurological tests 189
Modified Ashworth scale 192
Neurological assessment 192
References and further reading 195

Section 4 Respiratory 197

Respiratory anatomy illustrations 198
Respiratory volumes and capacities 201
Chest X-rays 203
Auscultation 206
Percussion note 208
Interpreting blood gas values 208
Respiratory failure 210
Nasal cannula 211
Sputum analysis 211

Contents

Preface ix
Acknowledgements xi

Section 1 Neuromusculoskeletal anatomy 1

Musculoskeletal anatomy illustrations 2
Brachial plexus 29
Lumbosacral plexus 30
Peripheral nerve motor innervation 31
Peripheral nerve sensory innervation 37
Dermatomes 39
Myotomes 40
Reflexes 40
Common locations for palpation of pulses 43
References and further reading 44

Section 2 Musculoskeletal 47

Muscle innervation chart 49
Muscles listed by function 54
Alphabetical listing of muscles 57
The Medical Research Council scale for muscle power 84
Trigger points 85
Normal joint range of movement 97
Average range of segmental movement 99
Close packed positions and capsular patterns for selected joints 101
Common postures 103
Beighton hypermobility score 108
Beighton criteria: diagnostic criteria for benign joint hypermobility syndrome 109

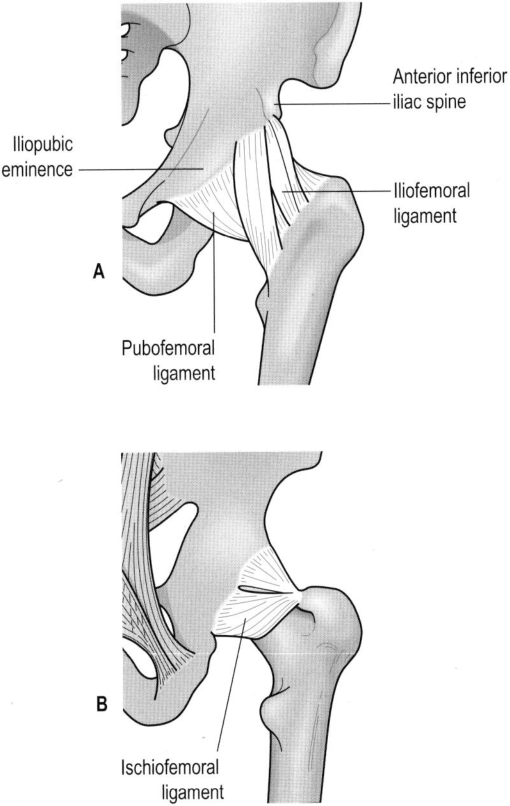
Anterior inferior
iliac spine
Iliopubic
eminence
Iliofemoral
ligament
A
Pubofemoral
ligament
B
Ischiofemoral
ligament

Figure 1.23 Ligaments of the hip joint. **A** Anterior. **B** Posterior.

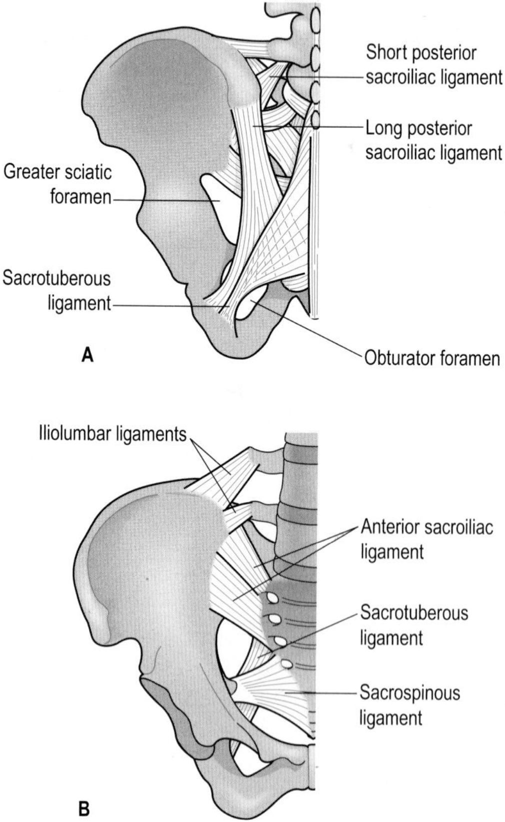
Short posterior sacroiliac ligament
Long posterior sacroiliac ligament
Greater sciatic foramen
Sacrotuberous ligament
A
Obturator foramen
Iliolumbar ligaments
Anterior sacroiliac ligament
Sacrotuberous ligament
Sacrospinous ligament
B

Figure 1.22 Ligaments of the sacroiliac joint. **A** Posterior. **B** Anterior.

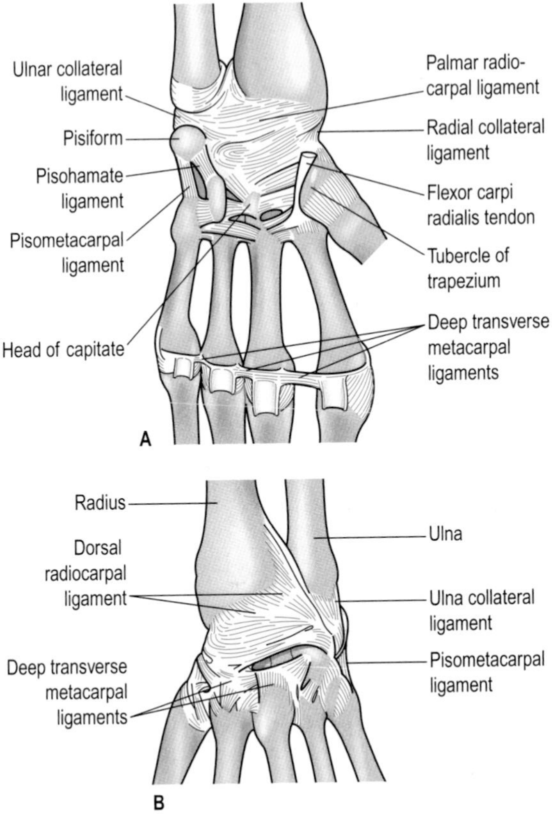
Ulnar collateral ligament
Pisiform
Pisohamate ligament
Pisometacarpal ligament
Head of capitate
Palmar radio-carpal ligament
Radial collateral ligament
Flexor carpi radialis tendon
Tubercle of trapezium
Deep transverse metacarpal ligaments
A
Radius
Dorsal radiocarpal ligament
Deep transverse metacarpal ligaments
Ulna
Ulna collateral ligament
Pisometacarpal ligament
B

Figure 1.21 Ligaments of the wrist and hand joints. **A** Anterior. **B** Posterior.

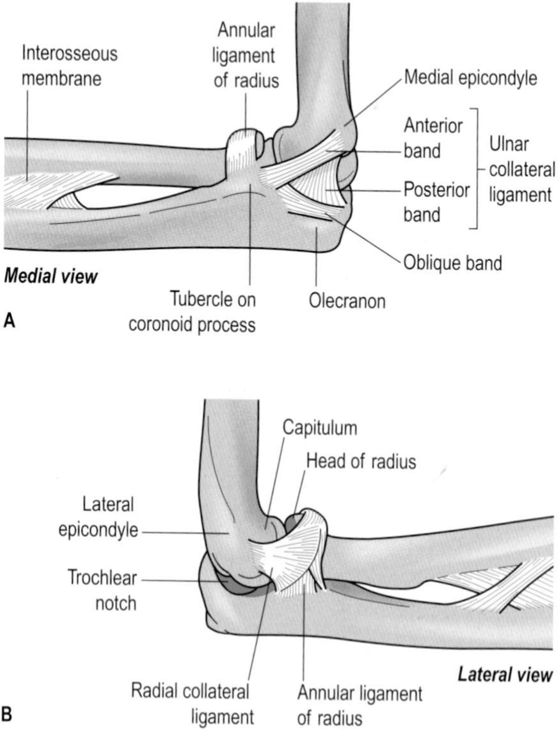
Interosseous membrane
Annular ligament of radius
Medial epicondyle
Anterior band
Posterior band
Ulnar collateral ligament
Oblique band
Medial view
Tubercle on coronoid process
Olecranon
A
Capitulum
Head of radius
Lateral epicondyle
Trochlear notch
Lateral view
Radial collateral ligament
Annular ligament of radius
B

Figure 1.20 Ligaments of the elbow joint. **A** Medial. **B** Lateral.

Peripheral nerve sensory innervation

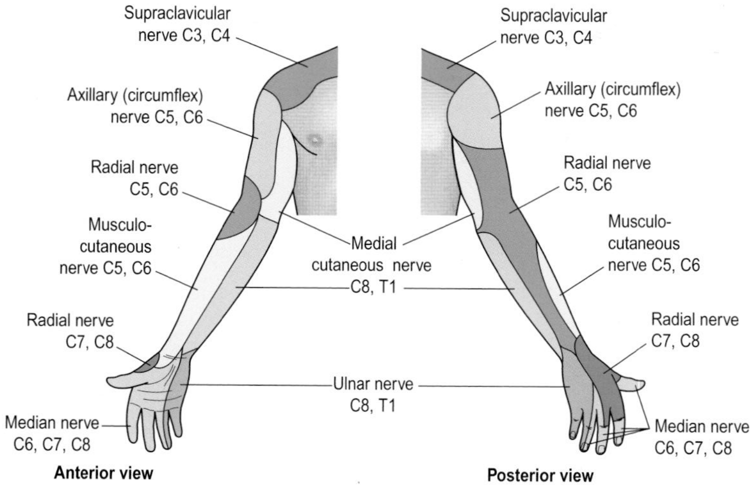
Supraclavicular
nerve C3, C4
Axillary (circumflex)
nerve C5, C6
Radial nerve
C5, C6
Musculo-
cutaneous
nerve C5, C6
Radial nerve
C7, C8
Median nerve
C6, C7, C8
Anterior view
Medial
cutaneous nerve
C8, T1
Ulnar nerve
C8, T1
Supraclavicular
nerve C3, C4
Axillary (circumflex)
nerve C5, C6
Radial nerve
C5, C6
Musculo-
cutaneous
nerve C5, C6
Radial nerve
C7, C8
Median nerve
C6, C7, C8
Posterior view

Figure 1.37 Cutaneous distribution of the upper limb.

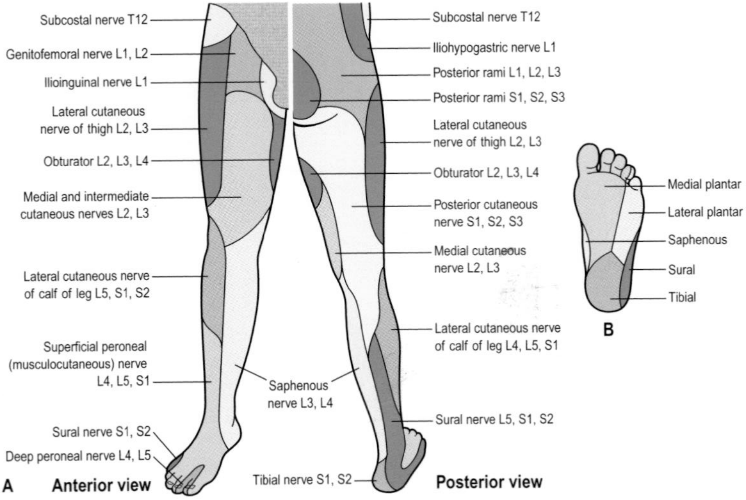
Subcostal nerve T12
Genitofemoral nerve L1, L2
Ilioinguinal nerve L1
Lateral cutaneous nerve of thigh L2, L3
Obturator L2, L3, L4
Medial and intermediate cutaneous nerves L2, L3
Lateral cutaneous nerve of calf of leg L5, S1, S2
Superficial peroneal (musculocutaneous) nerve L4, L5, S1
Sural nerve S1, S2
Deep peroneal nerve L4, L5
A
Anterior view
Saphenous nerve L3, L4
Tibial nerve S1, S2
Subcostal nerve T12
Iliohypogastric nerve L1
Posterior rami L1, L2, L3
Posterior rami S1, S2, S3
Lateral cutaneous nerve of thigh L2, L3
Obturator L2, L3, L4
Posterior cutaneous nerve S1, S2, S3
Medial cutaneous nerve L2, L3
Lateral cutaneous nerve of calf of leg L4, L5, S1
Sural nerve L5, S1, S2
Posterior view
Medial plantar
Lateral plantar
Saphenous
Sural
Tibial
B

Figure 1.38 Cutaneous distribution of (**A**) the lower limb and (**B**) the foot.

Extensors: latissimus dorsi, teres major, pectoralis major, deltoid (posterior fibres), triceps (long head)
Abductors: supraspinatus, deltoid (middle fibres)
Adductors: coracobrachialis, pectoralis major, latissimus dorsi, teres major
Medial rotators: subscapularis, teres major, latissimus dorsi, pectoralis major, deltoid (anterior fibres)
Lateral rotators: teres minor, infraspinatus, deltoid (posterior fibres)

Elbow

Flexors: biceps brachii, brachialis, brachioradialis, pronator teres
Extensors: triceps brachii, anconeus
Pronators: pronator teres, pronator quadratus
Supinators: supinator, biceps brachii

Wrist

Flexors: flexor carpi ulnaris, flexor carpi radialis, palmaris longus, flexor digitorum superficialis, flexor digitorum profundus, flexor pollicis longus
Extensors: extensor carpi radialis longus, extensor carpi radialis brevis, extensor carpi ulnaris, extensor digitorum, extensor indicis, extensor digiti minimi, extensor pollicis longus, extensor pollicis brevis
Ulnar deviation: flexor carpi ulnaris, extensor carpi ulnaris
Radial deviation: flexor carpi radialis, extensor carpi radialis longus, extensor carpi radialis brevis, abductor pollicis longus, extensor pollicis longus, extensor pollicis brevis

Fingers

Flexors: flexor digitorum superficialis, flexor digitorum profundus, lumbricals, flexor digiti minimi brevis
Extensors: extensor digitorum, extensor digiti minimi, extensor indicis, interossei, lumbricals
Abductors: dorsal interossei, abductor digiti minimi, opponens digiti minimi
Adductors: palmar interossei

Thumb

Flexors: flexor pollicis longus, flexor pollicis brevis
Extensors: extensor pollicis longus, extensor pollicis brevis, abductor pollicis longus
Abductors: abductor pollicis longus, abductor pollicis brevis
Adductors: adductor pollicis
Opposition: opponens pollicis

Hip

Flexors: psoas major, iliacus, rectus femoris, sartorius, pectineus
Extensors: gluteus maximus, semitendinosus, semimembranosus, biceps femoris
Abductors: gluteus maximus, gluteus medius, gluteus minimus, tensor fascia lata, sartorius, piriformis
Adductors: adductor magnus, adductor longus, adductor brevis, gracilis, pectineus
Medial rotators: gluteus medius, gluteus minimus, tensor fascia lata
Lateral rotators: gluteus maximus, piriformis, obturator internus, gemellus superior, gemellus inferior, quadratus femoris, obturator externus, sartorius

Knee

Flexors: semitendinosus, semimembranosus, biceps femoris, gastrocnemius, gracilis, sartorius, plantaris, popliteus
Extensors: rectus femoris, vastus lateralis, vastus intermedius, vastus medialis, tensor fascia lata
Tibial lateral rotators: biceps femoris
Tibial medial rotators: semitendinosus, semimembranosus, gracilis, sartorius, popliteus

Ankle

Plantarflexors: gastrocnemius, soleus, plantaris, peroneus longus, tibialis posterior, flexor digitorum longus, flexor hallucis longus, peroneus brevis
Dorsiflexors: tibialis anterior, extensor digitorum longus, extensor hallucis longus, peroneus tertius

Invertors: tibialis anterior, tibialis posterior
Evertors: peroneus longus, peroneus tertius, peroneus brevis

Toes

Flexors: flexor digitorum longus, flexor digitorum accessorius, flexor digitorum brevis, flexor hallucis longus, flexor hallucis brevis, flexor digiti minimi brevis, interossei, lumbricals, abductor hallucis
Extensors: extensor hallucis longus, extensor digitorum longus, extensor digitorum brevis, lumbricals, interossei
Abductors: abductor hallucis, abductor digiti minimi, dorsal interossei
Adductors: adductor hallucis, plantar interossei

Alphabetical listing of muscles

Abductor digiti minimi (foot)

Action: abducts fifth toe
Origin: calcaneal tuberosity, plantar aponeurosis, intermuscular septum
Insertion: lateral side of base of proximal phalanx of fifth toe
Nerve: lateral plantar nerve (S1–S3)

Abductor digiti minimi (hand)

Action: abducts little finger
Origin: pisiform, tendon of flexor carpi ulnaris, pisohamate ligament
Insertion: ulnar side of base of proximal phalanx of little finger
Nerve: ulnar nerve (C8, T1)

Abductor hallucis

Action: abducts and flexes great toe
Origin: flexor retinaculum, calcaneal tuberosity, plantar aponeurosis, intermuscular septum
Insertion: medial side of base of proximal phalanx of great toe
Nerve: medial plantar nerve (S1, S2)

Abductor pollicis brevis

Action: abducts thumb
Origin: flexor retinaculum, tubercles of scaphoid and trapezium, tendon of abductor pollicis longus
Insertion: radial side of base of proximal phalanx of thumb
Nerve: median nerve (C8, T1)

Abductor pollicis longus

Action: abducts and extends thumb, abducts wrist
Origin: upper part of posterior surface of ulna, middle third of posterior surface of radius, interosseous membrane
Insertion: radial side of first metacarpal base, trapezium
Nerve: posterior interosseous nerve (C7, C8)

Adductor brevis

Action: adducts hip
Origin: external aspect of body and inferior ramus of pubis
Insertion: upper half of linea aspera
Nerve: obturator nerve (L2, L3)

Adductor hallucis

Action: adducts great toe
Origin: oblique head – bases of second to fourth metatarsal, sheath of peroneus longus tendon; transverse head – plantar metatarsophalangeal ligaments of lateral three toes
Insertion: lateral side of base of proximal phalanx of great toe
Nerve: lateral plantar nerve (S2, S3)

Adductor longus

Action: adducts thigh
Origin: front of pubis
Insertion: middle third of linea aspera
Nerve: anterior division of obturator nerve (L2–L4)

Adductor magnus

Action: adducts thigh
Origin: inferior ramus of pubis, conjoined ischial ramus, inferolateral aspect of ischial tuberosity

Insertion: linea aspera, proximal part of medial supracondylar line
Nerve: obturator nerve and tibial division of sciatic nerve (L2–L4)

Adductor pollicis

Action: adducts thumb
Origin: oblique head – palmar ligaments of carpus, flexor carpi radialis tendon, base of second to fourth metacarpals, capitate; transverse head – palmar surface of third metacarpal
Insertion: base of proximal phalanx of thumb
Nerve: ulnar nerve (C8, T1)

Anconeus

Action: extends elbow
Origin: posterior surface of lateral epicondyle of humerus
Insertion: lateral surface of olecranon, upper quarter of posterior surface of ulna
Nerve: radial nerve (C6–C8)

Biceps brachii

Action: flexes shoulder and elbow, supinates forearm
Origin: long head – supraglenoid tubercle of scapula and glenoid labrum; short head – apex of coracoid process
Insertion: posterior part of radial tuberosity, bicipital aponeurosis into deep fascia over common flexor origin
Nerve: musculocutaneous nerve (C5, C6)

Biceps femoris

Action: flexes knee and extends hip, laterally rotates tibia on femur
Origin: long head – ischial tuberosity, sacrotuberous ligament; short head – lower half of lateral lip of linea aspera, lateral supracondylar line of femur, lateral intermuscular septum
Insertion: head of fibula, lateral tibial condyle
Nerve: sciatic nerve (L5–S2). Long head – tibial division; short head – common peroneal division

Brachialis

Action: flexes elbow
Origin: lower half of anterior surface of humerus, intermuscular septum
Insertion: coronoid process and tuberosity of ulna
Nerve: musculocutaneous nerve (C5, C6), radial nerve (C7)

Brachioradialis

Action: flexes elbow
Origin: upper two-thirds of lateral supracondylar ridge of humerus, lateral intermuscular septum
Insertion: lateral side of radius above styloid process
Nerve: radial nerve (C5, C6)

Coracobrachialis

Action: adducts shoulder and acts as weak flexor
Origin: apex of coracoid process
Insertion: midway along medial border of humerus
Nerve: musculocutaneous nerve (C5–C7)

Deltoid

Action: anterior fibres – flex and medially rotate shoulder; middle fibres – abduct shoulder; posterior fibres – extend and laterally rotate shoulder
Origin: anterior fibres – anterior border of lateral third of clavicle; middle fibres – lateral margin of acromion process; posterior fibres – lower edge of crest of spine of scapula
Insertion: deltoid tuberosity of humerus
Nerve: axillary nerve (C5, C6)

Diaphragm

Action: draws central tendon inferiorly. Changes volume and pressure of thoracic and abdominal cavities
Origin: posterior surface of xiphoid process, lower six costal cartilages and adjoining ribs on each side, medial and lateral arcuate ligaments, anterolateral aspect of bodies of lumbar vertebrae

Insertion: central tendon
Nerve: phrenic nerves (C3–5)

Dorsal interossei (foot)

Action: abducts toes, flexes metatarsophalangeal joints
Origin: proximal half of sides of adjacent metatarsals
Insertion: bases of proximal phalanges and dorsal digital expansion (first attaches medially to second toe; second, third and fourth attach laterally to second, third and fourth toes, respectively)
Nerve: lateral plantar nerve (S2, S3)

Dorsal interossei (hand)

Action: abducts index, middle and ring fingers, flexes metacarpophalangeal joints and extends interphalangeal joints
Origin: adjacent sides of two metacarpal bones (four bipennate muscles)
Insertion: bases of proximal phalanges and dorsal digital expansions (first attaches laterally to index finger; second and third attach to both sides of middle finger; fourth attaches medially to ring finger)
Nerve: ulnar nerve (C8, T1)

Erector spinae

See iliocostalis, longissimus and spinalis

Extensor carpi radialis brevis

Action: extends and abducts wrist
Origin: lateral epicondyle via common extensor tendon
Insertion: posterior surface of base of third metacarpal
Nerve: posterior interosseous branch of radial nerve (C7, C8)

Extensor carpi radialis longus

Action: extends and abducts wrist
Origin: lower third of lateral supracondylar ridge of humerus, intermuscular septa
Insertion: posterior surface of base of second metacarpal
Nerve: radial nerve (C6, C7)

Extensor carpi ulnaris

Action: extends and adducts wrist
Origin: lateral epicondyle via common extensor tendon
Insertion: medial side of fifth metacarpal base
Nerve: posterior interosseous nerve (C7, C8)

Extensor digiti minimi

Action: extends fifth digit and wrist
Origin: lateral epicondyle via common extensor tendon, intermuscular septa
Insertion: dorsal digital expansion of fifth digit
Nerve: posterior interosseous nerve (C7, C8)

Extensor digitorum

Action: extends fingers and wrist
Origin: lateral epicondyle via common extensor tendon, intermuscular septa
Insertion: lateral and dorsal surfaces of second to fifth digits
Nerve: posterior interosseous branch of radial nerve (C7, C8)

Extensor digitorum brevis

Action: extends great toe and adjacent three toes
Origin: superolateral surface of calcaneus, inferior extensor retinaculum, interosseous talocalcaneal ligament
Insertion: base of proximal phalanx of great toe, lateral side of dorsal hood of adjacent three toes
Nerve: deep peroneal nerve (L5, S1)

Extensor digitorum longus

Action: extends lateral four toes, ankle dorsiflexor
Origin: upper three-quarters of medial surface of fibula, interosseous membrane, lateral tibial condyle
Insertion: middle and distal phalanges of four lateral toes
Nerve: deep peroneal nerve (L5, S1)

Extensor hallucis longus

Action: extends great toe, ankle dorsiflexor
Origin: middle half of medial surface of fibula, interosseous membrane

Insertion: base of distal phalanx of great toe
Nerve: deep peroneal nerve (L5)

Extensor indicis

Action: extends index finger and wrist
Origin: lower part of posterior surface of ulna, interosseous membrane
Insertion: dorsal digital expansion on back of proximal phalanx of index finger
Nerve: posterior interosseous nerve (C7, C8)

Extensor pollicis brevis

Action: extends thumb and wrist, abducts wrist
Origin: posterior surface of radius, interosseous membrane
Insertion: dorsolateral base of proximal phalanx of thumb
Nerve: posterior interosseous nerve (C7, C8)

Extensor pollicis longus

Action: extends thumb and wrist, abducts wrist
Origin: middle third of posterior surface of ulna, interosseous membrane
Insertion: dorsal surface of distal phalanx of thumb
Nerve: posterior interosseous nerve (C7, C8)

External oblique

Action: flexes, laterally flexes and rotates trunk
Origin: outer borders of lower eight ribs and their costal cartilages
Insertion: outer lip of anterior two-thirds of iliac crest, abdominal aponeurosis to linea alba stretching from xiphoid process to symphysis pubis
Nerve: ventral rami of lower six thoracic nerves (T7–T12)

Flexor carpi radialis

Action: flexes and abducts wrist
Origin: medial epicondyle via common flexor tendon
Insertion: front of base of second and third metacarpals
Nerve: median (C6, C7)

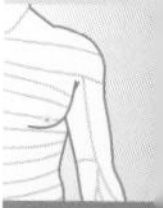

Flexor carpi ulnaris

Action: flexes and adducts wrist
Origin: humeral head – medial epicondyle via common flexor tendon; ulnar head – medial border of olecranon and upper two-thirds of border of ulna
Insertion: pisiform, hook of hamate and base of fifth metacarpal
Nerve: ulnar nerve (C7–T1)

Flexor digiti minimi brevis (foot)

Action: flexes fifth metatarsophalangeal joint, supports lateral longitudinal arch
Origin: plantar aspect of base of fifth metatarsal, sheath of peroneus longus tendon
Insertion: lateral side of base of proximal phalanx of fifth toe
Nerve: lateral plantar nerve (S2, S3)

Flexor digiti minimi brevis (hand)

Action: flexes little finger
Origin: hook of hamate, flexor retinaculum
Insertion: ulnar side of base of proximal phalanx of little finger
Nerve: ulnar nerve (C8, T1)

Flexor digitorum accessorius

Action: flexes distal phalanges of lateral four toes
Origin: medial head – medial tubercle of calcaneus; lateral head – lateral tubercle of calcaneus and long plantar ligament
Insertion: flexor digitorum longus tendon
Nerve: lateral plantar nerve (S1–S3)

Flexor digitorum brevis

Action: flexes proximal interphalangeal joints and metatarsophalangeal joints of lateral four toes
Origin: calcaneal tuberosity, plantar aponeurosis, intermuscular septa
Insertion: tendons divide and attach to both sides of base of middle phalanges of second to fifth toes
Nerve: medial plantar nerve (S1, S2)

Flexor digitorum longus

Action: flexes lateral four toes, plantarflexes ankle
Origin: medial part of posterior surface of tibia, deep transverse fascia
Insertion: plantar aspect of base of distal phalanges of second to fifth toes
Nerve: tibial nerve (L5–S2)

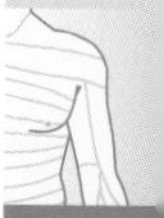

Flexor digitorum profundus

Action: flexes fingers and wrist
Origin: medial side of coronoid process of ulna, upper three-quarters of anterior and medial surfaces of ulna, interosseous membrane
Insertion: base of palmar surface of distal phalanx of second to fifth digits
Nerve: medial part – ulnar nerve (C8, T1); lateral part – anterior interosseous branch of median nerve (C8, T1)

Flexor digitorum superficialis

Action: flexes fingers and wrist
Origin: humeroulnar head – medial epicondyle via common flexor tendon, medial part of coronoid process of ulna, ulnar collateral ligament, intermuscular septa; radial head – upper two-thirds of anterior border of radius
Insertion: tendons divide and insert into sides of shaft of middle phalanx of second to fifth digits
Nerve: median (C8, T1)

Flexor hallucis brevis

Action: flexes metatarsophalangeal joint of great toe
Origin: medial side of plantar surface of cuboid, lateral cuneiform
Insertion: medial and lateral side of base of proximal phalanx of great toe
Nerve: medial plantar nerve (S1, S2)

Flexor hallucis longus

Action: flexes great toe, plantarflexes ankle

Origin: lower two-thirds of posterior surface of fibula, interosseous membrane, intermuscular septum
Insertion: plantar surface of base of distal phalanx of great toe
Nerve: tibial nerve (L5–S2)

Flexor pollicis brevis

Action: flexes metacarpophalangeal joint of thumb
Origin: flexor retinaculum, tubercle of trapezium, capitate, trapezoid
Insertion: base of proximal phalanx of thumb
Nerve: median nerve (C8–T1). Sometimes also supplied by ulnar nerve (C8–T1)

Flexor pollicis longus

Action: flexes thumb and wrist
Origin: anterior surface of radius, interosseous membrane
Insertion: palmar surface of distal phalanx of thumb
Nerve: anterior interosseous branch of median nerve (C7, C8)

Gastrocnemius

Action: plantarflexes ankle, flexes knee
Origin: medial head – posterior part of medial femoral condyle; lateral head – lateral surface of lateral femoral condyle
Insertion: posterior surface of calcaneus
Nerve: tibial nerve (S1, S2)

Gemellus inferior

Action: laterally rotates hip
Origin: upper part of ischial tuberosity
Insertion: with obturator internus tendon into medial surface of greater trochanter
Nerve: nerve to quadratus femoris (L5, S1)

Gemellus superior

Action: laterally rotates hip
Origin: gluteal surface of ischial spine
Insertion: with obturator internus tendon into medial surface of greater trochanter
Nerve: nerve to obturator internus (L5, S1)

Gluteus maximus

Action: extends, laterally rotates and abducts hip
Origin: posterior gluteal line of ilium, posterior border of ilium and adjacent part of iliac crest, aponeurosis of erector spinae, posterior aspect of sacrum, side of coccyx, sacrotuberous ligament, gluteal aponeurosis
Insertion: iliotibial tract of fascia lata, gluteal tuberosity of femur
Nerve: inferior gluteal nerve (L5–S2)

Gluteus medius

Action: abducts and medially rotates hip
Origin: gluteal surface of ilium between posterior and anterior gluteal lines
Insertion: superolateral side of greater trochanter
Nerve: superior gluteal nerve (L4–S1)

Gluteus minimus

Action: abducts and medially rotates hip
Origin: gluteal surface of ilium between anterior and inferior gluteal lines
Insertion: anterolateral ridge on greater trochanter
Nerve: superior gluteal nerve (L4–S1)

Gracilis

Action: flexes knee, adducts hip, medially rotates tibia on femur
Origin: lower half of body and inferior ramus of pubis, adjacent ischial ramus
Insertion: upper part of medial surface of tibia
Nerve: obturator nerve (L2, L3)

Iliacus

Action: flexes hip and trunk
Origin: superior two-thirds of iliac fossa, inner lip of iliac crest, ala of sacrum, anterior sacroiliac and iliolumbar ligaments

Insertion: blends with insertion of psoas major into lesser trochanter
Nerve: femoral nerve (L2, L3)

Iliocostalis cervicis

Action: extends and laterally flexes vertebral column
Origin: angles of third to sixth ribs
Insertion: posterior tubercles of transverse processes of C4 to C6
Nerve: dorsal rami

Iliocostalis lumborum

Action: extends and laterally flexes vertebral column
Origin: medial and lateral sacral crests, spines of T11, T12 and lumbar vertebrae and their supraspinous ligaments, medial part of iliac crest
Insertion: angles of lower six or seven ribs
Nerve: dorsal rami

Iliocostalis thoracis

Action: extends and laterally flexes vertebral column
Origin: angles of lower six ribs
Insertion: angles of upper six ribs, transverse process of C7
Nerve: dorsal rami

Inferior oblique

Action: rotates atlas and head
Origin: lamina of axis
Insertion: transverse process of atlas
Nerve: dorsal ramus (C1)

Infraspinatus

Action: laterally rotates shoulder
Origin: medial two-thirds of infraspinous fossa and infraspinous fascia
Insertion: middle facet on greater tubercle of humerus, posterior aspect of capsule of shoulder joint
Nerve: suprascapular nerve (C5, C6)

Intercostales externi

Action: elevate rib below towards rib above to increase thoracic cavity volume for inspiration
Origin: lower border of rib above
Insertion: upper border of rib below
Nerve: intercostal nerves

Intercostales interni

Action: draw ribs downwards to decrease thoracic cavity volume for expiration
Origin: lower border of costal cartilage and costal groove of rib above
Insertion: upper border of rib below
Nerve: intercostal nerves

Internal oblique

Action: flexes, laterally flexes and rotates trunk
Origin: lateral two-thirds of inguinal ligament, anterior two-thirds of intermediate line of iliac crest, thoracolumbar fascia
Insertion: lower four ribs and their cartilages, crest of pubis, abdominal aponeurosis to linea alba
Nerve: ventral rami of lower six thoracic nerves, first lumbar nerve

Interspinales

Action: extend and stabilize vertebral column
Origin and insertion: extend between adjacent spinous processes (best developed in cervical and lumbar regions – sometimes absent in thoracic)
Nerve: dorsal rami of spinal nerves

Intertransversarii

Action: laterally flex lumbar and cervical spine, stabilize vertebral column
Origin: transverse processes of cervical and lumbar vertebrae
Insertion: transverse process of vertebra superior to origin
Nerve: ventral and dorsal rami of spinal nerves

Latissimus dorsi

Action: extends, adducts and medially rotates shoulder
Origin: spinous processes of lower six thoracic and all lumbar and sacral vertebrae, intervening supra- and interspinous ligaments, outer lip of iliac crest, outer surfaces of lower three or four ribs, inferior angle of scapula
Insertion: intertubercular sulcus of humerus
Nerve: thoracodorsal nerve (C6–C8)

Levator scapulae

Action: elevates, medially rotates and retracts scapula, extends and laterally flexes neck
Origin: transverse processes of C1–C3/4
Insertion: medial border of scapula between superior angle and base of spine
Nerve: ventral rami (C3, C4), dorsal scapular nerve (C5)

Longissimus capitis

Action: extends, laterally flexes and rotates head
Origin: transverse processes of T1–T4/5, articular processes of C4/5–C7
Insertion: posterior aspect of mastoid process
Nerve: dorsal rami

Longissimus cervicis

Action: extends and laterally flexes vertebral column
Origin: transverse processes of T1–T4/5
Insertion: transverse processes of C2–C6
Nerve: dorsal rami

Longissimus thoracis

Action: extends and laterally flexes vertebral column
Origin: transverse and accessory processes of lumbar vertebrae and thoracolumbar fascia
Insertion: transverse processes of T1–T12 and lower nine or ten ribs
Nerve: dorsal rami

Longus capitis

Action: flexes neck
Origin: occipital bone
Insertion: anterior tubercles of transverse processes of C3–C6
Nerve: anterior primary rami (C1–C3)

Longus colli

Action: flexes neck
Origin: inferior oblique part – front of bodies of T1–T2/3; vertical intermediate part – front of bodies of T1–T3 and C5–C7; superior oblique part – anterior tubercles of transverse processes of C3–C5
Insertion: inferior oblique part – anterior tubercles of transverse processes of C5 and C6; vertical intermediate part – front of bodies of C2–C4; superior oblique part – anterior tubercle of atlas
Nerve: anterior primary rami (C2–C6)

Lumbricals (foot)

Action: flexes metatarsophalangeal joints and extends interphalangeal joints of lateral four toes
Origin: tendons of flexor digitorum longus
Insertion: medial side of extensor hood and base of proximal phalanx of lateral four toes
Nerve: first lumbrical – medial plantar nerve (S2, S3); lateral three lumbricals – lateral plantar nerve (S2, S3)

Lumbricals (hand)

Action: flexes metacarpophalangeal joints and extends interphalangeal joints of fingers
Origin: tendons of flexor digitorum profundus
Insertion: lateral margin of dorsal digital expansion of extensor digitorum
Nerve: first and second – median nerve (C8, T1); third and fourth – ulnar nerve (C8, T1)

Multifidus

Action: extends, rotates and laterally flexes vertebral column
Origin: back of sacrum, aponeurosis of erector spinae, posterior superior iliac spine, dorsal sacroiliac ligaments,

mamillary processes in lumbar region, all thoracic transverse processes, articular processes of lower four cervical vertebrae

Insertion: spines of all vertebrae from L5 to axis (deep layer attaches to vertebrae above; middle layer attaches to second or third vertebrae above; outer layer attaches to third or fourth vertebrae above)

Nerve: dorsal rami of spinal nerves

Obturator externus

Action: laterally rotates hip

Origin: outer surface of obturator membrane and adjacent bone of pubic and ischial rami

Insertion: trochanteric fossa of femur

Nerve: posterior branch of obturator nerve (L3, L4)

Obturator internus

Action: laterally rotates hip

Origin: internal surface of obturator membrane and surrounding bony margin

Insertion: medial surface of greater trochanter

Nerve: nerve to obturator internus (L5, S1)

Opponens digiti minimi

Action: abducts fifth digit, pulls it forwards and rotates it laterally

Origin: hook of hamate, flexor retinaculum

Insertion: medial border of fifth metacarpal

Nerve: ulnar nerve (C8, T1)

Opponens pollicis

Action: rotates thumb into opposition with fingers

Origin: flexor retinaculum, tubercles of scaphoid and trapezium, abductor pollicis longus tendon

Insertion: radial side of base of proximal phalanx of thumb

Nerve: median nerve (C8, T1)

Palmar interossei

Action: adducts thumb, index, ring and little finger
Origin: shaft of metacarpal of digit on which it acts
Insertion: dorsal digital expansion and base of proximal phalanx of same digit
Nerve: ulnar nerve (C8, T1)

Palmaris longus

Action: flexes wrist
Origin: medial epicondyle via common flexor tendon
Insertion: flexor retinaculum, palmar aponeurosis
Nerve: median (C7, C8)

Pectineus

Action: flexes and adducts hip
Origin: pecten pubis, iliopectineal eminence, pubic tubercle
Insertion: along a line from lesser trochanter to linea aspera
Nerve: femoral nerve (L2, L3), occasionally accessory obturator (L3)

Pectoralis major

Action: adducts, medially rotates, flexes and extends shoulder
Origin: clavicular attachment – sternal half of anterior surface of clavicle; sternocostal attachment – anterior surface of manubrium, body of sternum, upper six costal cartilages, sixth rib, aponeurosis of external oblique muscle
Insertion: lateral lip of intertubercular sulcus of humerus
Nerve: medial and lateral pectoral nerves (C5–T1)

Pectoralis minor

Action: protracts and medially rotates scapula
Origin: outer surface of third to fifth ribs and adjoining intercostal fascia
Insertion: upper surface and medial border of coracoid process
Nerve: medial and lateral pectoral nerves (C5–T1)

Peroneus brevis

Action: everts and plantarflexes ankle
Origin: lower two-thirds of lateral surface of fibula, intermuscular septa

Insertion: lateral side of base of fifth metatarsal
Nerve: superficial peroneal nerve (L5, S1)

Peroneus longus

Action: everts and plantarflexes ankle
Origin: lateral tibial condyle, upper two-thirds of lateral surface of fibula, intermuscular septa
Insertion: lateral side of base of first metatarsal, medial cuneiform
Nerve: superficial peroneal nerve (L5, S1)

Peroneus tertius

Action: everts and dorsiflexes ankle
Origin: distal third of medial surface of fibula, interosseous membrane, intermuscular septum
Insertion: medial aspect of base of fifth metatarsal
Nerve: deep peroneal nerve (L5, S1)

Piriformis

Action: laterally rotates and abducts hip
Origin: front of second to fourth sacral segments, gluteal surface of ilium, pelvic surface of sacrotuberous ligament
Insertion: medial side of greater trochanter
Nerve: anterior rami of sacral plexus (L5–S2)

Plantar interossei

Action: adduct third to fifth toes, flex metatarsophalangeal joints of lateral three toes
Origin: base and medial side of lateral three toes
Insertion: medial side of base of proximal phalanx of same toes and dorsal digital expansions
Nerve: lateral plantar nerve (S2, S3)

Plantaris

Action: plantarflexes ankle, flexes knee
Origin: lateral supracondylar ridge, oblique popliteal ligament

Insertion: tendo calcaneus
Nerve: tibial nerve (S1, S2)

Popliteus

Action: medially rotates tibia, flexes knee
Origin: outer surface of lateral femoral condyle
Insertion: posterior surface of tibia above soleal line
Nerve: tibial nerve (L4–S1)

Pronator quadratus

Action: pronates forearm
Origin: lower quarter of anterior surface of ulna
Insertion: lower quarter of anterior surface of radius
Nerve: anterior interosseous branch of median nerve (C7, C8)

Pronator teres

Action: pronates forearm, flexes elbow
Origin: humeral head – medial epicondyle via common flexor tendon, intermuscular septum, antebrachial fascia; ulnar head – medial part of coronoid process
Insertion: middle of lateral surface of radius
Nerve: median nerve (C6, C7)

Psoas major

Action: flexes hip and lumbar spine
Origin: bodies of T12 and all lumbar vertebrae, bases of transverse processes of all lumbar vertebrae, lumbar intervertebral discs
Insertion: lesser trochanter
Nerve: anterior rami of lumbar plexus (L1–L3)

Psoas minor (not always present)

Action: flexes trunk (weak)
Origin: bodies of T12 and L1 vertebrae and intervertebral discs
Insertion: pecten pubis, iliopubic eminence, iliac fascia
Nerve: anterior primary ramus (L1)

Quadratus femoris

Action: laterally rotates hip
Origin: ischial tuberosity
Insertion: quadrate tubercle midway down intertrochanteric crest
Nerve: nerve to quadratus femoris (L5, S1)

Quadratus lumborum

Action: laterally flexes trunk, extends lumbar vertebrae, steadies twelfth rib during deep inspiration
Origin: iliolumbar ligament, posterior part of iliac crest
Insertion: lower border of twelfth rib, transverse processes of L1–L4
Nerve: ventral rami of T12 and L1–L3/4

Rectus abdominis

Action: flexes trunk
Origin: symphysis pubis, pubic crest
Insertion: fifth to seventh costal cartilages, xiphoid process
Nerve: ventral rami of T6/7–T12

Rectus capitis anterior

Action: flexes neck
Origin: anterior surface of lateral mass of atlas and root of its transverse process
Insertion: occipital bone
Nerve: anterior primary rami (C1, C2)

Rectus capitis lateralis

Action: laterally flexes neck
Origin: transverse process of atlas
Insertion: jugular process of occipital bone
Nerve: ventral rami (C1, C2)

Rectus capitis posterior major

Action: extends and rotates neck
Origin: spinous process of axis
Insertion: lateral part of inferior nuchal line of occipital bone
Nerve: dorsal ramus (C1)

Rectus capitis posterior minor

Action: extends neck
Origin: posterior tubercle of atlas
Insertion: medial part of inferior nuchal line of occipital bone
Nerve: dorsal ramus (C1)

Rectus femoris

Action: extends knee, flexes hip
Origin: straight head – anterior inferior iliac spine; reflected head – area above acetabulum, capsule of hip joint
Insertion: base of patella, then forms part of patellar ligament
Nerve: femoral nerve (L2–L4)

Rhomboid major

Action: retracts and medially rotates scapula
Origin: spines and supraspinous ligaments of T2–T5
Insertion: medial border of scapula between root of spine and inferior angle
Nerve: dorsal scapular nerve (C4, C5)

Rhomboid minor

Action: retracts and medially rotates scapula
Origin: spines and supraspinous ligaments of C7–T1, lower part of ligamentum nuchae
Insertion: medial end of spine of scapula
Nerve: dorsal scapular nerve (C4, C5)

Rotatores

Action: extends vertebral column and rotates thoracic region
Origin: transverse process of each vertebra
Insertion: lamina of vertebra above
Nerve: dorsal rami of spinal nerves

Sartorius

Action: flexes hip and knee, laterally rotates and abducts hip, medially rotates tibia on femur
Origin: anterior superior iliac spine and area just below
Insertion: upper part of medial side of tibia
Nerve: femoral nerve (L2, L3)

Scalenus anterior

Action: flexes, laterally flexes and rotates neck, raises first rib during respiration
Origin: anterior tubercles of transverse processes of C3–C6
Insertion: scalene tubercle on inner border of first rib
Nerve: ventral rami (C4–C6)

Scalenus medius

Action: laterally flexes neck, raises first rib during respiration
Origin: transverse processes of atlas and axis, posterior tubercles of transverse processes of C3–C7
Insertion: upper surface of first rib
Nerve: ventral rami (C3–C8)

Scalenus posterior

Action: laterally flexes neck, raises second rib during respiration
Origin: posterior tubercles of transverse processes of C4–C6
Insertion: outer surface of second rib
Nerve: ventral rami (C6–C8)

Semimembranosus

Action: flexes knee, extends hip and medially rotates tibia on femur
Origin: ischial tuberosity
Insertion: posterior aspect of medial tibial condyle
Nerve: tibial division of sciatic nerve (L5–S2)

Semispinalis capitis

Action: extends and rotates head
Origin: transverse processes of C7–T6/7, articular processes of C4–C6
Insertion: between superior and inferior nuchal lines of occipital bone
Nerve: dorsal rami of spinal nerves

Semispinalis cervicis

Action: extends and rotates vertebral column
Origin: transverse processes of T1–T5/6

Insertion: spinous processes of C2–C5
Nerve: dorsal rami of spinal nerves

Semispinalis thoracis

Action: extends and rotates vertebral column
Origin: transverse processes of T6–T10
Insertion: spinous processes of C6–T4
Nerve: dorsal rami of spinal nerves

Semitendinosus

Action: flexes knee, extends hip and medially rotates tibia on femur
Origin: ischial tuberosity
Insertion: upper part of medial surface of tibia
Nerve: tibial division of sciatic nerve (L5–S2)

Serratus anterior

Action: protracts and laterally rotates scapula
Origin: outer surfaces and superior borders of upper eight, nine or ten ribs and intervening intercostal fascia
Insertion: costal surface of medial border of scapula
Nerve: long thoracic nerve (C5–C7)

Soleus

Action: plantarflexes ankle
Origin: soleal line and middle third of medial border of tibia, posterior surface of head and upper quarter of fibula, fibrous arch between tibia and fibula
Insertion: posterior surface of calcaneus
Nerve: tibial nerve (S1, S2)

Spinalis (capitis*, cervicis*, thoracis)

Action: extends vertebral column
Origin: spinalis thoracis – spinous processes of T11–L2
Insertion: spinalis thoracis – spinous processes of upper four to eight thoracic vertebrae
*Spinalis capitis and spinalis cervicis are poorly developed and blend with adjacent muscles
Nerve: dorsal rami

Splenius capitis

Action: extends, laterally flexes and rotates neck
Origin: lower half of ligamentum nuchae, spinous processes of C7–T3/4 and their supraspinous ligaments
Insertion: mastoid process of temporal bone, lateral third of superior nuchal line of occipital bone
Nerve: dorsal rami (C3–C5)

Splenius cervicis

Action: laterally flexes, rotates and extends neck
Origin: spinous processes of T3–T6
Insertion: posterior tubercles of transverse processes of C1–C3/4
Nerve: dorsal rami (C5–C7)

Sternocleidomastoid

Action: laterally flexes and rotates neck; anterior fibres flex neck, posterior fibres extend neck
Origin: sternal head – anterior surface of manubrium sterni; clavicular head – upper surface of medial third of clavicle
Insertion: mastoid process of temporal bone, lateral half of superior nuchal line of occipital bone
Nerve: accessory nerve (XI)

Subscapularis

Action: medially rotates shoulder
Origin: medial two-thirds of subscapular fossa and tendinous intramuscular septa
Insertion: lesser tubercle of humerus, anterior capsule of shoulder joint
Nerve: upper and lower subscapular nerves (C5, C6)

Superior oblique

Action: extends neck
Origin: upper surface of transverse process of atlas
Insertion: superior and inferior nuchal lines of occipital bone
Nerve: dorsal ramus (C1)

Supinator

Action: supinates forearm
Origin: inferior aspect of lateral epicondyle, radial collateral ligament, annular ligament, supinator crest and fossa of ulna
Insertion: posterior, lateral and anterior aspects of upper third of radius
Nerve: posterior interosseous nerve (C6, C7)

Supraspinatus

Action: abducts shoulder
Origin: medial two-thirds of supraspinous fossa and supraspinous fascia
Insertion: capsule of shoulder joint, greater tubercle of humerus
Nerve: suprascapular nerve (C5, C6)

Tensor fascia lata

Action: extends knee, abducts and medially rotates hip
Origin: outer lip of iliac crest between iliac tubercle and anterior superior iliac spine
Insertion: iliotibial tract
Nerve: superior gluteal nerve (L4–S1)

Teres major

Action: extends, adducts and medially rotates shoulder
Origin: dorsal surface of inferior scapular angle
Insertion: medial lip of intertubercular sulcus of humerus
Nerve: lower subscapular nerve (C5–C7)

Teres minor

Action: laterally rotates shoulder
Origin: upper two-thirds of dorsal surface of scapula
Insertion: lower facet on greater tuberosity of humerus, lower posterior surface of capsule of shoulder joint
Nerve: axillary nerve (C5, C6)

Tibialis anterior

Action: dorsiflexes and inverts ankle
Origin: lateral tibial condyle and upper two-thirds of lateral surface of tibia, interosseous membrane

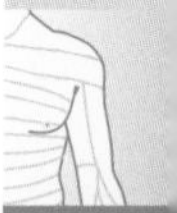

Insertion: medial and inferior surface of medial cuneiform, base of first metatarsal
Nerve: deep peroneal nerve (L4, L5)

Tibialis posterior

Action: plantarflexes and inverts ankle
Origin: lateral aspect of posterior surface of tibia below soleal line, interosseous membrane, upper half of posterior surface of fibula, deep transverse fascia
Insertion: tuberosity of navicular, medial cuneiform, sustentaculum tali, intermediate cuneiform, base of second to fourth metatarsals
Nerve: tibial nerve (L4, L5)

Transversus abdominis

Action: compresses abdominal contents, raises intra-abdominal pressure
Origin: lateral third of inguinal ligament, anterior two-thirds of inner lip of iliac crest, thoracolumbar fascia between iliac crest and twelfth rib, lower six costal cartilages where it interdigitates with diaphragm
Insertion: abdominal aponeurosis to linea alba
Nerve: ventral rami of lower six thoracic and first lumbar spinal nerve

Trapezius

Action: upper fibres elevate scapula, middle fibres retract scapula, lower fibres depress scapula, upper and lower fibres together laterally rotate scapula. Also extends and laterally flexes head and neck
Origin: medial third of superior nuchal line, external occipital protuberance, ligamentum nuchae, spinous processes and supraspinous ligaments of C7–T12
Insertion: upper fibres – posterior border of lateral third of clavicle; middle fibres – medial border of acromion,

superior lip of crest of spine of scapula; lower fibres – tubercle at medial end of spine of scapula
Nerve: accessory nerve (XI), ventral rami (C3, C4)

Triceps brachii

Action: extends elbow and shoulder
Origin: long head – infraglenoid tubercle of scapula, shoulder capsule; lateral head – above and lateral to spiral groove on posterior surface of humerus; medial head – below and medial to spiral groove on posterior surface of humerus
Insertion: upper surface of olecranon, deep fascia of forearm
Nerve: radial nerve (C6–C8)

Vastus intermedius

Action: extends knee
Origin: upper two-thirds of anterior and lateral surfaces of femur, lower part of lateral intermuscular septum
Insertion: deep surface of quadriceps tendon, lateral border of patella, lateral tibial condyle
Nerve: femoral nerve (L2–L4)

Vastus lateralis

Action: extends knee
Origin: intertrochanteric line, greater trochanter, gluteal tuberosity, lateral lip of linea aspera
Insertion: tendon of rectus femoris, lateral border of patella
Nerve: femoral nerve (L2–L4)

Vastus medialis

Action: extends knee
Origin: intertrochanteric line, spiral line, medial lip of linea aspera, medial supracondylar line, medial intermuscular septum, tendons of adductor longus and adductor magnus
Insertion: tendon of rectus femoris, medial border of patella, medial tibial condyle
Nerve: femoral nerve (L2–L4)

The Medical Research Council scale for muscle power

Grade	Response
0	No movement
1	Flicker of contraction
2	Active movement with gravity eliminated
3	Active movement against gravity
4	Active movement against resistance but not to full strength
5	Normal power

In addition, grade 4 movements may be subdivided into:

4− movement against slight resistance
4 movement against moderate resistance
4+ movement against strong resistance.

Trigger points

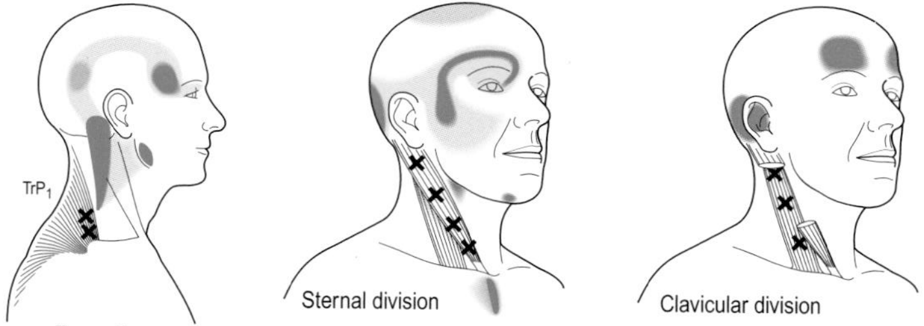
TrP1
Sternal division
Clavicular division

Trapezius

Sternocleidomastoid

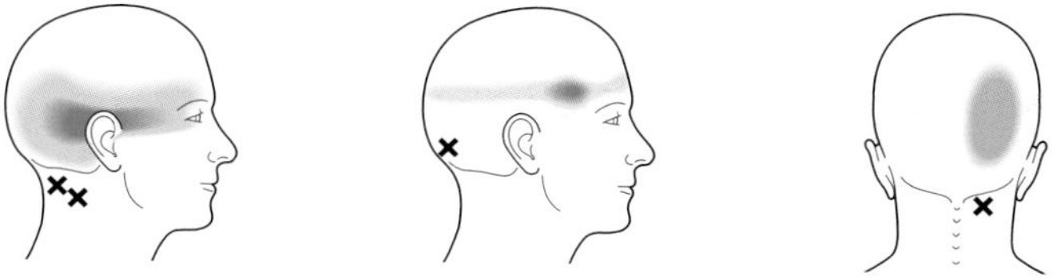

Suboccipital

Semispinalis capitis

Semispinalis cervicis

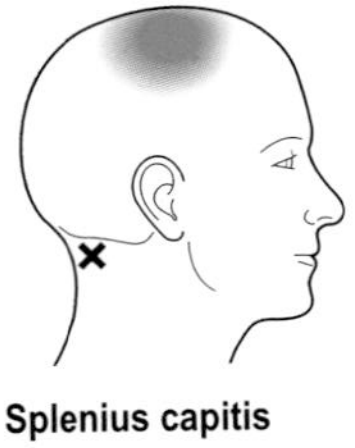
Splenius capitis

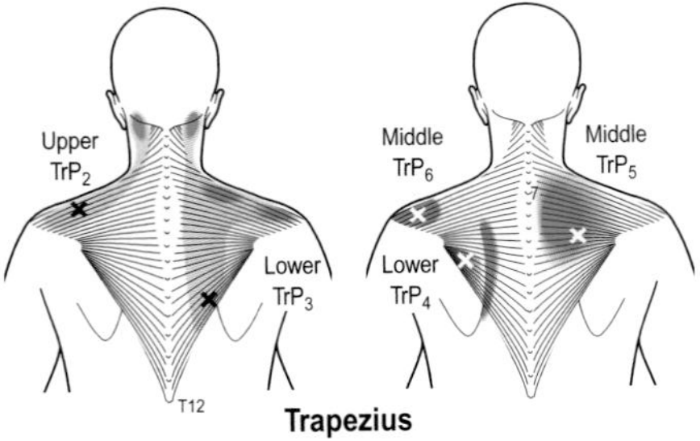
Upper
TrP_2
Lower
TrP_3
T12
Middle
TrP_6
Middle
TrP_5
Lower
TrP_4
Trapezius

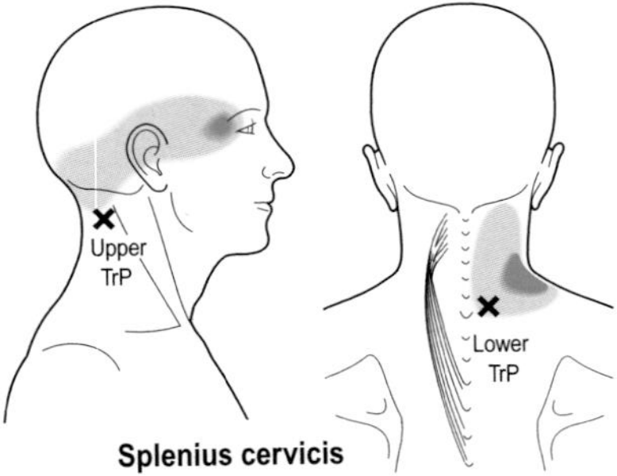
Upper
TrP
Lower
TrP
Splenius cervicis

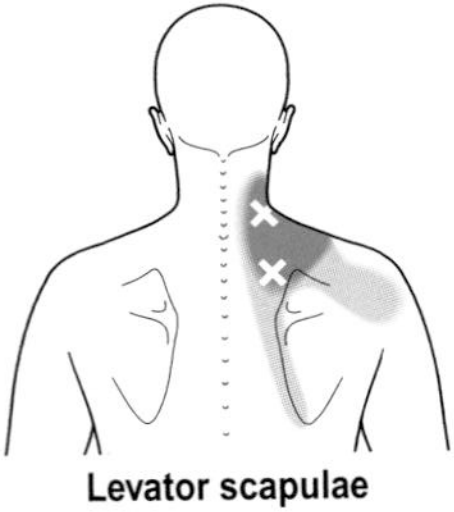
Levator scapulae

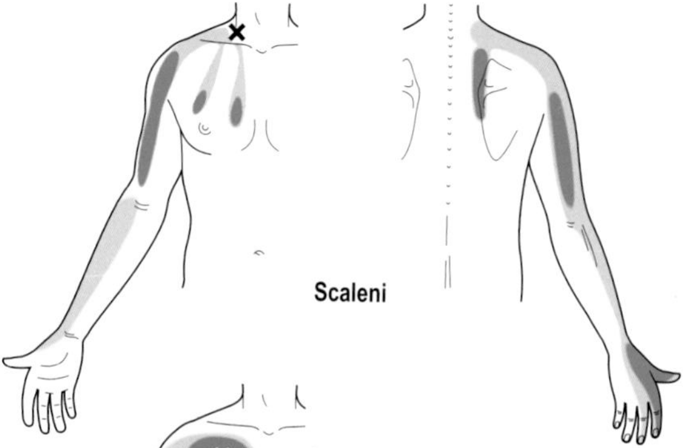

Scaleni

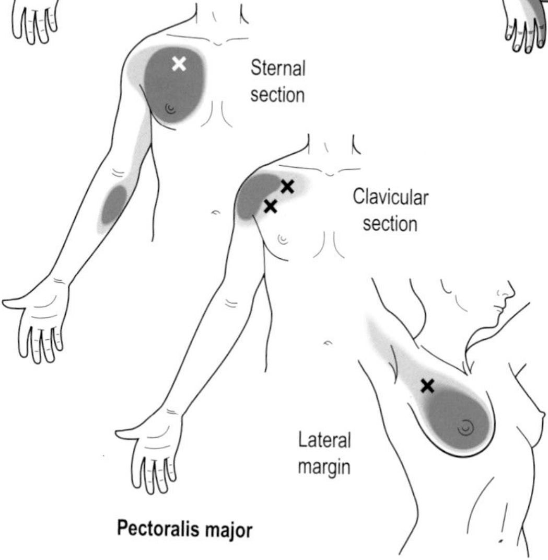
Sternal section
Clavicular section
Lateral margin

Pectoralis major

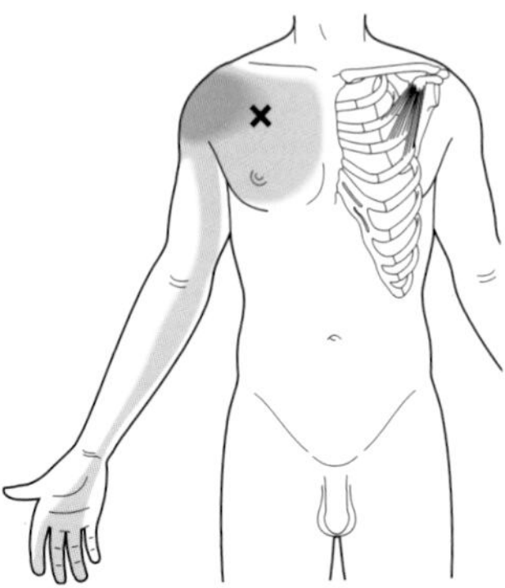

Pectoralis minor

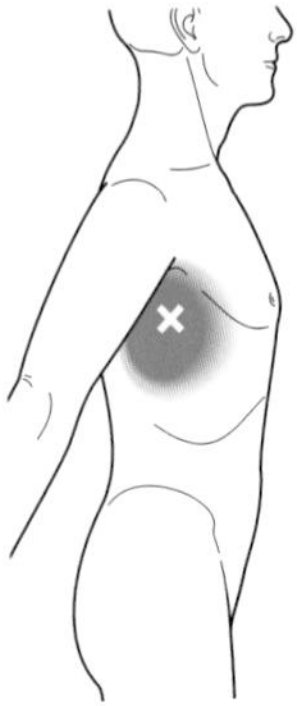

Serratus anterior

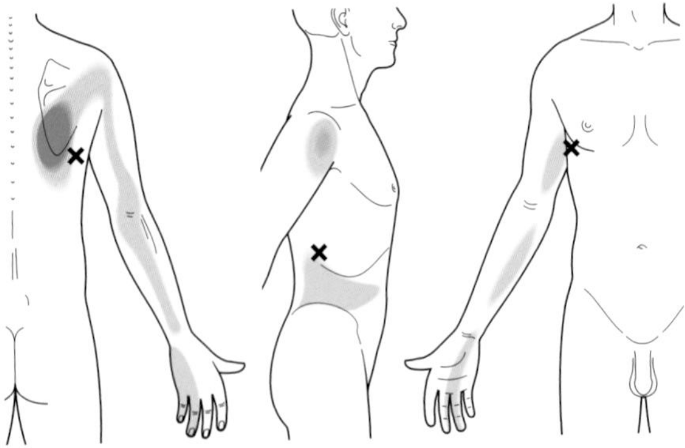

Latissimus dorsi

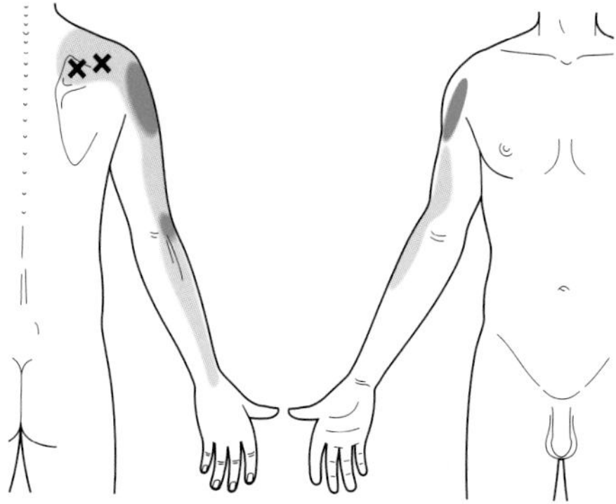

Supraspinatus

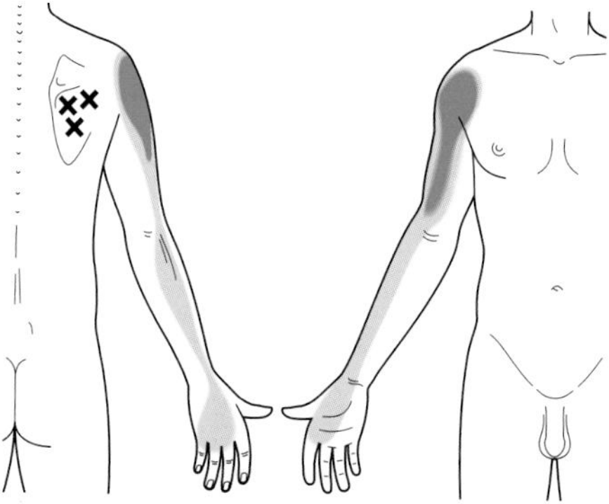

Infraspinatus

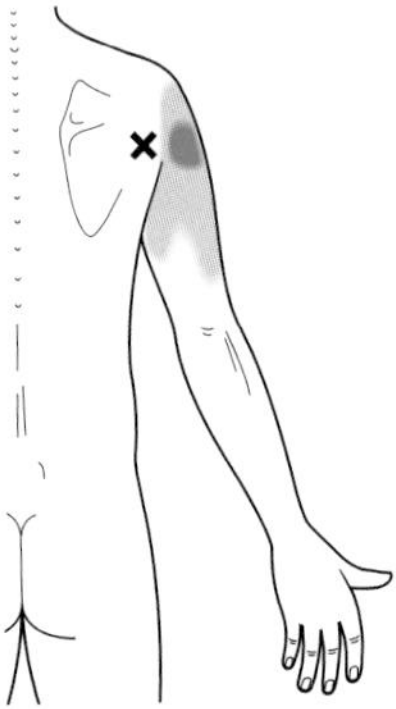

Teres minor

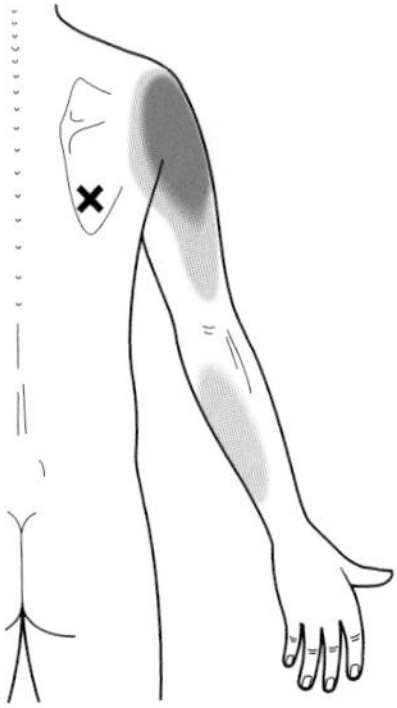

Teres major

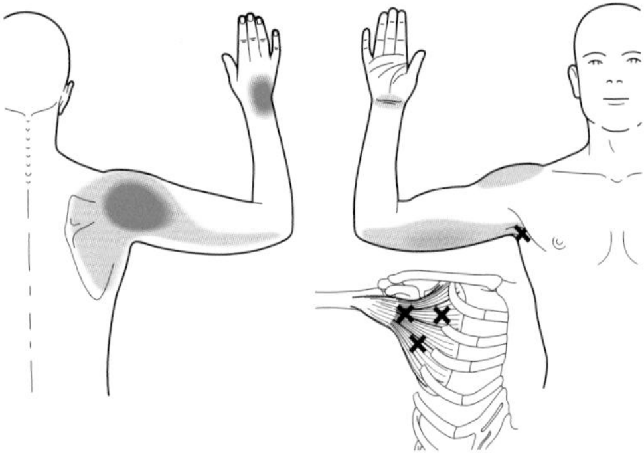

Subscapularis

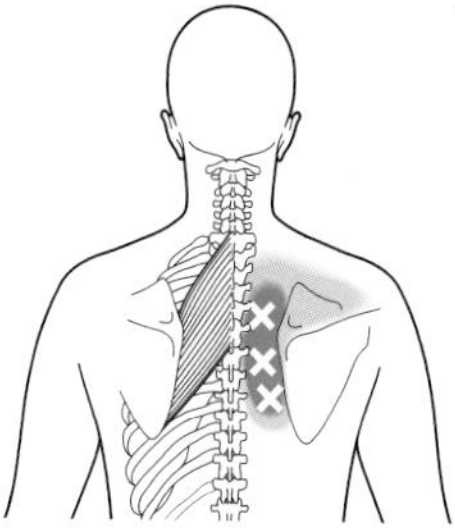

Rhomboideus

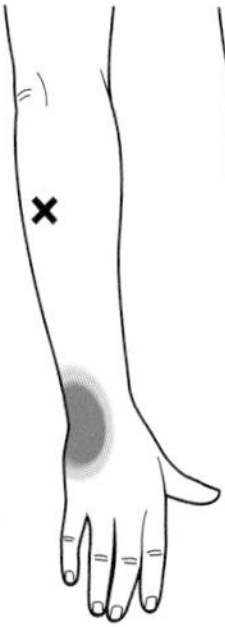

Extensor carpi ulnaris

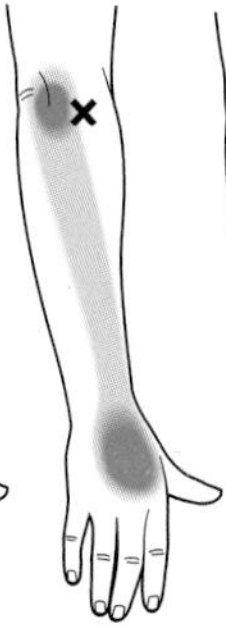

Extensor carpi radialis longus

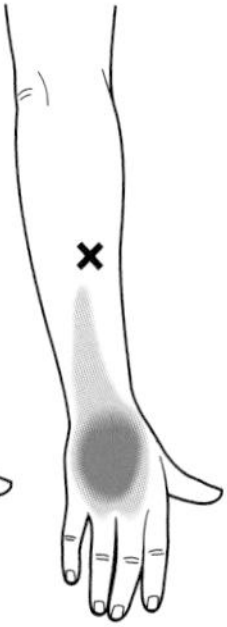

Extensor carpi radialis brevis

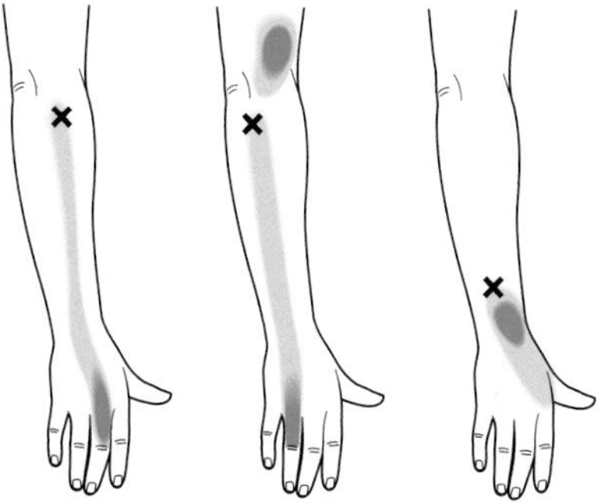

Middle finger

Ring finger

Extensor indicis

Finger extensors

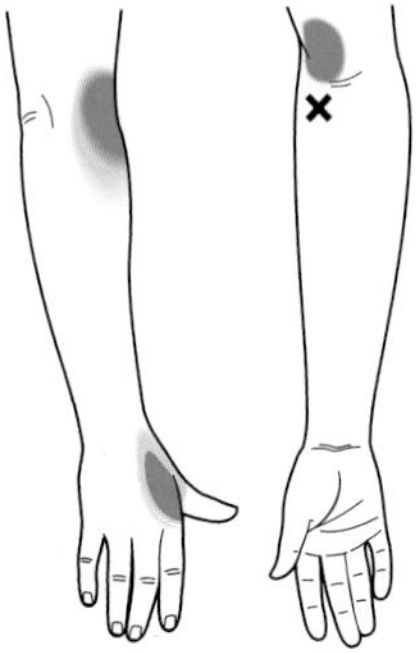

Supinator

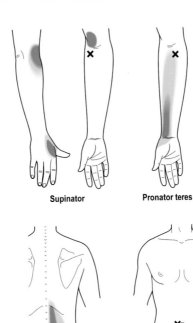

Pronator teres

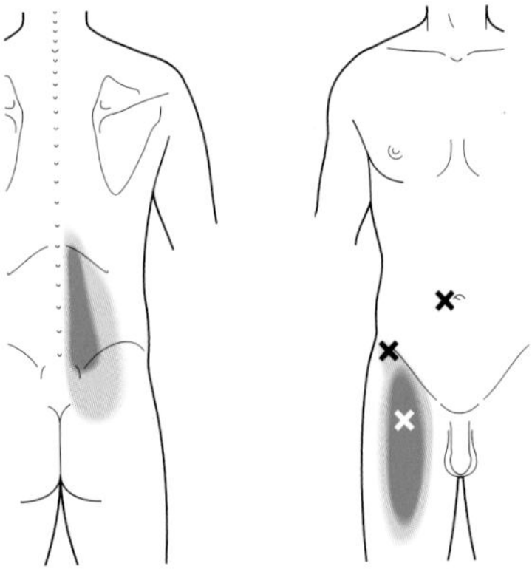

Iliopsoas

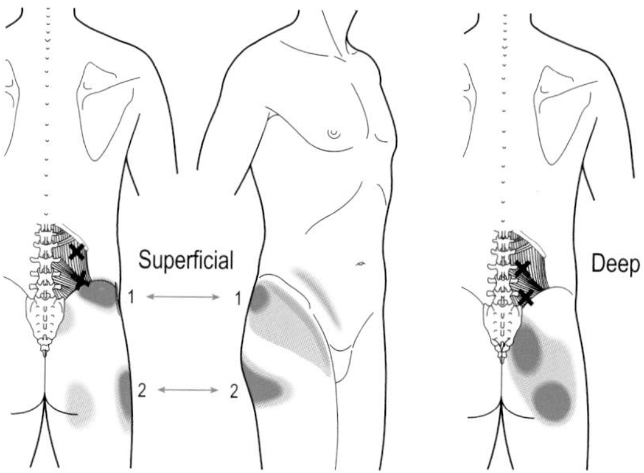
Superficial
Deep
1
1
2
2

Quadratus lumborum

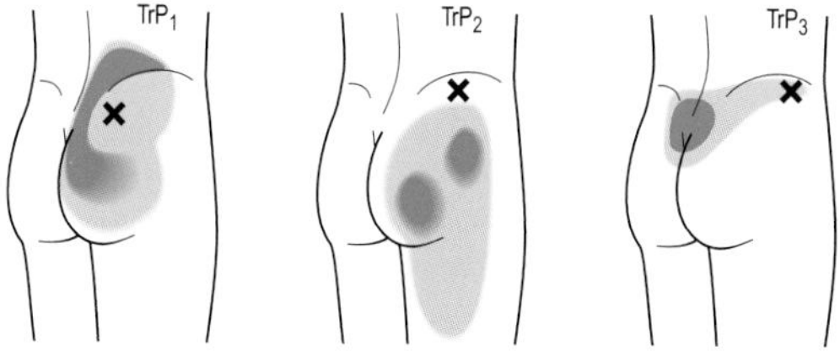
TrP1
TrP2
TrP3

Gluteus medius

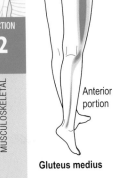

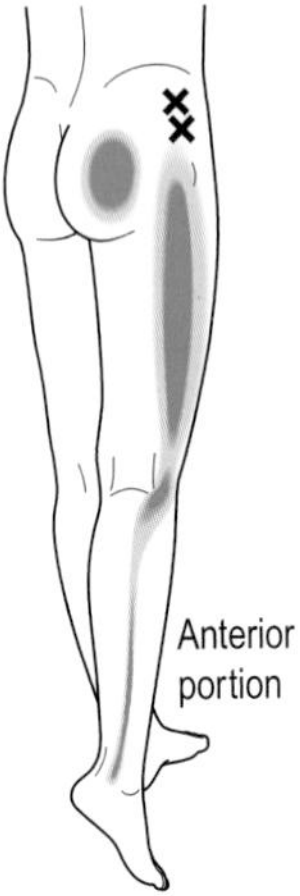
Anterior
portion

Gluteus medius

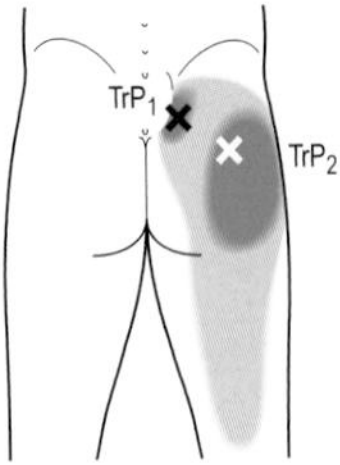
TrP1
TrP2

Piriformis

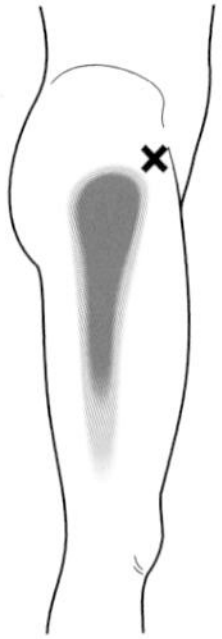

Tensor fasciae latae

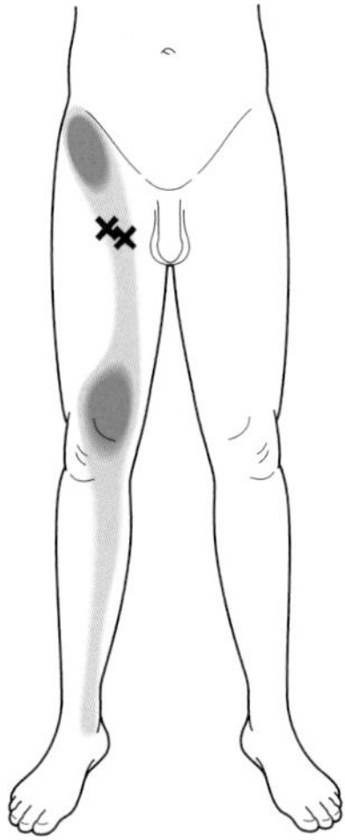

Adductor brevis

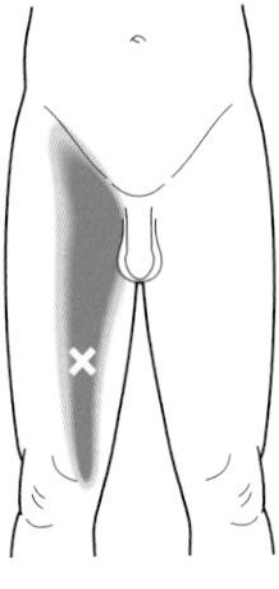

Adductor magnus

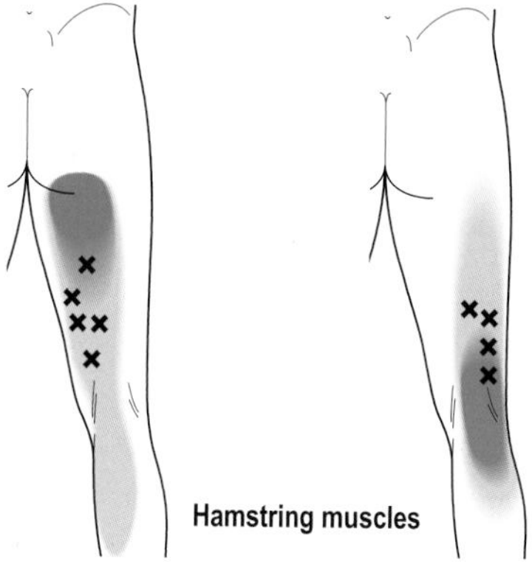
Hamstring muscles

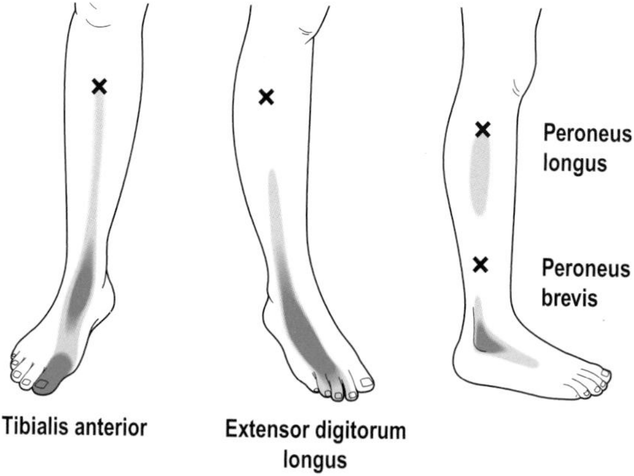
Peroneus longus
Peroneus brevis
Tibialis anterior
Extensor digitorum longus

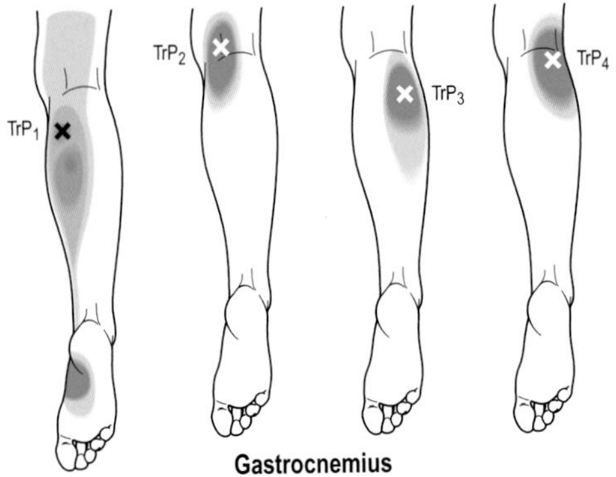
TrP1
TrP2
TrP3
TrP4

Gastrocnemius

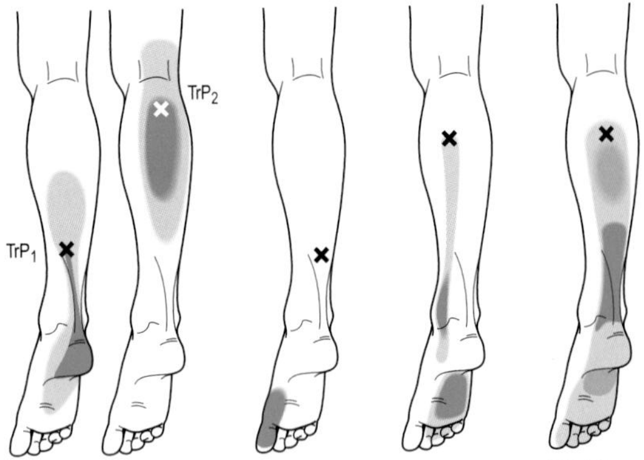
TrP2
TrP1

Soleus

Flexor hallucis longus

Flexor digitorum longus

Tibialis posterior

Normal joint range of movement

Shoulder

Flexion	160–180°
Extension	50–60°
Abduction	170–180°
Medial rotation	70–90°
Lateral rotation	80–100°

Elbow

Flexion	140–150°
Extension	0°
Pronation	80–90°
Supination	80–90°

Wrist

Flexion	70–80°
Extension	60–80°
Radial deviation	15–25°
Ulnar deviation	30–40°

Hip

Flexion	120–125°
Extension	15–30°
Abduction	30–50°
Adduction	20–30°
Medial rotation	25–40°
External rotation	40–50°

Knee

Flexion	130–140°
Extension	0°

Ankle

Dorsiflexion	15–20°
Plantarflexion	50–60°
Inversion	30–40°
Eversion	15–20°

Normal ranges of movement vary greatly between individuals. The above figures represent average ranges of movement.

Average range of segmental movement (Middleditch & Oliver 2005, with permission)

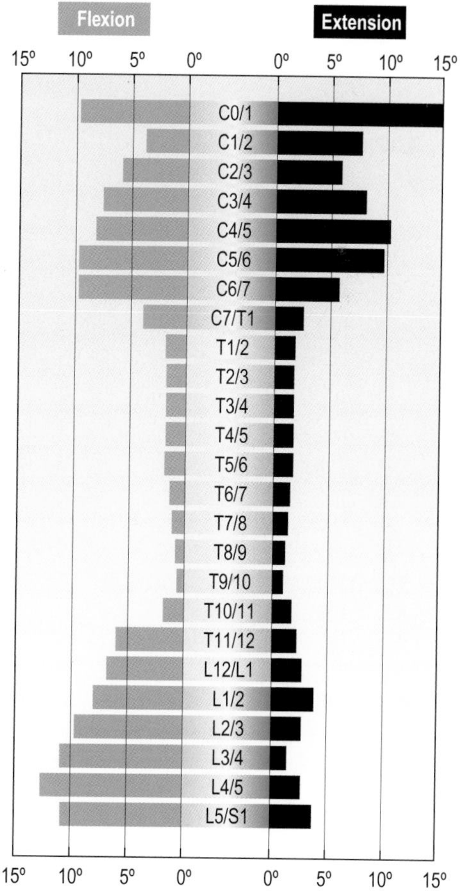
Flexion
Extension
15° 10° 5° 0°
0° 5° 10° 15°
C0/1
C1/2
C2/3
C3/4
C4/5
C5/6
C6/7
C7/T1
T1/2
T2/3
T3/4
T4/5
T5/6
T6/7
T7/8
T8/9
T9/10
T10/11
T11/12
L12/L1
L1/2
L2/3
L3/4
L4/5
L5/S1
15° 10° 5° 0°
0° 5° 10° 15°

Figure 2.1 Spinal flexion and extension.

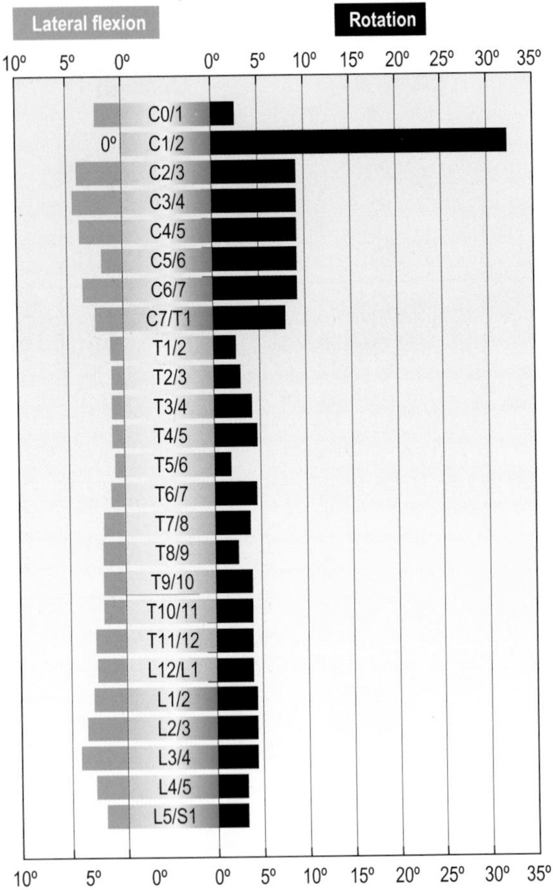
Lateral flexion
Rotation
10° 5° 0° 0° 5° 10° 15° 20° 25° 30° 35°
C0/1
0° C1/2
C2/3
C3/4
C4/5
C5/6
C6/7
C7/T1
T1/2
T2/3
T3/4
T4/5
T5/6
T6/7
T7/8
T8/9
T9/10
T10/11
T11/12
L12/L1
L1/2
L2/3
L3/4
L4/5
L5/S1
10° 5° 0° 0° 5° 10° 15° 20° 25° 30° 35°

Figure 2.2 Spinal lateral flexion and rotation.

Close packed positions and capsular patterns for selected joints

Joint	Close packed position	Capsular pattern*
Temporomandibular	Clenched teeth	Opening mouth
Cervical spine	Extension (also applies to thoracic and lumbar spine)	Side flexion and rotation equally limited; flexion is full but painful, extension is limited
Glenohumeral	Abduction and lateral rotation	Lateral rotation then abduction then medial rotation
Humeroulnar	Extension	Flexion then extension
Radiocarpal	Extension with radial deviation	Flexion and extension equally limited
Trapeziometacarpal	None	Abduction and extension, full flexion
Metacarpophalangeal interphalangeal	*Metacarpophalangeal* Flexion (fingers) Opposition (thumb) *Interphalangeal* Extension	Flexion then extension
Hip	Extension and medial rotation	Flexion, abduction and medial rotation (order may vary) Extension is slightly limited
Knee	Extension and lateral rotation of tibia	Flexion then extension

Joint	Close packed position	Capsular pattern*
Talocrural	Dorsiflexion	Plantarflexion then dorsiflexion
Subtalar	Inversion	Inversion
Mid-tarsal	Inversion (also applies to tarsometatarsal)	Dorsiflexion, plantarflexion, adduction and medial rotation
First metatarsophalangeal	*Metatarsophalangeal* Extension *Interphalangeal* Extension	Extension then flexion

*Movements are listed in order of restriction, from the most limited to the least limited.
Data from Cyriax (1982) and Magee (2008).

Common postures (from Kendall et al 2005, with permission of Lippincott Williams & Wilkins)

Ideal alignment: side view (Fig. 2.3)

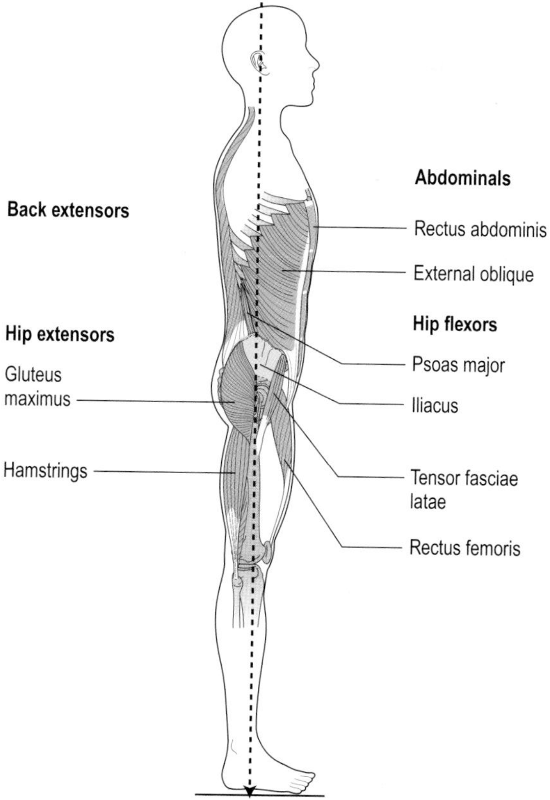
Back extensors
Hip extensors
Gluteus maximus
Hamstrings
Abdominals
Rectus abdominis
External oblique
Hip flexors
Psoas major
Iliacus
Tensor fasciae latae
Rectus femoris

Figure 2.3 Ideal alignment (side view).

Anteriorly, the abdominal muscles pull upward and the hip flexors pull downward. Posteriorly, the back muscles pull upward and the hip extensors pull downward. Thus, the abdominal and hip extensor muscles work together to tilt the pelvis posteriorly; the back and hip flexor muscles work together to tilt the pelvis anteriorly.

Ideal alignment: posterior view (Fig. 2.4)

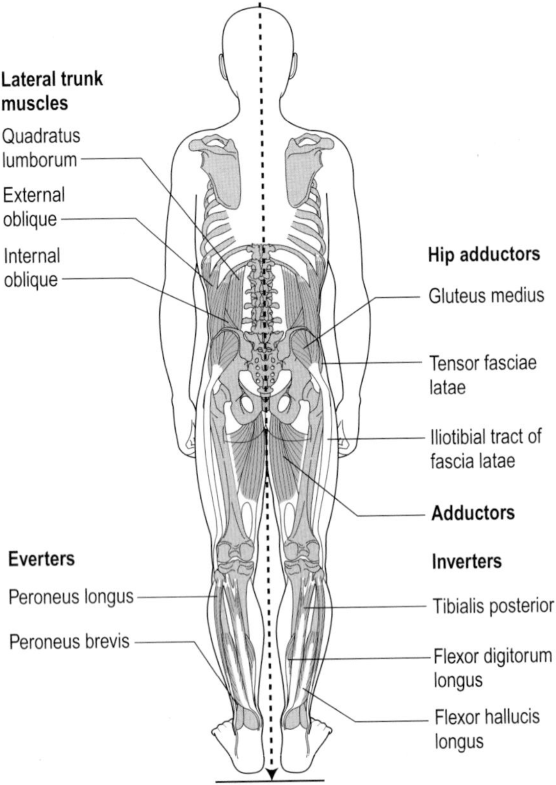
Lateral trunk muscles
Quadratus lumborum
External oblique
Internal oblique
Hip adductors
Gluteus medius
Tensor fasciae latae
Iliotibial tract of fascia latae
Adductors
Everters
Peroneus longus
Peroneus brevis
Inverters
Tibialis posterior
Flexor digitorum longus
Flexor hallucis longus

Figure 2.4 Ideal alignment (posterior view).

Laterally, the following groups of muscles work together in stabilizing the trunk, pelvis and lower extremities:

- Right lateral trunk flexors
- Right hip adductors
- Left hip abductors
- Right tibialis posterior
- Right flexor hallucis longus
- Right flexor digitorum longus
- Left peroneus longus and brevis
- Left lateral trunk flexors
- Left hip adductors
- Right hip abductors
- Left tibialis posterior
- Left flexor hallucis longus
- Left flexor digitorum longus
- Right peroneus longus and brevis

Kyphosis–lordosis posture (Fig. 2.5)

Short and strong: neck extensors and hip flexors. The low back is strong and may or may not develop shortness.

Elongated and weak: neck flexors, upper back erector spinae and external oblique. Hamstrings are slightly elongated but may or may not be weak.

Sway-back posture (Fig. 2.6)

Short and strong: hamstrings and upper fibres of internal oblique. Strong but not short: lumbar erector spinae.

Elongated and weak: one-joint hip flexors, external oblique, upper back extensors and neck flexors.

Flat-back posture (Fig. 2.7)

Short and strong: hamstrings and often the abdominals.

Elongated and weak: one-joint hip flexors.

Faulty alignment: posterior view (Fig. 2.8)

Short and strong: right lateral trunk muscles, left hip abductors, right hip adductors, left peroneus longus and brevis, right tibialis posterior, right flexor hallucis longus, right

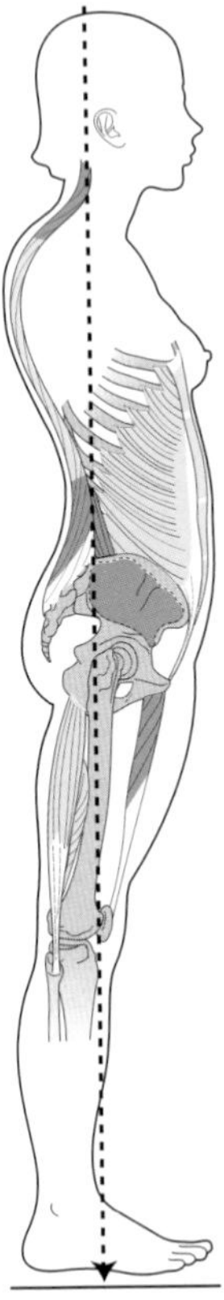

Figure 2.5 Kyphosis–lordosis posture.

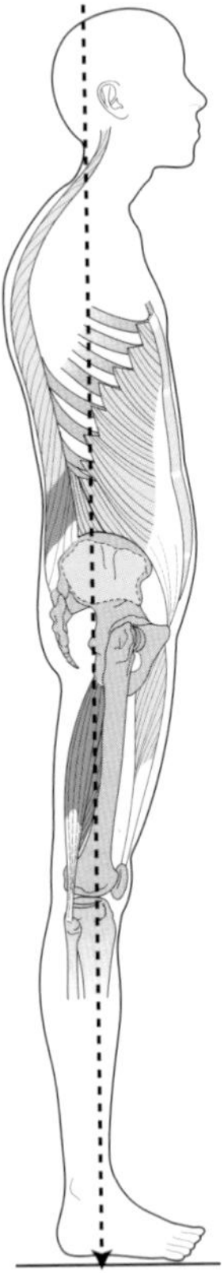

Figure 2.6 Sway-back posture.

flexor digitorum longus. The left tensor fascia lata is usually strong and there may be tightness in the iliotibial band.

Elongated and weak: left lateral trunk muscles, right hip abductors (especially posterior gluteus medius), left hip

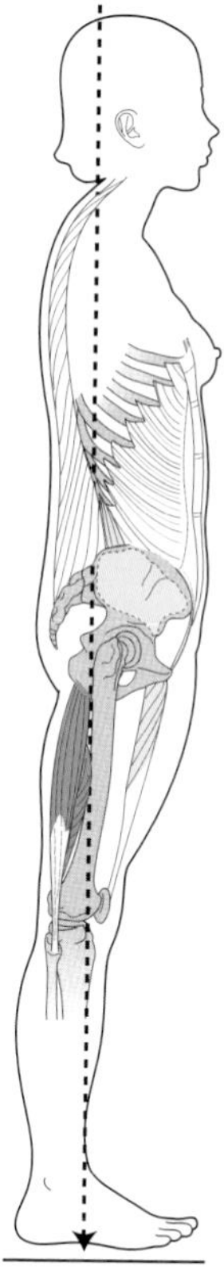

Figure 2.7 Flat-back posture.

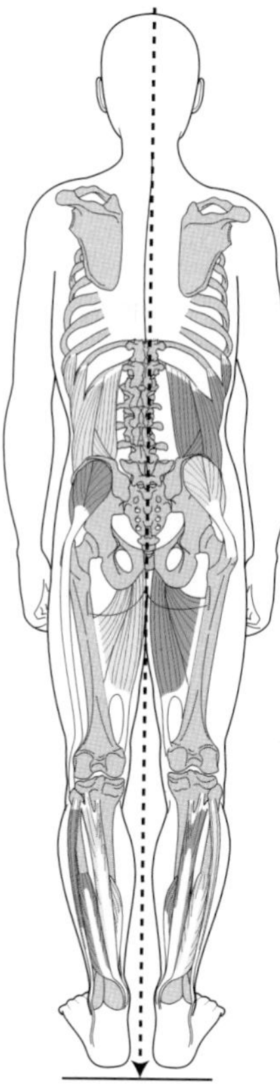

Figure 2.8 Faulty alignment (posterior view). Typical of right-handed individuals.

adductors, right peroneus longus and brevis, left tibialis posterior, left flexor hallucis longus, left flexor digitorum longus. The right tensor fascia lata may or may not be weak.

Beighton hypermobility score

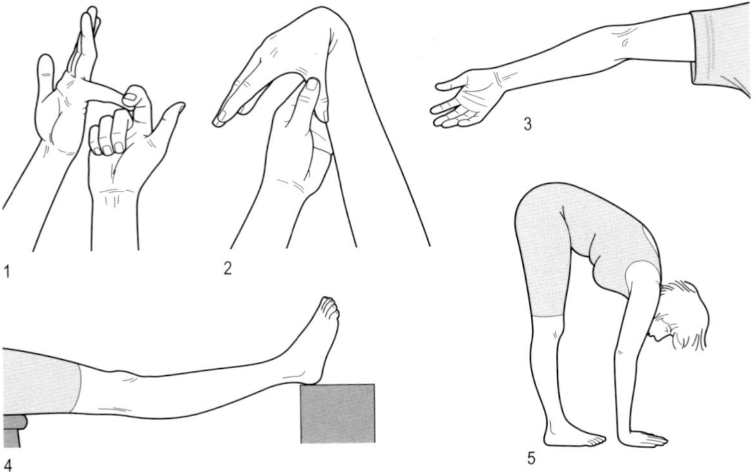
1
2
3
4
5

Figure 2.9 Beighton score for joint hypermobility.

Nine-point Beighton hypermobility score

The ability to:		Right	Left
1	Passively extend the fifth metacarpophalangeal joint to ≥90°	1	1
2	Passively appose the thumb to the anterior aspect of the forearm	1	1
3	Passively hyperextend the elbow to ≥10°	1	1
4	Passively hyperextend the knee to ≥10°	1	1
5	Actively place hands flat on the floor without bending the knees	1	
TOTAL		9	

One point is given for each side for manoeuvres 1–4 so that the hypermobility score will have a maximum of 9 points if all are positive.

It is generally considered that hypermobility is present if 4 out of 9 points are scored.

Brighton criteria: diagnostic criteria for benign joint hypermobility syndrome (from Grahame et al 2000, with permission)

Major criteria

1. A Beighton score of 4/9 or greater (either currently or historically)
2. Arthralgia for longer than 3 months in four or more joints

Minor criteria

1. A Beighton score of 1, 2 or 3/9 (0, 1, 2 or 3 if aged 50+)
2. Arthralgia (≥3 months) in 1–3 joints, or back pain (≥3 months), spondylosis, spondylolysis/spondylolisthesis
3. Dislocation/subluxation in more than one joint, or in one joint on more than one occasion
4. Soft tissue rheumatism ≥3 lesions (e.g. epicondylitis, tenosynovitis, bursitis)

5. Marfanoid habitus: tall, slim, span : height ratio >1.03, upper : lower segment ratio <0.89, arachnodactyly (positive Steinberg/wrist signs)
6. Abnormal skin: striae, hyperextensibility, thin skin, papyraceous scarring
7. Eye signs: drooping eyelids or myopia or anti-mongoloid slant
8. Varicose veins or hernia or uterine/rectal prolapse

Benign joint hypermobility syndrome (BJHS) is diagnosed in the presence of **two** major criteria, or **one** major and **two** minor criteria, or **four** minor criteria. **Two** minor criteria will suffice where there is an unequivocally affected first-degree relative. BJHS is excluded by the presence of Marfan or Ehlers–Danlos syndrome (EDS) (other than the EDS hypermobility type – formerly EDS III). Criteria Major 1 and Minor 1 are mutually exclusive, as are Major 2 and Minor 2.

Common classifications of fractures

Proximal humeral fractures: Neer's classification

Group I
All proximal humeral fractures where there is minimal displacement or angulation.

Group II
Displaced fractures of the anatomical neck (>1 cm).

Group III
Severely displaced or angled fractures of the surgical neck. These may be impacted or comminuted.

Group IV
Displaced fractures of the greater tuberosity.

Group V
Displaced fractures of the lesser tuberosity.

Group VI
Fracture-dislocations.

Radial head fractures: Hotchkiss modification of Mason's classification

Type 1

Small vertical split with minimal displacement (<2 mm). Stability and rotation largely uncompromised.

Type 2

Displaced single fragment fracture (<2 mm), usually distally. Any fracture that restricts rotation. Any comminuted fracture that can be internally fixated.

Type 3

Highly comminuted fractures that cannot be internally fixated.

Fractures of the radius and ulna

Monteggia fracture-dislocation

Fracture of the ulna associated with dislocation of the radial head.

Galeazzi fracture-dislocation

Fracture of the distal third of the radius associated with dislocation of the inferior radioulnar joint.

Colles' fracture

Transverse fracture of the distal radius with dorsal (posterior) displacement of the distal fragment.

Smith's fracture

Transverse fracture of the distal radius with volar (anterior) displacement of the distal fragment (often called a 'reversed Colles').

Barton's fracture

The true Barton's fracture is a form of Smith's fracture associated with volar subluxation of the carpus. However, dorsal subluxation of the carpus can also occur, which is sometimes called a 'dorsal Barton's fracture'.

Fractures of the thumb metacarpal

Bennett's fracture

Oblique fracture of the first metacarpal extending into the trapeziometacarpal joint associated with dislocation of the carpometacarpal joint.

Rolando's fracture

Intra-articular comminuted fracture of the base of the first metacarpal.

Scaphoid fractures: Herbert classification

A1 Fracture of the tubercle (stable)
A2 Hairline fracture of the waist (stable)
B1 Oblique fracture of distal third (unstable)
B2 Displaced fracture of the waist (unstable)
B3 Proximal pole fracture (unstable)
B4 Fracture associated with carpal dislocation (unstable)
B5 Comminuted fracture (unstable)

Pelvic fractures: Tile classification

Type A (stable)

- A1: fractures of the pelvis not involving the pelvic ring
- A2: stable, minimally displaced fractures of the pelvic ring

Type B (rotationally unstable but vertically stable)

- B1: anteroposterior compression fractures (open book fractures)
- B2: lateral compression fractures, ipsilateral
- B3: lateral compression fractures, contralateral

Type C (rotationally and vertically unstable)

- C1: unilateral
- C2: bilateral
- C3: associated with acetabular fracture

Intracapsular fractures of the neck of femur: Garden classification

Type I

Incomplete fracture of the neck of femur with angulation of the trabecular lines.

Type II

Complete fracture without displacement of the neck of femur. The trabecular lines are interrupted but not angulated.

Type III

Complete fracture with partial displacement of the neck of femur.

Type IV

Complete fracture with total displacement of the neck of femur.

Tibial plateau fractures: Schatzker classification

Type I

Split or wedge fracture of the lateral tibial condyle.

Type II

Split or wedge fracture of the lateral tibial condyle combined with depression of the adjacent remaining load-bearing portion of the lateral plateau.

Type III

Pure depression fracture of the lateral tibial plateau without an associated split or wedge fracture.

Type IV

Fracture of the medial tibial plateau. May be a split or a split depression fracture.

Type V

Split fracture of both the medial and lateral tibial condyles.

Type VI

Combined condylar and subcondylar fractures that separate the tibial shaft from the tibial condyles.

Ankle fractures: Weber's classification

Fibular fractures are classified into three types:

Type A

Fracture below the tibiofibular syndesmosis.

Type B

Fracture at the level of the tibial plafond, which often spirals upwards. The syndesmosis is usually involved; however, it remains intact.

Type C

Fracture above the tibiofibular syndesmosis. The syndesmosis is ruptured.

Classification of ligament and muscle sprains

Ligament sprains

Grade I/mild sprain

Few ligament fibres torn, stability maintained.

Grade II/moderate sprain

Partial rupture, increased laxity but no gross instability.

Grade III/severe sprain

Complete rupture, gross instability.

Muscle strains

Grade I/mild strain

Few muscle fibres torn, minimum loss of strength and pain on muscle contraction.

Grade II/moderate strain

Approximately half of muscle fibres torn, significant muscle weakness and loss of function. Moderate to severe pain on isometric contraction.

Grade III/severe strain

Complete tear of the muscle, significant muscle weakness and severe loss of function. Minimum to no pain on isometric contraction.

Common musculoskeletal tests

A brief description of each test is given below. For a fuller description of how each test is performed, please refer to a musculoskeletal assessment textbook (e.g. Magee 2008, Malanga & Nadler 2006, Petty 2006).

Cervical spine

Spurling's test

Tests: nerve root compression.

Procedure: patient sitting. Extend neck and rotate head. Apply downward pressure to head.

Positive sign: radiating pain into shoulder or arm on side to which the head is rotated.

Distraction test

Tests: nerve root compression.

Procedure: patient in sitting. Place one hand under chin and other hand under occiput. Gently lift patient's head.

Positive sign: relief or decrease in pain.

Shoulder

Active compression test (O'Brien)

Tests: labral pathology, acromioclavicular joint pathology.

Procedure: patient upright with elbow in extension and shoulder in 90° flexion, 10–15° adduction and medial rotation. Stand behind patient and apply downward force to arm. Repeat with arm in lateral rotation.

Positive sign: pain/increased pain with medial rotation and decreased pain with lateral rotation. Pain inside the glenohumeral joint indicates labral abnormality. Pain over the acromioclavicular joint indicates acromioclavicular joint abnormality.

Anterior drawer test

Tests: anterior shoulder stability.

Procedure: patient supine. Place shoulder in 80–120° abduction, 0–20° forward flexion and 0–30° lateral rotation. Stabilize scapula. Draw humerus anteriorly.

Positive sign: click and/or apprehension.

Anterior slide test

Tests: labral pathology.

Procedure: patient upright with hands on hips, thumbs facing posteriorly. Stand behind patient and stabilize scapula and clavicle with one hand. With the other, apply an antero-superior force to elbow while instructing the patient to gently push back against the force.

Positive sign: pain/reproduction of symptoms/click.

Apprehension test

Tests: glenohumeral joint stability.

Procedure: patient in standing or supine. Abduct shoulder to 90°. Move it into maximum lateral rotation. If movement well tolerated, apply a posteroanterior force to humeral head.

Positive sign: apprehension and pain.

Biceps load test I

Tests: superior labral pathology.

Procedure: patient supine with shoulder in 90° abduction, elbow in 90° flexion and forearm supinated. Laterally rotate shoulder until patient becomes apprehensive. Maintain this position. Resist elbow flexion.

Positive sign: pain/apprehension remains unchanged or increases during resisted elbow flexion.

Biceps load test II

Tests: superior labral pathology.

Procedure: patient supine with shoulder in 120° abduction and maximum lateral rotation, elbow in 90° flexion and forearm supinated. Resist elbow flexion.

Positive sign: increased pain during resisted elbow flexion.

Clunk test

Tests: tear of glenoid labrum.

Procedure: patient supine. Abduct shoulder over patient's head. Apply anterior force to posterior aspect of humeral head while rotating humerus laterally.

Positive sign: a clunk or grinding sound and/or apprehension if anterior instability present.

Crank test

Tests: labral pathology.

Procedure: patient sitting or supine with shoulder in 160° flexion in scapular plane. Hold elbow and apply a longitudinal compressive force to humerus while rotating it medially and laterally.

Positive sign: pain/reproduction of symptoms, with or without click, usually during lateral rotation.

Crossed-arm adduction test (Apley scarf test)

Tests: acromioclavicular joint pathology.

Procedure: patient upright. Horizontally adduct the arm as far as possible.

Positive sign: pain around acromioclavicular joint.

Drop test (external rotation lag sign)

Tests: infraspinatus and supraspinatus integrity.

Procedure: patient upright with shoulder in 20° abduction (in the scapular plane) with elbow in 90° flexion. Place shoulder in full lateral rotation. Support elbow and ask patient to hold position.

Positive sign: arm drops into medial rotation.

Hawkins–Kennedy impingement test

Tests: impingement of supraspinatus tendon.

Procedure: patient sitting or standing. Forward flex shoulder to 90° and flex elbow to 90°. Apply passive medial rotation.

Positive sign: reproduction of symptoms.

Hornblower's sign

Tests: teres minor integrity.

Procedure: patient sitting or standing with arms by side. Patient lifts hands up to mouth.

Positive sign: inability to lift the hand to the mouth without abducting arm first (this compensatory manoeuvre on the affected side is the hornblower's sign).

Jerk test

Tests: posterior shoulder stability.

Procedure: patient sitting. Place shoulder in 90° forward flexion and medial rotation. Apply longitudinal cephalad force to humerus and move arm into horizontal adduction.

Positive sign: sudden jerk or clunk.

Lift-off test

Tests: subscapularis integrity.

Procedure: patient upright with arm medially rotated behind back. Patient lifts hand away from back.

Positive sign: inability to lift arm indicates tendon rupture.

Load and shift test

Tests: anterior and posterior shoulder stability.

Procedure: patient sitting. Stabilize scapula by fixing coracoid process and spine of scapula. Grasp humeral head and apply a medial, compressive force to seat it in the glenoid fossa (load). Glide the humeral head anteriorly and posteriorly (shift).

Positive sign: increased anterior or posterior glide indicates anterior or posterior instability.

Neer impingement test

Tests: impingement of supraspinatus tendon and/or biceps tendon.

Procedure: patient sitting or standing. Passively elevate arm through forward flexion and medial rotation.

Positive sign: reproduction of symptoms.

Patte's test

Tests: infraspinatus and teres minor integrity.

Procedure: patient sitting. Place shoulder in 90° flexion in the scapular plane and elbow in 90° flexion. Patient rotates arm laterally against resistance.

Positive sign: resistance with pain indicates tendinopathy. Inability to resist with gradual lowering of the arm or forearm indicates tendon rupture.

Posterior drawer test

Tests: posterior shoulder stability.

Procedure: patient supine. Place shoulder in 100–120° abduction and 20–30° forward flexion with elbow flexed to 120°. Stabilize scapula. Medially rotate and forward flex shoulder between 60° and 80° while pushing head of humerus posteriorly.

Positive sign: significant posterior displacement and/or patient apprehension.

Relocation test (Fowler's sign)

Tests: differentiates between anterior shoulder stability and primary impingement.

Procedure: perform the apprehension test in supine. At the point where the patient feels pain or apprehension apply an anteroposterior force to humeral head.

Positive sign: persistence of pain or apprehension indicates primary impingement. Decrease in pain or apprehension and increased lateral rotation indicates instability and secondary impingement.

Speed's test

Tests: biceps tendon pathology.

Procedure: patient sitting or standing. Forward flex shoulder, supinate forearm and extend elbow. Resist patient's attempt to flex shoulder.

Positive sign: increased pain in bicipital groove.

Sulcus sign

Tests: inferior shoulder stability.

Procedure: patient standing or sitting, arm by side. Grip arm below elbow and pull distally.

Positive sign: reproduction of symptoms and/or appearance of sulcus under acromion.

Supraspinatus (empty can) test

Tests: supraspinatus tendon pathology; suprascapular nerve neuropathy.

Procedure: patient sitting or standing. Abduct shoulder to 90°. Horizontally flex to 30° and medially rotate so thumbs point downwards. Resist patient's attempt to abduct.

Positive sign: reproduction of symptoms or weakness.

Yergason's test

Tests: biceps tendon pathology; subacromial impingement.

Procedure: patient sitting or standing with elbow in 90° flexion and forearm pronated. Resist patient's attempts to supinate.

Positive sign: increased pain in bicipital groove.

Elbow

Elbow flexion test

Tests: cubital tunnel (ulnar nerve) syndrome.

Procedure: patient standing or sitting. Fully flex elbows with wrist extended. Hold for 5 minutes.

Positive sign: tingling or paraesthesia in ulnar nerve distribution.

Lateral epicondylitis (tennis elbow) test: method 1

Tests: lateral epicondylitis.

Procedure: passively extend elbow, pronate forearm and flex wrist and fingers while palpating lateral epicondyle.

Positive sign: reproduction of symptoms.

Lateral epicondylitis (tennis elbow) test: method 2

Tests: lateral epicondylitis.

Procedure: resist extension of middle finger distal to PIP (proximal interphalangeal) joint.

Positive sign: reproduction of symptoms.

Medial epicondylitis (golfer's elbow) test

Tests: medial epicondylitis.

Procedure: passively extend elbow, supinate forearm and extend wrist and fingers while palpating medial epicondyle.

Positive sign: reproduction of symptoms.

Pinch grip test

Tests: anterior interosseous (median) nerve entrapment.

Procedure: patient pinches tips of index finger and thumb together.

Positive sign: inability to pinch tip to tip.

Tinel's sign (at elbow)

Tests: point of regeneration of sensory fibres of ulnar nerve.

Procedure: tap ulnar nerve in groove between olecranon and medial epicondyle.

Positive sign: tingling sensation in ulnar distribution of forearm and hand. Furthest point at which abnormal sensation felt indicates point to which the nerve has regenerated.

Valgus stress test

Tests: stability of medial collateral ligament.

Procedure: patient in sitting. Stabilize upper arm with elbow in 20–30° flexion and humerus in full lateral rotation. Apply abduction/valgus force to forearm.

Positive sign: increased laxity or reproduction of symptoms.

Varus stress test

Tests: stability of lateral collateral ligament.

Procedure: patient in sitting. Stabilize upper arm with elbow in 20–30° flexion and humerus in full medial rotation. Apply adduction/varus force to forearm.

Positive sign: excessive laxity or reproduction of symptoms.

Wrist and hand

Finkelstein test

Tests: tenosynovitis of abductor pollicis longus and extensor pollicis brevis tendons (de Quervain's tenosynovitis).

Procedure: patient makes a fist with thumb inside. Passively move wrist into ulnar deviation.

Positive sign: reproduction of symptoms.

Froment's sign

Tests: ulnar nerve paralysis.

Procedure: grip piece of paper between index finger and thumb. Pull paper away.

Positive sign: flexion of IP (interphalangeal) thumb joint as paper pulled away.

Ligamentous instability test for the fingers

Tests: stability of collateral ligaments.

Procedure: apply valgus and varus force to PIP (proximal interphalangeal) or DIP (distal interphalangeal) joint.

Positive sign: increased laxity.

Linburg's sign

Tests: tendon pathology at interconnection between flexor pollicis longus and flexor indicis.

Procedure: thumb flexion onto hypothenar eminence and index finger extension.

Positive sign: limited extension and reproduction of symptoms.

Lunotriquetral ballottement (Reagan's) test

Tests: stability of lunotriquetral ligament.

Procedure: stabilize lunate and apply posterior and anterior glide to triquetrum and pisiform.

Positive sign: reproduction of symptoms, crepitus or laxity.

Phalen's (wrist flexion) test

Tests: median nerve pathology; carpal tunnel syndrome.

Procedure: place dorsal aspect of hands together with wrists flexed. Hold for 1 minute.

Positive sign: tingling in distribution of median nerve.

Reverse Phalen's test

Tests: median nerve pathology.

Procedure: place palms of hands together with wrists extended. Hold for 1 minute.

Positive sign: tingling in distribution of median nerve.

Sweater finger sign

Tests: rupture of flexor digitorum profundus tendon.

Procedure: patient makes a fist.

Positive sign: loss of DIP joint flexion of one of the fingers.

Tinel's sign (at the wrist)

Tests: median nerve pathology; carpal tunnel syndrome.

Procedure: tap over carpal tunnel.

Positive sign: tingling or paraesthesia in median distribution in hand. Furthest point at which abnormal sensation felt indicates point to which the nerve has regenerated.

Triangular fibrocartilage complex (TFCC) load test

Tests: triangular fibrocartilage complex integrity.

Procedure: hold forearm. With other hand hold wrist in ulnar deviation then move it through supination and pronation while applying a compressive force.

Positive sign: pain, clicking, crepitus.

Watson (scaphoid shift) test

Tests: stability of scaphoid.

Procedure: hold wrist in full ulnar deviation and slight extension. With other hand apply pressure to scaphoid tubercle (palmar aspect) and move wrist into radial deviation and slight flexion.
Positive sign: pain and/or subluxation of scaphoid.

Pelvis

Compression test

Tests: sprain of posterior sacroiliac joint or ligaments.
Procedure: patient supine or side lying. Push right and left ASIS (anterior superior iliac spine) towards each other.
Positive sign: reproduction of symptoms.

Gapping test (distraction)

Tests: sprain of anterior sacroiliac joint or ligaments.
Procedure: patient supine. Push right and left ASIS apart.
Positive sign: reproduction of symptoms.

Femoral shear test

Tests: sacroiliac joint pathology.
Procedure: patient supine with knee flexed and hip in slight flexion, abduction and 45° lateral rotation. Apply a graded longitudinal cephalad force along the femoral axis.
Positive sign: pain.

Gillet's test

Tests: sacroiliac joint dysfunction.
Procedure: patient standing. Palpate PSIS (posterior superior iliac spine) and sacrum at same level. Patient flexes hip and knee on side being palpated while standing on opposite leg. Repeat test on other side and compare.
Positive sign: if the PSIS on the side tested does not move downwards in relation to the sacrum it indicates hypomobility on that side.

Piedallu's sign (sitting flexion)

Tests: movement of sacrum on ilia.
Procedure: patient sitting. Left and right PSIS are palpated while patient forward flexes.
Positive sign: one side moves higher than the other, indicating hypomobility on that side.

Standing flexion

Tests: movement of ilia on sacrum.

Procedure: patient standing. Left and right PSIS are palpated while patient forward flexes.

Positive sign: one side moves higher than the other, indicating hypomobility on that side.

Supine to sit (long sitting) test

Tests: sacroiliac joint dysfunction caused by pelvic torsion or rotation.

Procedure: patient supine. Note level of inferior borders of medial malleoli. Patient sits up and relative position of malleoli noted.

Positive sign: one leg moves up more than the other.

Hip

Faber's test (Patrick's test)

Tests: hip joint or sacroiliac joint dysfunction; spasm of iliopsoas muscle.

Procedure: patient supine. Place foot of test leg on opposite knee. Gently lower knee of test leg.

Positive sign: knee remains above the opposite leg; pain or spasm.

Leg length test

Tests: leg-length discrepancy.

Procedure: patient supine. Measure between the anterior superior iliac spine and the medial or lateral malleolus.

Positive sign: a difference of more than 1.3 cm is considered significant.

Ober's sign

Tests: tensor fascia lata and iliotibial band contractures.

Procedure: patient in side lying with hip and knee of lower leg flexed. Stabilize pelvis. Passively abduct and extend upper leg with knee extended or flexed to 90°, then allow it to drop towards plinth.

Positive sign: upper leg remains abducted and does not lower to plinth.

Piriformis test

Tests: piriformis involvement in sciatic pain.

Procedure: patient side lying on edge of bed with test leg uppermost. Flex hip to 60° with knee flexed. Stabilize hip and apply downward pressure to knee.

Positive sign: localized pain indicates tight piriformis. Pain with radiation indicates sciatic nerve involvement.

Quadrant test

Tests: intra-articular hip joint pathology.

Procedure: patient supine. Place hip in full flexion and adduction. Abduct hip in a circular arc, maintaining full flexion, while applying a longitudinal compressive force.

Positive sign: pain, locking, crepitus, clicking, apprehension.

Rectus femoris contracture test

Tests: rectus femoris contracture.

Procedure: patient supine with test knee flexed to 90° over edge of plinth. Patient hugs other knee to chest.

Positive sign: knee over edge of plinth extends.

Thomas test

Tests: hip flexion contracture.

Procedure: patient supine. Patient hugs one knee to chest.

Positive sign: opposite leg lifts off plinth.

Trendelenburg's sign

Tests: stability of the hip, strength of hip abductors (gluteus medius).

Procedure: patient stands on one leg.

Positive sign: pelvis on opposite side drops.

Weber–Barstow manoeuvre

Tests: leg length asymmetry.

Procedure: patient supine with hips and knees flexed. Hold patient's feet, palpating medial malleoli with thumbs. Patient lifts pelvis off bed and returns to starting position. Passively extend legs and compare relative position of medial malleoli.

Positive sign: leg length asymmetry.

Knee

Abduction (valgus) stress test

Tests: full knee extension: anterior cruciate ligament, medial quadriceps expansion, semimembranosus muscle, medial collateral ligaments, posterior oblique ligament, posterior cruciate ligament, posteromedial capsule.

20–30° flexion: medial collateral ligament, posterior oblique ligament, posterior cruciate ligament, posteromedial capsule.

Procedure: patient supine. Stabilize ankle and apply medial pressure (valgus stress) to knee joint at 0° and then at 20–30° extension.

Positive sign: excessive movement compared with opposite knee.

Adduction (varus) stress test

Tests: full knee extension: cruciate ligaments, lateral gastrocnemius muscle, lateral collateral ligament, arcuate–popliteus complex, posterolateral capsule, iliotibial band, biceps femoris tendon.

20–30° flexion: lateral collateral ligament, arcuate–popliteus complex, posterolateral capsule, iliotibial band, biceps femoris tendon.

Procedure: patient supine. Stabilize ankle. Apply lateral pressure (varus stress) to knee joint at 0° and then at 20–30° extension.

Positive sign: excessive movement compared to opposite knee.

Anterior drawer test

Tests: anterior cruciate ligament, posterior oblique ligament, arcuate–popliteus complex, posteromedial and posterolateral capsules, medial collateral ligament, iliotibial band.

Procedure: patient supine with hips flexed to 45° and knee flexed to 90°. Stabilize foot. Apply posteroanterior force to tibia.

Positive sign: tibia moves more than 6 mm on the femur.

Apley's test

Tests: distraction for ligamentous injury; compression for meniscus injury.

Procedure: patient prone with knee flexed to 90°. Medially and laterally rotate tibia – first with distraction and then compression.
Positive sign: pain.

Brush test

Tests: mild effusion.
Procedure: stroke medial side of patella from just below joint line up to suprapatellar pouch two or three times. Use opposite hand to stroke down lateral side of patella.
Positive sign: fluid travels to medial side and appears as bulge below distal border of patella.

External rotation recurvatum test

Tests: posterolateral rotary stability in knee extension.
Procedure: patient supine. Hold heel and place knee in 30° flexion. Slowly extend knee while palpating posterolateral aspect of knee.
Positive sign: excessive hyperextension and lateral rotation palpated.

Fairbanks' apprehension test

Tests: patellar subluxation or dislocation.
Procedure: patient supine with knee in 30° flexion and quads relaxed. Passively glide patella laterally.
Positive sign: patient apprehension or excessive movement.

Hughston plica test

Tests: inflammation of suprapatellar plica.
Procedure: patient supine. Flex and medially rotate knee while applying medial glide to patella and palpating medial femoral condyle. Passively extend and flex knee.
Positive sign: popping of plica band over femoral condyle, tenderness.

Lachman's test

Tests: anterior cruciate ligament, posterior oblique ligament, arcuate–popliteus complex.
Procedure: patient supine with knee flexed 0–30°. Stabilize femur. Apply posteroanterior force to tibia.
Positive sign: soft end feel or excessive movement.

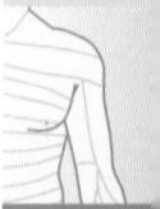

McConnell test for chondromalacia patellae

Tests: chondromalacia patellae.

Procedure: patient in high sitting with femur laterally rotated. Isometric quad contractions are performed at 0°, 30°, 60°, 90° and 120° of knee flexion for 10 seconds. If pain is produced with any of these movements, repeat test with patella pushed medially.

Positive sign: decrease in symptoms with medial glide.

McMurray test

Tests: medial meniscus and lateral meniscus injury.

Procedure: patient supine with test knee completely flexed. To test the medial meniscus, laterally rotate knee and passively extend to 90° while palpating joint line. To test the lateral meniscus, repeat test with the knee in medial rotation.

Positive sign: a snap or click.

Posterior drawer test

Tests: posterior cruciate ligament, arcuate–popliteus complex, posterior oblique ligament, anterior cruciate ligament.

Procedure: patient supine with hips flexed to 45° and knee flexed to 90°. Stabilize foot. Apply anteroposterior force to tibia.

Positive sign: excessive movement.

Posterior sag sign

Tests: posterior cruciate ligament, arcuate–popliteus complex, posterior oblique ligament, anterior cruciate ligament.

Procedure: patient supine with hips flexed to 45° and knee flexed to 90° with feet on plinth.

Positive sign: tibia drops posteriorly.

Slocum test for anterolateral rotary instability

Tests: anterior and posterior cruciate ligaments, posterolateral capsule, arcuate–popliteus complex, lateral collateral ligaments, iliotibial band.

Procedure: patient supine with hips flexed to 45° and knee flexed to 90°. Place foot in 30° medial rotation and stabilize. Apply posteroanterior force to tibia.

Positive sign: excessive movement on lateral side when compared with other knee.

Slocum test for anteromedial rotary instability

Tests: medial collateral ligament, posterior oblique ligament, posteromedial capsule, anterior cruciate ligament.

Procedure: patient supine with hips flexed to 45° and knee flexed to 90°. Place foot in 15° lateral rotation and stabilize. Apply posteroanterior force to tibia.

Positive sign: excessive movement on medial side when compared with other knee.

Ankle and foot

Anterior drawer sign

Tests: medial and lateral ligament integrity.

Procedure: patient prone with knee flexed. Apply posteroanterior force to talus with ankle in dorsiflexion and then plantarflexion.

Positive sign: excessive anterior movement (both ligaments affected) or movement on one side only (ligament on that side affected).

Talar tilt

Tests: adduction: mainly integrity of calcaneofibular ligament but also anterior talofibular ligament. Abduction: integrity of deltoid ligament.

Procedure: patient prone, supine or side lying with knee flexed. Tilt talus into abduction and adduction with patient's foot in neutral.

Positive sign: excessive movement.

Thompson's test

Tests: Achilles tendon rupture.

Procedure: patient prone with feet over edge of plinth. Squeeze calf muscles.

Positive sign: absence of plantarflexion.

Common vascular tests

Adson's manoeuvre

Tests: thoracic outlet syndrome.

Procedure: patient sitting. Patient turns head towards test arm and extends head. Laterally rotate and extend shoulder

and arm while palpating radial pulse. Patient takes a deep breath and holds it.
Positive sign: disappearance of radial pulse.

Homan's test

Tests: deep vein thrombophlebitis.
Procedure: patient supine. Passive dorsiflexion of ankle with knee extended.
Positive sign: pain in the calf.

Provocation elevation test

Tests: thoracic outlet syndrome.
Procedure: patient standing with arms above head. Opens and closes hands 15 times.
Positive sign: fatigue, cramp, tingling.

Neurodynamic tests (from Petty & Moore 2001, with permission)

Upper limb neurodynamic tests

When conducting the upper limb neurodynamic tests (ULNT) the sequence of the test movements is relatively unimportant and may be adapted to suit the patient's condition. However, if the tests are to be of value as an assessment tool, the order used for a particular patient must be the same each time the patient is tested.

ULNT 1

ULNT 1 (Fig. 2.10) consists of:

- Fixing shoulder to prevent shoulder elevation during abduction [1]
- Shoulder joint abduction [2]
- Wrist and finger extension [3]
- Forearm supination [3]
- Shoulder lateral rotation [4]
- Elbow extension [5]

Sensitizing test: cervical lateral flexion away from the symptomatic side [6].

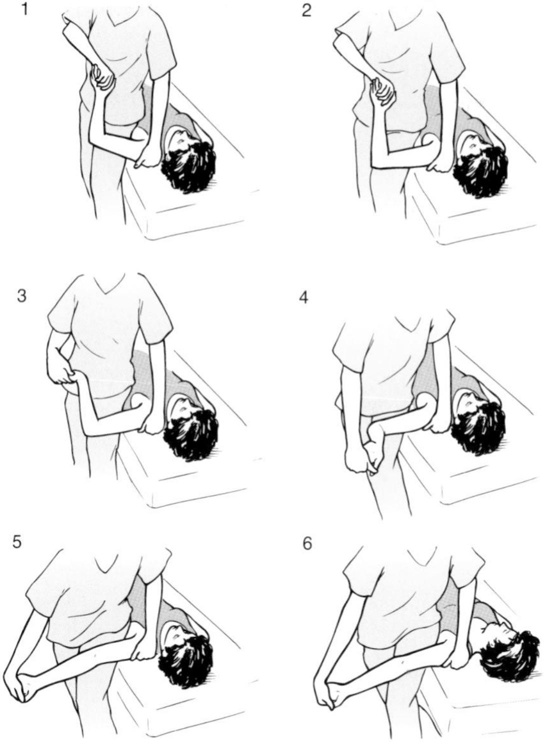
1
2
3
4
5
6

Figure 2.10 (1–6) Upper limb neurodynamic test 1.

Desensitizing test: cervical lateral flexion towards the symptomatic side.

ULNT 2a

ULNT 2a (Fig. 2.11) consists of:

- Shoulder girdle depression [1, 2]
- Elbow extension [3]
- Lateral rotation of whole arm [4]

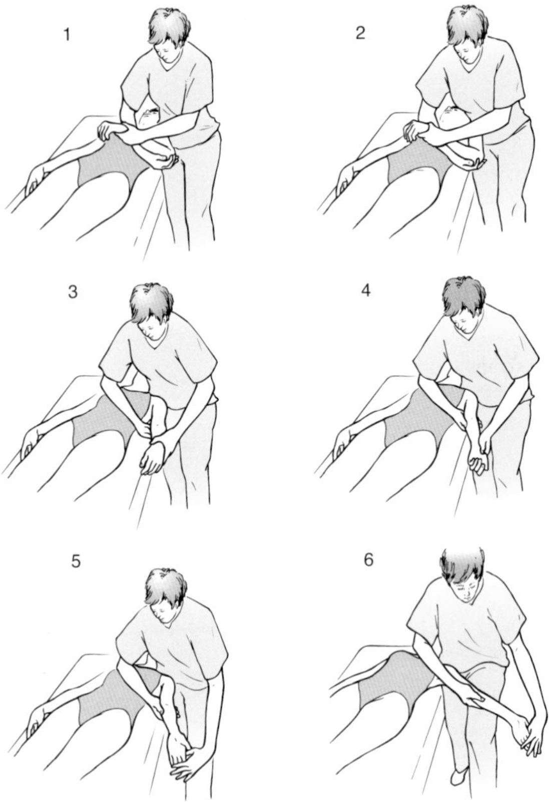
1
2
3
4
5
6

Figure 2.11 (1–6) Upper limb neurodynamic test 2a. Median nerve bias.

- Wrist, finger and thumb extension [5]
- Abduction of shoulder [6]

Sensitizing test: cervical lateral flexion away from the symptomatic side.

Desensitizing tests: cervical lateral flexion towards the symptomatic side or release of the shoulder girdle depression.

ULNT 2b

ULNT 2b (Fig. 2.12) consists of:

- Shoulder girdle depression [1]
- Elbow extension [2]
- Medial rotation of whole arm [3]
- Wrist and finger flexion [4]
- Shoulder abduction

Sensitizing test: cervical lateral flexion away from the symptomatic side.

Desensitizing tests: cervical lateral flexion towards the symptomatic side or release of the shoulder girdle depression.

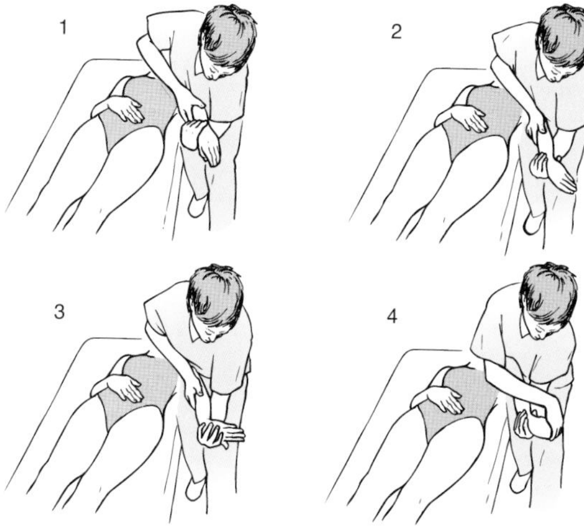
1
2
3
4

Figure 2.12 (1–4) Upper limb neurodynamic test 2b. Radial nerve bias.

ULNT 3

ULNT 3 (Fig. 2.13) consists of:

- Shoulder girdle depression [1]
- Wrist and finger extension [1]
- Forearm pronation [2]
- Elbow flexion [3]
- Shoulder lateral rotation [4]
- Shoulder abduction [5]

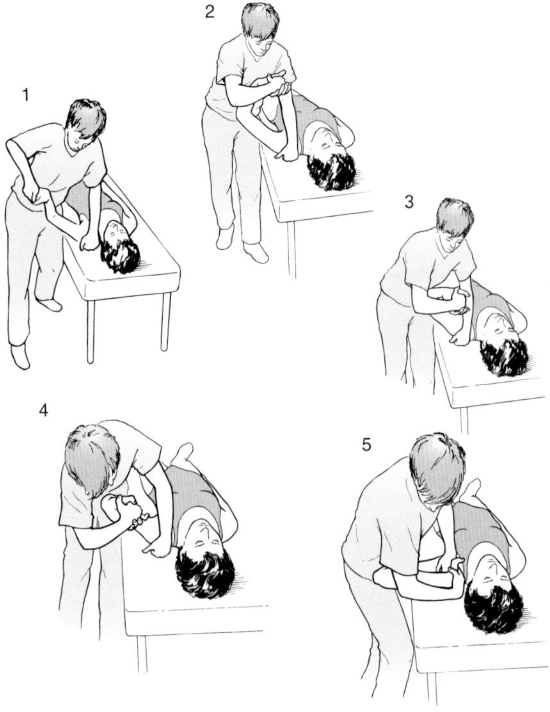
1
2
3
4
5

Figure 2.13 (1–5) Upper limb neurodynamic test 3. Ulnar nerve bias.

Sensitizing test: cervical lateral flexion away from the symptomatic side.

Desensitizing tests: cervical lateral flexion towards the symptomatic side or release of the shoulder girdle depression.

For all the upper limb neurodynamic tests you may wish to place the patient's head in contralateral cervical flexion before you do the test and then instruct them to bring their head back to midline at the end of the sequence.

Slump test (Fig. 2.14)

Starting position: patient sits upright with knee crease at the edge of plinth and hands behind back [1].

The slump test consists of:

- Spinal slump [2]
- Neck flexion [3]

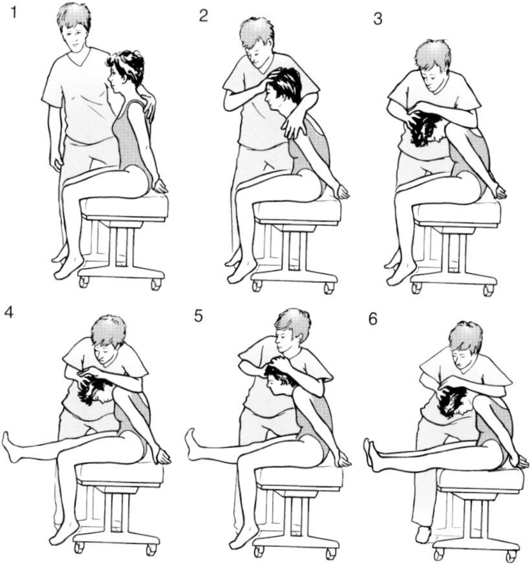

1
2
3
4
5
6

Figure 2.14 (1–6) Slump test.

- Knee extension [4]
- Release neck flexion [5]

The steps can be performed in any order.

Additional movements: add dorsiflexion or plantarflexion with knee extension; bilateral knee extension [6], hip abduction (obturator nerve bias).

Straight leg raise

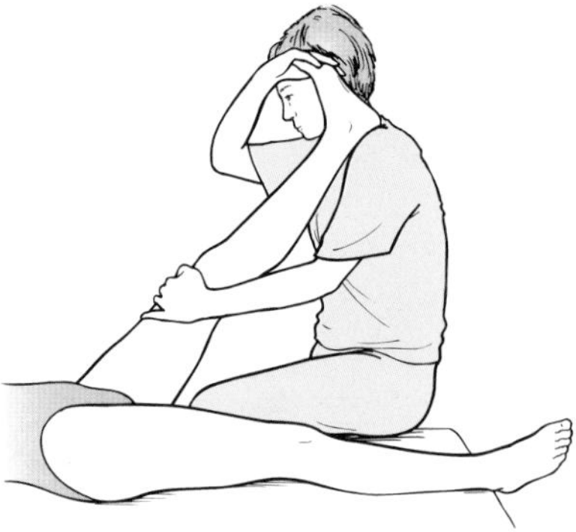

Figure 2.15 Straight leg raise.

The test consists of passive hip flexion with the knee extended.

Sensitizing tests: dorsiflexion, hip adduction, hip medial rotation, neck flexion and spinal lateral flexion.

Additional sensitizing tests: Add ankle dorsiflexion and eversion (tibial nerve bias), plantarflexion and inversion (superficial peroneal nerve bias), dorsiflexion and inversion (sural nerve bias).

Passive neck flexion

The test consists of passive neck flexion.

Sensitizing tests: straight leg raise, upper limb neurodynamic tests.

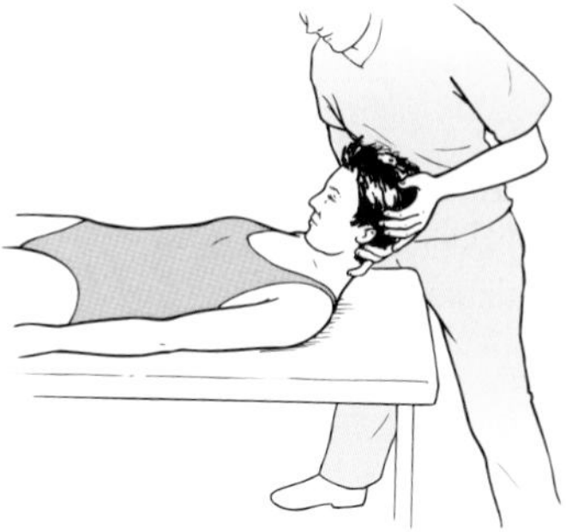

Figure 2.16 Passive neck flexion.

Slump knee bend

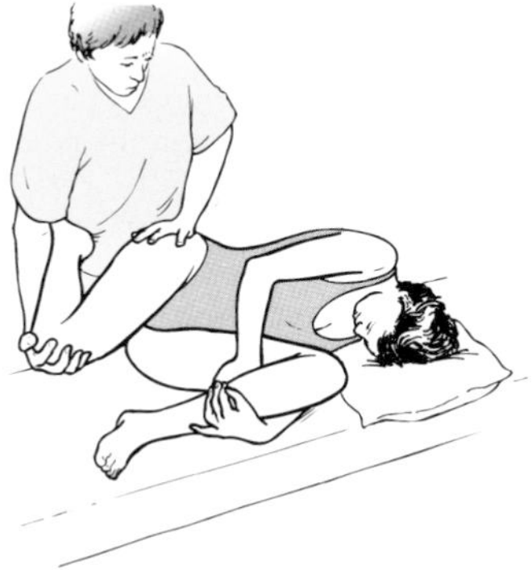

Figure 2.17 Slump knee bend.

Starting position: patient in side lying. Holds bottom knee to chest and flexes neck.

The slump knee bend consists of:

1. Flex uppermost knee
2. Hip extension

Desensitizing test: cervical extension.

Precautions with physical neural examination and management (from Butler 2000 *The Sensitive Nervous System*, Noigroup Press, with permission of Noigroup Publications)

- Patients with suspected 'red flags' need to be identified and managed accordingly.
- Take care with elongation and pinching manoeuvres with acute nerve root disorders.
- Watch that repeated movements do not aggravate a central sensitivity state.
- Be careful in acute states, when clinical pictures such as disc trauma or compartment syndrome suggest that nerve irritation/compression could occur.
- Take care with recent apparent peripheral severe nerve injury that may, initially, be clinically silent. Wait for a few days to see what the clinical expression will be.
- There are some states where peripheral nerves appear tethered and will not move with various physical therapies. Repeated attempts will just worsen the problem. A surgical opinion is necessary.
- Take care with disorders such as diabetes, rheumatoid arthritis and Guillain–Barré. However, programmes including graded mobilization and fitness may be useful for symptomatic relief and to minimize complications.
- Where there are hard upper motor neurone signs, as could occur after trauma or with tethered cord syndrome, seek specialist medical opinion.

Nerve pathways

Brachial plexus

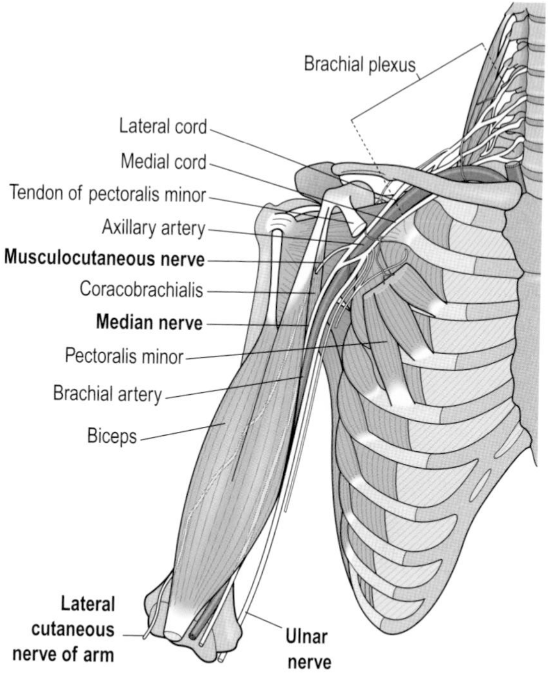

Brachial plexus
Lateral cord
Medial cord
Tendon of pectoralis minor
Axillary artery
Musculocutaneous nerve
Coracobrachialis
Median nerve
Pectoralis minor
Brachial artery
Biceps
Lateral cutaneous nerve of arm
Ulnar nerve

Figure 2.18 Brachial plexus.

SECTION 2

MUSCULOSKELETAL

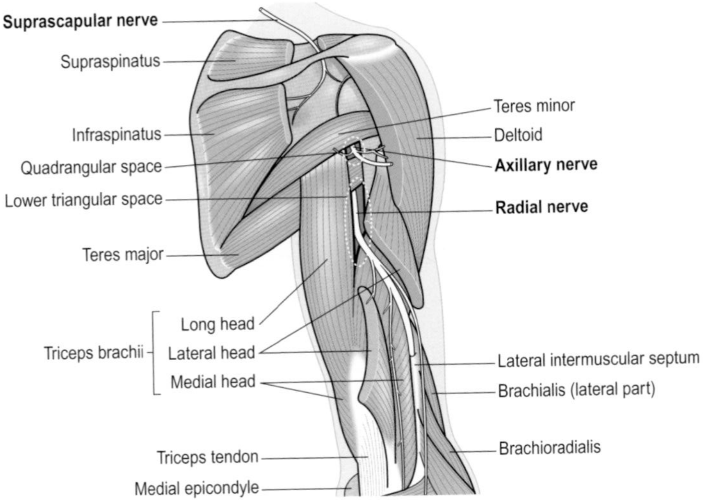
Suprascapular nerve
Supraspinatus
Infraspinatus
Quadrangular space
Lower triangular space
Teres major
Triceps brachii
Long head
Lateral head
Medial head
Triceps tendon
Medial epicondyle
Teres minor
Deltoid
Axillary nerve
Radial nerve
Lateral intermuscular septum
Brachialis (lateral part)
Brachioradialis

Figure 2.19 Axillary and radial nerves.

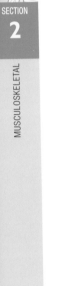

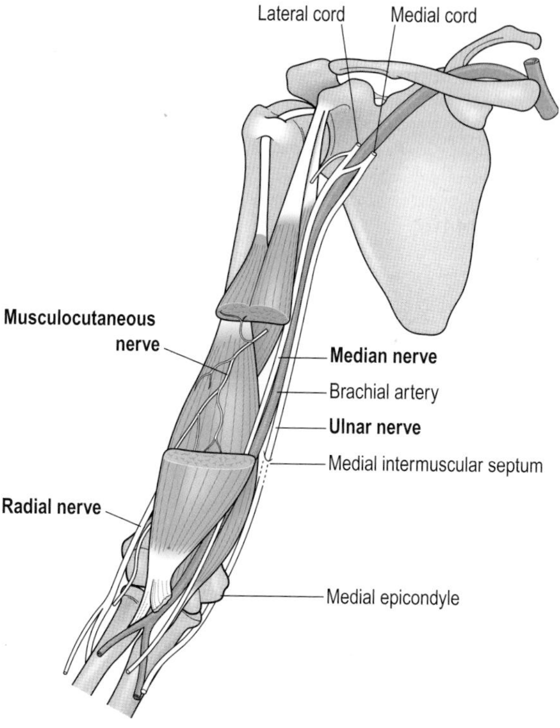
Lateral cord
Medial cord
Musculocutaneous nerve
Median nerve
Brachial artery
Ulnar nerve
Medial intermuscular septum
Radial nerve
Medial epicondyle

Figure 2.20 Musculocutaneous, median and ulnar nerves.

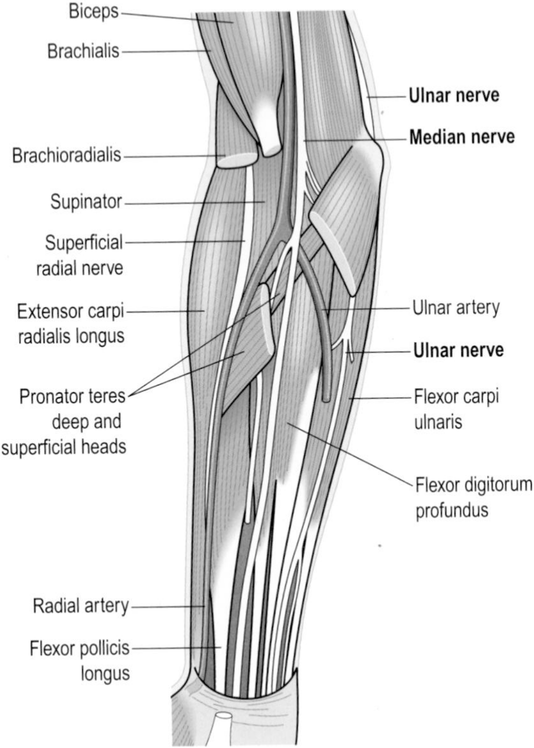
Biceps
Brachialis
Brachioradialis
Supinator
Superficial radial nerve
Extensor carpi radialis longus
Pronator teres deep and superficial heads
Radial artery
Flexor pollicis longus
Ulnar nerve
Median nerve
Ulnar artery
Ulnar nerve
Flexor carpi ulnaris
Flexor digitorum profundus

Figure 2.21 Ulnar and median nerves.

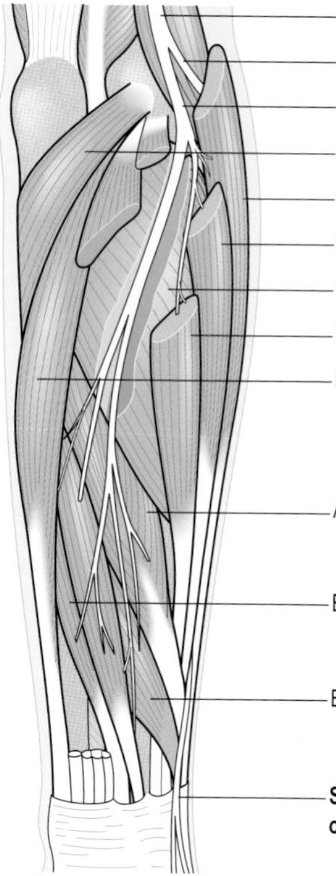

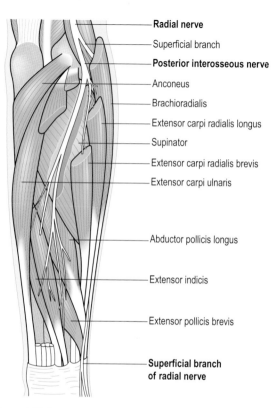

Radial nerve
Superficial branch
Posterior interosseous nerve
Anconeus
Brachioradialis
Extensor carpi radialis longus
Supinator
Extensor carpi radialis brevis
Extensor carpi ulnaris
Abductor pollicis longus
Extensor indicis
Extensor pollicis brevis
Superficial branch
of radial nerve

Figure 2.22 Radial nerve.

Axillary

Origin: Posterior cord (C5–C6)
Course:

- Descends laterally posterior to axillary artery and anterior to subscapularis
- Passes posteriorly at lower border of subscapularis together with posterior circumflex humeral vessels via quadrangular space
- Divides: anterior and posterior branches. Anterior branch winds around surgical neck of humerus and supplies anterior deltoid. Posterior branch supplies teres minor and posterior deltoid. Continues as upper lateral cutaneous nerve of the arm after passing around deltoid

Musculocutaneous nerve

Origin: Large terminal branch of lateral cord (C5–C7)
Course:

- Descends from lower border of pectoralis minor, lateral to axillary artery
- Pierces coracobrachialis and descends diagonally between biceps and brachialis to lateral side of arm
- Pierces deep fascia of antecubital fossa and continues as lateral cutaneous nerve of the forearm
- Divides: anterior and posterior branches

Ulnar nerve

Origin: Large terminal branch of the medial cord (C7, C8, T1)
Course:

- Descends medial to brachial artery and anterior to triceps as far as the insertion of coracobrachialis
- Penetrates medial intermuscular septum and enters posterior compartment to continue descent anterior to medial head of triceps
- Passes posterior to medial epicondyle
- Enters anterior compartment between humeral and ulnar heads of flexor carpi ulnaris

- Descends medially, anterior to flexor digitorum profundus and posterior to flexor carpi ulnaris
- Pierces deep fascia lateral to flexor carpi ulnaris and proximal to flexor retinaculum
- Passes anterior to flexor retinaculum and lateral to pisiform
- Crosses hook of hamate
- Divides: superficial and deep branches

Median nerve

Origin: Lateral cord (C5–C7) and medial cord (C8, T1)
Course:

- The two cords unite anterior to the third part of the axillary artery at the inferior margin of teres major
- Descends lateral to brachial artery and posterior to biceps, passing medial and anterior to brachial artery at the insertion of coracobrachialis
- Crosses front of elbow lying on brachialis and deep to bicipital aponeurosis
- Dives between the two heads of pronator teres and descends through flexor digitorum superficialis and profundus
- Becomes superficial near the wrist, passing between the tendons of flexor carpi radialis (lateral) and flexor digitorum superficialis (medial), deep to palmaris longus
- Passes through the carpal tunnel
- Divides: medial and lateral branches

Radial nerve

Origin: Posterior cord (C5–C8 (T1))
Course:

- Descends posterior to axillary and brachial arteries and anterior to tendons of subscapularis, latissimus dorsi and teres major
- Enters posterior compartment via lower triangular space together with profunda brachii artery
- Descends obliquely towards lateral humerus along spiral groove lying between lateral and medial head of triceps

- Enters anterior compartment via lateral intermuscular septum to lie between brachialis and brachioradialis
- Divides: superficial radial nerve (sensory) and posterior interosseous nerve (motor) anterior to lateral epicondyle

Posterior interosseous nerve

Course:

- Enters posterior compartment between two heads of supinator
- Descends between deep and superficial groups of extensors
- Ends in flattened expansion on interosseous membrane

Lumbosacral plexus

(See Figure 2.23)

Lower limb

(See Figure 2.24 to 2.28)

Sciatic nerve

Origin: Ventral rami L4–S3
Course:

- Forms anterior to piriformis. Leaves pelvis via greater sciatic foramen below piriformis
- Enters gluteal region approximately midway between ischial tuberosity and greater trochanter
- Descends on top of superior gemellus, obturator internus, inferior gemellus, quadratus femoris and adductor magnus and under gluteus maximus and long head of biceps femoris
- Divides: tibial and common peroneal nerves at approximately distal third of thigh

Tibial nerve

Origin: Medial terminal branch of sciatic nerve (L4–S3)
Course:

- Descends through popliteal fossa, passing laterally to medially across the popliteal vessels
- Passes under tendinous arch of soleus

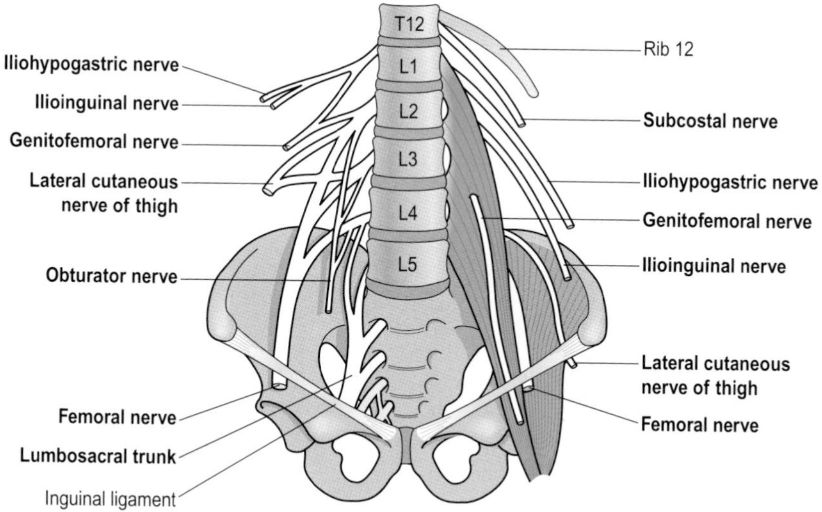
T12
L1
L2
L3
L4
L5
Iliohypogastric nerve
Ilioinguinal nerve
Genitofemoral nerve
Lateral cutaneous nerve of thigh
Obturator nerve
Femoral nerve
Lumbosacral trunk
Inguinal ligament
Rib 12
Subcostal nerve
Iliohypogastric nerve
Genitofemoral nerve
Ilioinguinal nerve
Lateral cutaneous nerve of thigh
Femoral nerve

Figure 2.23 Lumbosacral plexus.

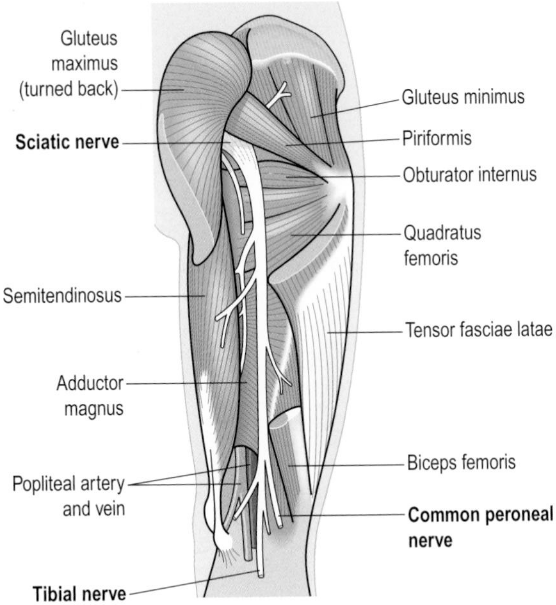
Gluteus maximus (turned back)
Sciatic nerve
Semitendinosus
Adductor magnus
Popliteal artery and vein
Tibial nerve
Gluteus minimus
Piriformis
Obturator internus
Quadratus femoris
Tensor fasciae latae
Biceps femoris
Common peroneal nerve

Figure 2.24 Sciatic nerve.

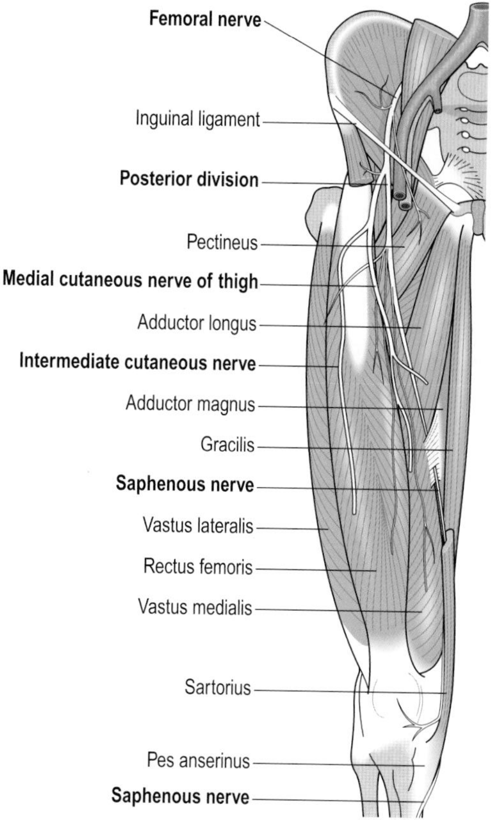

Femoral nerve
Inguinal ligament
Posterior division
Pectineus
Medial cutaneous nerve of thigh
Adductor longus
Intermediate cutaneous nerve
Adductor magnus
Gracilis
Saphenous nerve
Vastus lateralis
Rectus femoris
Vastus medialis
Sartorius
Pes anserinus
Saphenous nerve

Figure 2.25 Femoral nerve.

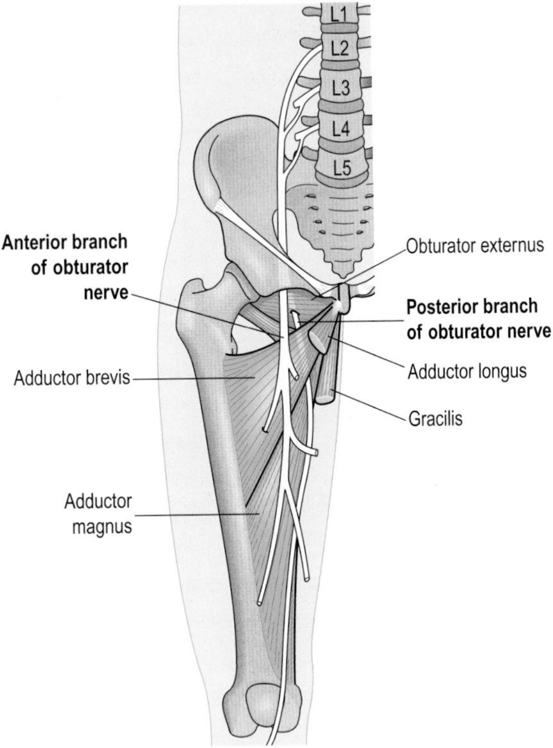
L1
L2
L3
L4
L5
Anterior branch of obturator nerve
Obturator externus
Posterior branch of obturator nerve
Adductor brevis
Adductor longus
Gracilis
Adductor magnus

Figure 2.26 Obturator nerve.

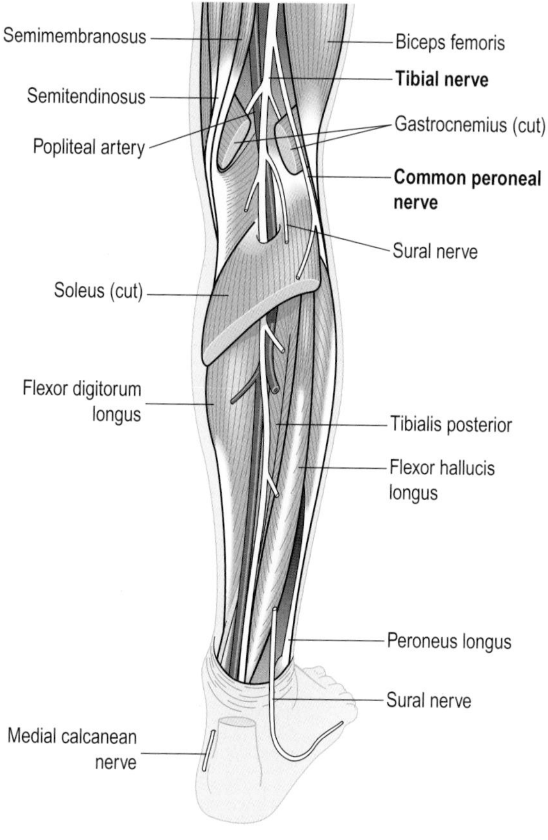
Semimembranosus
Biceps femoris
Tibial nerve
Semitendinosus
Gastrocnemius (cut)
Popliteal artery
Common peroneal nerve
Sural nerve
Soleus (cut)
Flexor digitorum longus
Tibialis posterior
Flexor hallucis longus
Peroneus longus
Sural nerve
Medial calcanean nerve

Figure 2.27 Tibial and common peroneal nerves.

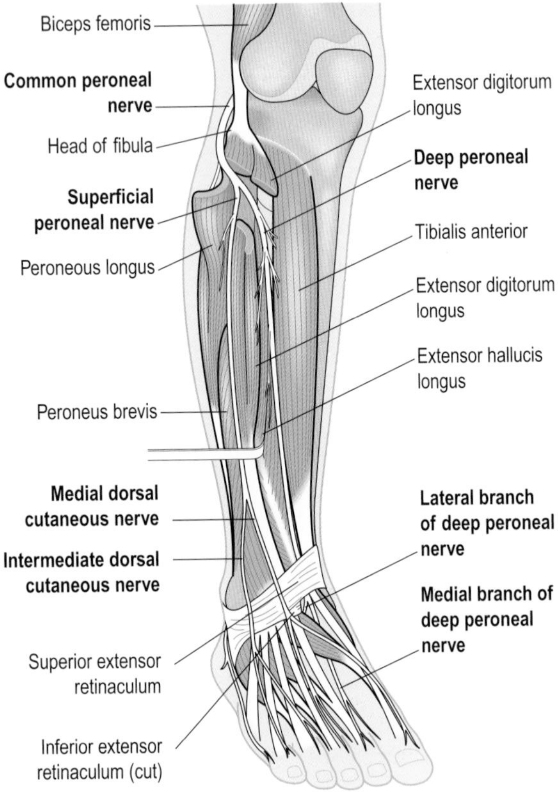

Biceps femoris
Common peroneal nerve
Head of fibula
Superficial peroneal nerve
Peroneous longus
Peroneus brevis
Medial dorsal cutaneous nerve
Intermediate dorsal cutaneous nerve
Superior extensor retinaculum
Inferior extensor retinaculum (cut)
Extensor digitorum longus
Deep peroneal nerve
Tibialis anterior
Extensor digitorum longus
Extensor hallucis longus
Lateral branch of deep peroneal nerve
Medial branch of deep peroneal nerve

Figure 2.28 Superficial and deep peroneal nerves.

- Descends inferomedially under soleus and gastrocnemius, lying on tibialis posterior and between flexor digitorum longus and flexor hallucis longus
- Passes through tarsal tunnel (formed by the flexor retinaculum, which extends from the medial malleolus to the medial calcaneus)

- Enters plantar aspect of foot
- Divides: medial and lateral plantar nerves

Common peroneal nerve

Origin: Lateral terminal branch of sciatic nerve (L4–S3)
Course:

- Descends along lateral side of popliteal fossa between biceps femoris and lateral head of gastrocnemius
- Passes anteriorly by winding around the neck of the fibula, deep to peroneus longus
- Divides: superficial and deep peroneal nerves

Superficial peroneal nerve

Course:

- Descends between extensor digitorum longus and peroneus longus, anterior to the fibula
- Pierces deep fascia halfway down the leg to become superficial
- Divides: medial and intermediate dorsal cutaneous nerves which enter foot via anterolateral aspect of ankle

Deep peroneal nerve

Course:

- Passes inferomedially into anterior compartment deep to extensor digitorum longus
- Descends on interosseous membrane deep to extensor hallucis longus and superior extensor retinaculum
- Crosses ankle deep to inferior extensor retinaculum and tendon of extensor hallucis longus and medial to tibialis anterior
- Enters dorsum of foot between tendons of extensor hallucis and digitorum longus
- Divides: medial and lateral branches

Obturator nerve

Origin: Anterior divisions of L2–L4
Course:

- Anterior divisions unite in psoas major
- Emerges from psoas major on lateral aspect of sacrum

- Crosses sacroiliac joint and obturator internus
- Enters obturator canal below superior pubic rami
- Exits obturator canal above obturator externus in medial compartment of thigh
- Divides: anterior and posterior branches (separated by obturator externus and adductor brevis)

Femoral nerve

Origin: Posterior divisions of L2–L4
Course:

- Posterior divisions unite in psoas major
- Emerges from lower lateral border of psoas major
- Descends in groove between psoas major and iliacus, deep to iliac fossa
- Passes posterior to inguinal ligament and lateral to femoral artery
- Enters femoral triangle
- Divides: number of anterior and posterior branches

Diagnostic triage for back pain (including red flags) (from Clinical Standards Advisory Group 1994, with permission)

The main diagnostic indicators for simple backache, nerve root pain and possible serious spinal pathology ('red flags') are outlined below:

Simple backache

- Onset generally age 20–55 years
- Lumbosacral region, buttocks and thighs
- Pain mechanical in nature
  - varies with physical activity
  - varies with time
- Patient well
- Prognosis good (90% recover from acute attack in 6 weeks)

Nerve root pain

- Unilateral leg pain > back pain
- Pain generally radiates to foot or toes
- Numbness and paraesthesia in the same distribution
- Nerve irritation signs
  - reduced straight leg raising which reproduces leg pain
- Motor, sensory or reflex change
  - limited to one nerve root
- Prognosis reasonable (50% recover from acute attack within 6 weeks)

Possible serious spinal pathology

Red flags

- Age of onset <20 or >55 years
- Violent trauma: e.g. fall from a height, road traffic accident
- Constant, progressive, non-mechanical pain
- Thoracic pain
- Previous medical history – carcinoma
- Systemic steroids
- Drug abuse, HIV
- Systemically unwell
- Weight loss
- Persisting severe restriction of lumbar flexion
- Widespread neurology
- Structural deformity

If there are suspicious clinical features, or if pain has not settled in 6 weeks, an ESR and plain X-ray should be considered.

Cauda equina syndrome/widespread neurological disorder

- Difficulty with micturition
- Loss of anal sphincter tone or faecal incontinence
- Saddle anaesthesia about the anus, perineum or genitals
- Widespread (more than one nerve root) or progressive motor weakness in the legs or gait disturbance

Inflammatory disorders (ankylosing spondylitis and related disorders)

- Gradual onset
- Marked morning stiffness
- Persisting limitation of spinal movements in all directions
- Peripheral joint involvement
- Iritis, skin rashes (psoriasis), colitis, urethral discharge
- Family history

Psychosocial yellow flags (Accident Compensation Corporation 2004, with permission)

Attitudes and beliefs about back pain

- Belief that pain is harmful or disabling, resulting in fear-avoidance behaviour, e.g. the development of guarding and fear of movement
- Belief that a pain must be abolished before attempting to return to work or normal activity
- Expectation of increased pain with activity or work, lack of ability to predict capability
- Catastrophizing, thinking the worst, misinterpreting bodily symptoms
- Belief that pain is uncontrollable
- Passive attitude to rehabilitation behaviours
- Use of extended rest, disproportionate 'downtime'
- Reduced activity level with significant withdrawal from activities of daily living
- Irregular participation or poor compliance with physical exercise, tendency for activities to be in a 'boom–bust' cycle
- Avoidance of normal activity and progressive substitution of lifestyle away from productive activity
- Report of extremely high intensity of pain, e.g. above 10, on a 0–10 visual analogue scale
- Excessive reliance on use of aids or appliances
- Sleep quality reduced since onset of back pain

- High intake of alcohol or other substances (possibly as self-medication), with an increase since onset of back pain
- Smoking

Compensation issues

- Lack of financial incentive to return to work
- Delay in accessing income support and treatment cost, disputes over eligibility
- History of claim/s due to other injuries or pain problems
- History of extended time off work due to injury or other pain problem (e.g. more than 12 weeks)
- History of previous back pain, with a previous claim/s and time off work
- Previous experience of ineffective case management (e.g. absence of interest, perception of being treated punitively)

Diagnosis and treatment

- Health professional sanctioning disability, not providing interventions that will improve function
- Experience of conflicting diagnoses or explanations for back pain, resulting in confusion
- Diagnostic language leading to catastrophizing and fear (e.g. fear of ending up in a wheelchair)
- Dramatization of back pain by health professional producing dependency on treatments, and continuation of passive treatment
- Number of visits to health professional in previous year (excluding the present episode of back pain)
- Expectation of a 'techno-fix', e.g. requests to treat as if body were a machine
- Lack of satisfaction with previous treatment for back pain
- Advice to withdraw from job

Emotions

- Fear of increased pain with activity or work
- Depression (especially long-term low mood), loss of sense of enjoyment
- More irritable than usual

- Anxiety about and heightened awareness of body sensations (includes sympathetic nervous system arousal)
- Feeling under stress and unable to maintain sense of control
- Presence of social anxiety or lack of interest in social activity
- Feeling useless and not needed

Family

- Over-protective partner/spouse, emphasizing fear of harm or encouraging catastrophizing (usually well intentioned)
- Solicitous behaviour from spouse (e.g. taking over tasks)
- Socially punitive responses from spouse (e.g. ignoring, expressing frustration)
- Extent to which family members support any attempt to return to work
- Lack of support person to talk to about problems

Work

- History of manual work, notably from the following occupational groups:
  - Fishing, forestry and farming workers
  - Construction, including carpenters and builders
  - Nurses
  - Truck drivers
  - Labourers
- Work history, including patterns of frequent job changes, experiencing stress at work, job dissatisfaction, poor relationships with peers or supervisors, lack of vocational direction
- Belief that work is harmful; that it will do damage or be dangerous
- Unsupportive or unhappy current work environment
- Low educational background, low socioeconomic status
- Job involves significant bio-mechanical demands, such as lifting, manual handling of heavy items, extended sitting, extended standing, driving, vibration, maintenance of constrained or sustained postures, inflexible work schedule preventing appropriate breaks

- Job involves shift work or working unsociable hours
- Minimal availability of selected duties and graduated return to work pathways, with unsatisfactory implementation of these
- Negative experience of workplace management of back pain (e.g. absence of a reporting system, discouragement to report, punitive response from supervisors and managers)
- Absence of interest from employer

Remember the key question to bear in mind while conducting these clinical assessments is: **'What can be done to help this person experience less distress and disability?'**

How to judge if a person is at risk for long-term work loss and disability

A person may be at risk if:

- There is a cluster of a few very salient factors
- There is a group of several less important factors that combine cumulatively

There is good agreement that the following factors are important and consistently predict poor outcomes:

- Presence of a belief that back pain is harmful or potentially severely disabling
- Fear-avoidance behaviour (avoiding a movement or activity due to misplaced anticipation of pain) and reduced activity levels
- Tendency to low mood and withdrawal from social interaction
- An expectation that passive treatments rather than active participation will help

Suggested questions (to be phrased in treatment provider's own words):

- Have you had time off work in the past with back pain?
- What do you understand is the cause of your back pain?
- What are you expecting will help you?
- How is your employer responding to your back pain? Your co-workers? Your family?

- What are you doing to cope with back pain?
- Do you think that you will return to work? When?

Musculoskeletal assessment

Patients present with a variety of conditions, and assessments need to be adapted to suit their needs. This section provides a basic framework for the subjective and physical musculoskeletal assessment of a patient.

Subjective examination

Body chart

Location of current symptoms
Type of pain
Depth, quality, intensity of symptoms
Intermittent or constant
Abnormal sensation (e.g. pins and needles, numbness)
Relationship of symptoms
Check other relevant regions

Behaviour of symptoms

Aggravating factors
Easing factors
Severity
Irritability
Daily activities/functional limitations
24-hour behaviour (night pain)
Stage of the condition

Special questions

Red flags
Spinal cord or cauda equina symptoms
Bilateral extremity numbness/pins and needles
Dizziness or other symptoms of vertebrobasilar insufficiency (diplopia, drop attacks, dysarthria, dysphagia, nausea)

History of present condition

Mechanism of injury
History of each symptomatic area

Relationship of onset of each symptomatic area
Change of each symptom since onset
Recent X-rays or investigations

Past medical history

Relevant medical history
Previous episodes of present complaint
Previous treatment and outcome
General health
THREAD (**T**hyroid disorders, **H**eart problems, **R**heumatoid arthritis, **E**pilepsy, **A**sthma or other respiratory problems, **D**iabetes)

Drug history

Current medication
Steroids
Anticoagulants
Allergies

Social and family history

Age and gender
Home and work situation
Dependants
Hobbies and activities
Exercise
Yellow flags

Physical examination

Observation

Posture
Function
Gait
Structural abnormalities
Muscle bulk and tone
Soft tissues

Active and passive joint movements

Active and passive physiological movements
Joint effusion measurement

Muscle tests

Muscle strength
Muscle control and stability
Muscle length
Isometric muscle testing

Neurological tests

Integrity of the nervous system
- dermatomes
- reflexes
- myotomes

Mobility of the nervous system
- straight leg raise
- slump test
- slump knee bend
- passive neck flexion
- upper limb neurodynamic tests

Special tests (e.g. coordination)

Palpation

Skin and superficial soft tissue
Muscle and tendon
Nerve
Ligament
Joint
Bone

Joint integrity tests

Passive accessory movements

References and further reading

Accident Compensation Corporation 2004 New Zealand acute low back pain guide: incorporating the guide to assessing psychosocial yellow flags in acute low back pain. ACC, New Zealand (www.acc.co.nz)

Adams J C, Hamblen D L 2001 Outline of orthopaedics, 13th edn. Churchill Livingstone, Edinburgh

Baxter R 2003 Pocket guide to musculoskeletal assessment, 2nd edn. Saunders, St Louis

Brukner P, Khan K 2006 Clinical sports medicine, 3rd edn. McGraw-Hill, Sydney
Butler D S 2000 The sensitive nervous system. Noigroup Publications, Adelaide
Clinical Standards Advisory Group 1994 Back pain: report of a CSAG committee on back pain. HMSO, London
Cyriax J 1982 Textbook of orthopaedic medicine. Vol. 1: Diagnosis of soft tissue lesions, 8th edn. Baillière Tindall, London
Dandy D J, Edwards D J 2003 Essential orthopaedics and trauma, 4th edn. Churchill Livingstone, Edinburgh
Douglas G, Nicol F, Robertson C 2005 Macleod's clinical examination, 11th edn. Churchill Livingstone, Edinburgh
Drake R L, Vogl W, Mitchell A W M 2005 Gray's anatomy for students. Churchill Livingstone, Philadelphia
Grahame R, Bird H A, Child A, et al 2000 The British Society for Rheumatology special interest group on heritable disorders of connective tissue criteria for the benign joint hypermobility syndrome. The revised (Brighton 1998) criteria for the diagnosis of the BJHS. Journal of Rheumatology 27(7): 1777–1779
Greenhalgh S, Selfe J 2006 Red flags: a guide to identifying serious pathology of the spine. Churchill Livingstone, Edinburgh
Grieve G P 1991 Mobilisation of the spine: a primary handbook of clinical method, 5th edn. Churchill Livingstone, Edinburgh
Gross J, Fetto J, Rosen E 2002 Musculoskeletal examination, 2nd edn. Blackwell Science, Malden, MA
Hengeveld E, Banks K 2005 Maitland's peripheral manipulation, 4th edn. Butterworth Heinemann, Edinburgh
Hengeveld E, Banks K, English K 2005 Maitland's vertebral manipulation, 7th edn. Butterworth Heinemann, Edinburgh
Kendall F P, McCreary E K, Provance P G, et al 2005 Muscles: testing and function with posture and pain, 5th edn. Lippincott Williams & Wilkins, Baltimore
McRae R 2006 Pocketbook of orthopaedics and fractures, 2nd edn. Churchill Livingstone, Edinburgh
McRae R, Esser M 2008 Practical fracture treatment, 5th edn. Churchill Livingstone, Edinburgh
Magee D J 2008 Orthopaedic physical assessment, 5th edn. Saunders, St Louis
Malanga G A, Nadler S F 2006 Musculoskeletal physical examination: an evidence-based approach. Mosby, Philadelphia
Middleditch A, Oliver J 2005 Functional anatomy of the spine, 2nd edn. Butterworth Heinemann, Edinburgh

O'Brien M D 2000 Guarantors of 'Brain' 1999–2000 (prepared by O'Brian M D). Aids to the examination of the peripheral nervous system, 4th edn. W B Saunders, Edinburgh

Palastanga N, Field D, Soames R 2006 Anatomy and human movement: structure and function, 5th edn. Butterworth Heinemann, Oxford

Petty N J 2006 Neuromusculoskeletal examination and assessment: a handbook for therapists, 3rd edn. Churchill Livingstone, Edinburgh

Petty N J, Moore A P 2001 Neuromusculoskeletal examination and assessment: a handbook for therapists, 2nd edn. Churchill Livingstone, Edinburgh

Reese N B, Bandy W D 2002 Joint range of motion and muscle length testing. W B Saunders, Philadelphia

Shacklock M 2005 Clinical neurodynamics: a new system of musculoskeletal treatment. Butterworth Heinemann, Edinburgh

Simons D G, Travell J G, Simons L S 1998 Travell and Simons' Myofascial pain and dysfunction: the trigger point manual. Volume 1. Upper half of body, 2nd edn. Lippincott Williams & Wilkins, Baltimore

Soloman L, Warwick D J, Nayagam S 2001 Apley's system of orthopaedics and fractures, 8th edn. Arnold, London

Standring S 2004 Gray's anatomy, 39th edn. Churchill Livingstone, Edinburgh

Stone R J, Stone J A 2005 Atlas of skeletal muscles, 5th edn. McGraw-Hill, Boston

Thompson J C 2002 Netter's concise atlas of orthopaedic anatomy. Icon Learning Systems, Teterboro, NJ

Travell J G, Simons D G 1991 Myofascial pain and dysfunction: the trigger point manual. Volume 2. The lower extremities Lippincott Williams & Wilkins, Baltimore

Waddell G 2004 The back pain revolution, 2nd edn. Churchill Livingstone, Edinburgh

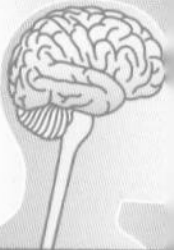

Neurology

Neuroanatomy illustrations **166**

Signs and symptoms of cerebrovascular lesions **171**

Signs and symptoms of injury to the lobes of the brain **175**

Signs and symptoms of haemorrhage to other areas of the brain **178**

Cranial nerves **179**

Key features of upper and lower motor neurone lesions **183**

Functional implications of spinal cord injury **184**

Glossary of neurological terms **187**

Neurological tests **189**

Modified Ashworth scale **192**

Neurological assessment **192**

References and further reading **195**

Neuroanatomy illustrations

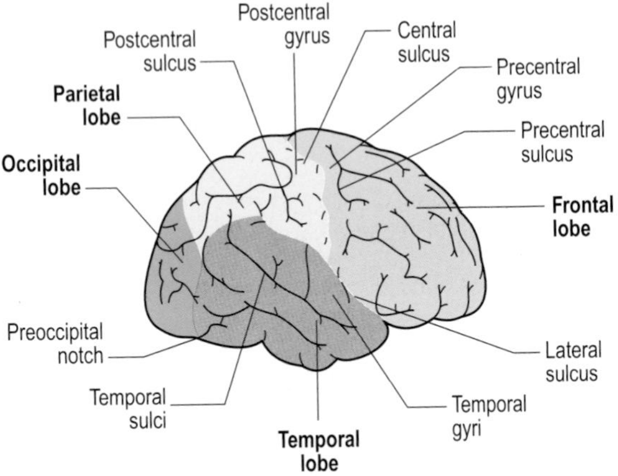
Postcentral
gyrus
Central
sulcus
Postcentral
sulcus
Precentral
gyrus
Parietal
lobe
Precentral
sulcus
Occipital
lobe
Frontal
lobe
Preoccipital
notch
Lateral
sulcus
Temporal
sulci
Temporal
gyri
Temporal
lobe

Figure 3.1 Lateral view of right cerebral hemisphere.

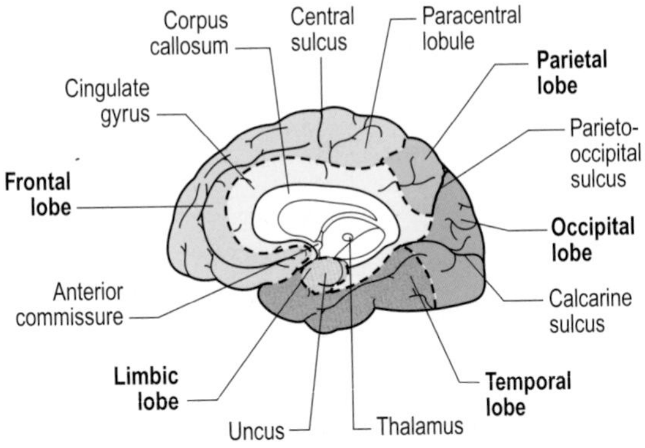
Corpus
callosum
Central
sulcus
Paracentral
lobule
Parietal
lobe
Cingulate
gyrus
Parieto-
occipital
sulcus
Frontal
lobe
Occipital
lobe
Anterior
commissure
Calcarine
sulcus
Limbic
lobe
Temporal
lobe
Uncus
Thalamus

Figure 3.2 Medial view of right cerebral hemisphere.

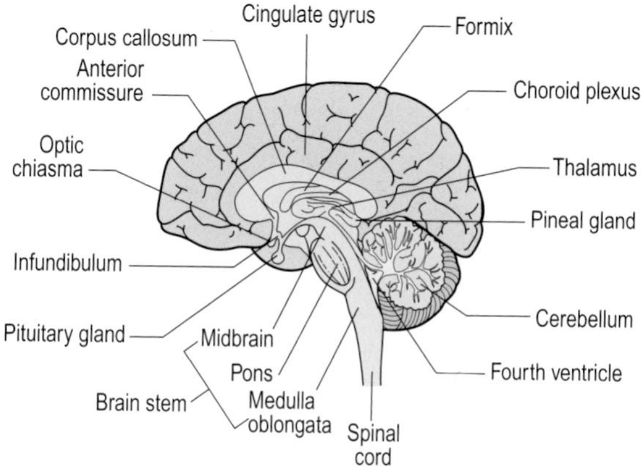
Cingulate gyrus
Corpus callosum
Formix
Anterior commissure
Choroid plexus
Optic chiasma
Thalamus
Pineal gland
Infundibulum
Cerebellum
Pituitary gland
Midbrain
Pons
Fourth ventricle
Brain stem
Medulla oblongata
Spinal cord

Figure 3.3 Mid-sagittal section of the brain.

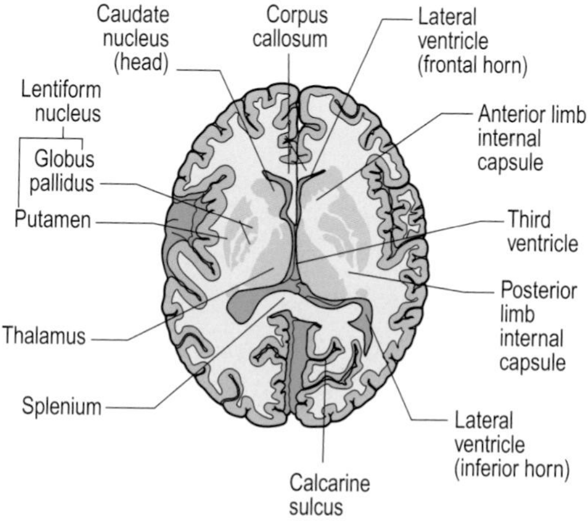
Caudate nucleus (head)
Corpus callosum
Lateral ventricle (frontal horn)
Lentiform nucleus
Anterior limb internal capsule
Globus pallidus
Putamen
Third ventricle
Posterior limb internal capsule
Thalamus
Splenium
Lateral ventricle (inferior horn)
Calcarine sulcus

Figure 3.4 Horizontal section through the brain.

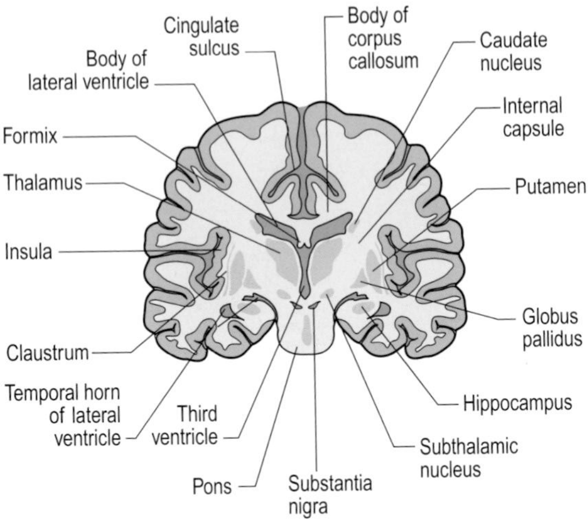
Cingulate sulcus
Body of corpus callosum
Caudate nucleus
Body of lateral ventricle
Internal capsule
Formix
Thalamus
Putamen
Insula
Globus pallidus
Claustrum
Temporal horn of lateral ventricle
Third ventricle
Hippocampus
Subthalamic nucleus
Pons
Substantia nigra

Figure 3.5 Coronal section of the brain.

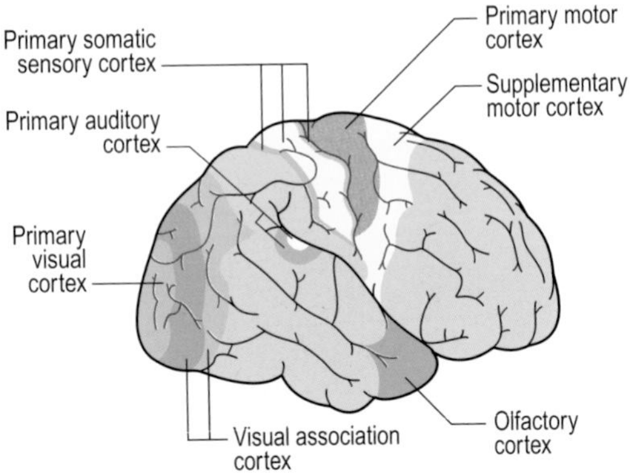
Primary motor cortex
Primary somatic sensory cortex
Supplementary motor cortex
Primary auditory cortex
Primary visual cortex
Visual association cortex
Olfactory cortex

Figure 3.6 Lateral view of sensory and motor cortical areas.

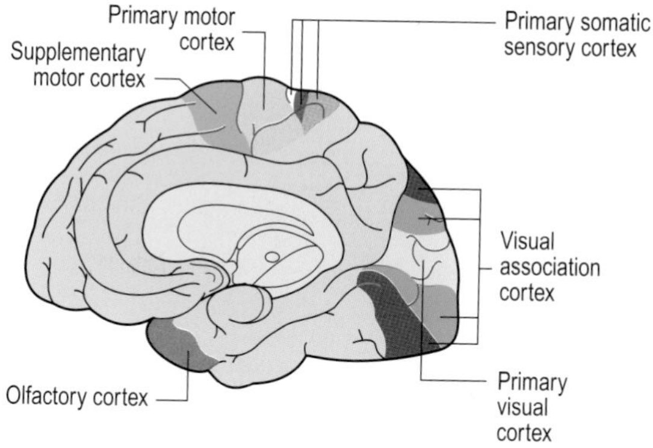
Primary motor cortex
Supplementary motor cortex
Primary somatic sensory cortex
Visual association cortex
Olfactory cortex
Primary visual cortex

Figure 3.7 Medial view of sensory and motor cortical areas.

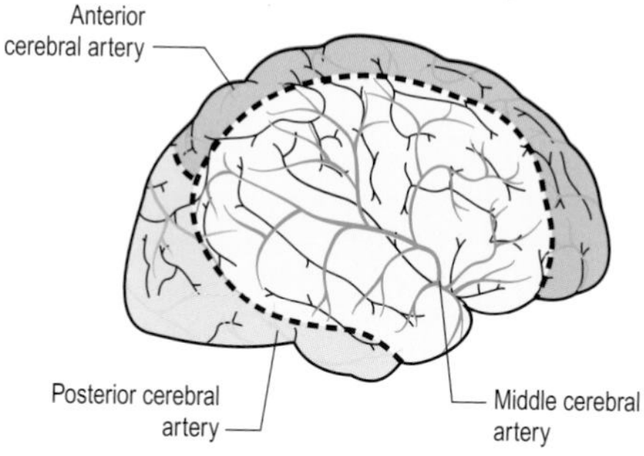
Anterior cerebral artery
Posterior cerebral artery
Middle cerebral artery

Figure 3.8 Lateral view of right hemisphere showing territories supplied by the cerebral arteries.

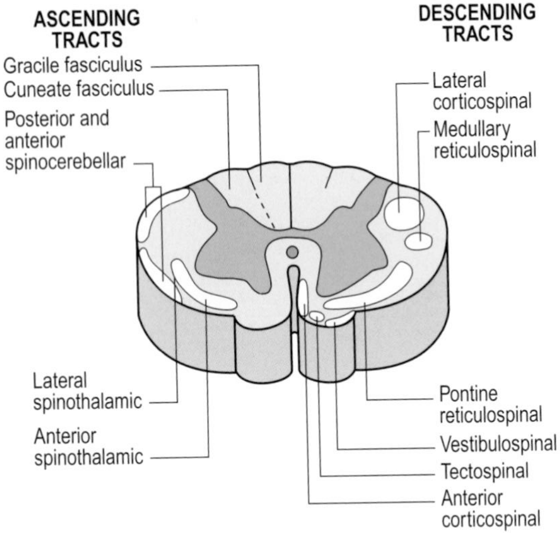
ASCENDING TRACTS
Gracile fasciculus
Cuneate fasciculus
Posterior and anterior spinocerebellar
Lateral spinothalamic
Anterior spinothalamic
DESCENDING TRACTS
Lateral corticospinal
Medullary reticulospinal
Pontine reticulospinal
Vestibulospinal
Tectospinal
Anterior corticospinal

Figure 3.9 Ascending and descending spinal cord tracts.

Ascending tracts	Descending tracts
Gracile fasciculus – proprioception and discriminative touch in legs and lower trunk	Lateral corticospinal – voluntary movements
Cuneate fasciculus – proprioception and discriminative touch in arms and upper trunk	Medullary retrospinal – locomotion and posture
Posterior and anterior spinocerebellar – reflex and proprioception	Pontine reticulospinal – locomotion and posture
Lateral spinothalamic – pain and temperature	Vestibulospinal – balance and antigravity muscles
Anterior spinothalamic – light touch	Tectospinal – orientates head to visual stimulation
	Anterior corticospinal – voluntary movements

Middle cerebral artery (MCA)

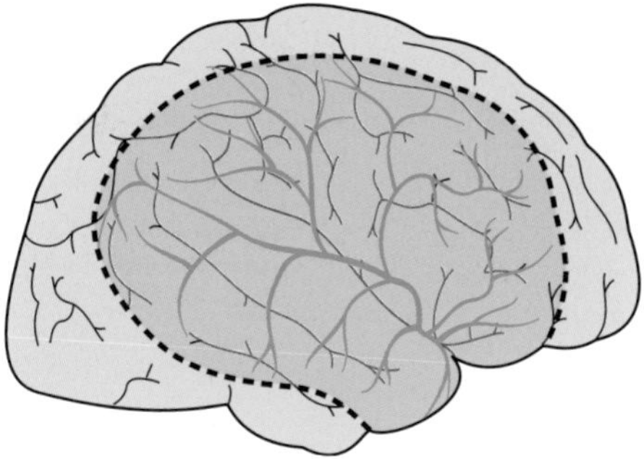

Figure 3.10 Middle cerebral artery.

The middle cerebral artery arises from the internal carotid artery. The proximal part supplies a large portion of the frontal, parietal and temporal lobes. The deep branches supply the basal ganglia (corpus striatum and globus pallidus), internal capsule and thalamus.

Signs and symptoms	Structures involved
Contralateral weakness/ paralysis of face, arm, trunk and leg	Motor cortex (precentral gyrus)
Contralateral sensory impairment/loss of face, arm, trunk and leg	Somatosensory cortex (postcentral gyrus)
Broca's dysphasia	Motor speech area of Broca (dominant frontal lobe)
Wernicke's dysphasia	Sensory speech area of Wernicke (dominant parietal/ temporal lobe)

Signs and symptoms	Structures involved
Neglect of contralateral side, dressing and constructional apraxia, geographical agnosia, anosognosia	Parietal lobe (non-dominant lobe)
Homonymous hemianopia (often upper homonymous quadrantanopia)	Optic radiation – temporal fibres
Ocular deviation	Frontal lobe
Gait disturbance	Frontal lobe (usually bilateral)
Pure motor hemiplegia	Posterior limb of internal capsule and adjacent corona radiata
Pure sensory syndrome	Ventral posterior nucleus of thalamus

Anterior cerebral artery (ACA)

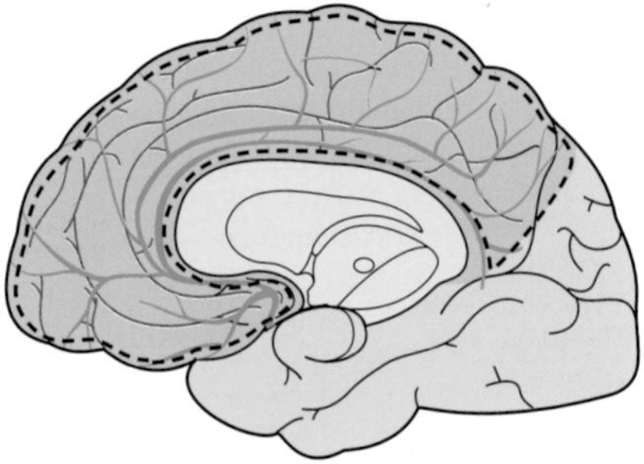

Figure 3.11 Anterior cerebral artery.

The anterior cerebral artery arises from the internal carotid artery and is connected by the anterior communicating artery. It follows the curve of the corpus callosum and supplies the medial aspect of the frontal and parietal lobes, corpus callosum, internal capsule and basal ganglia (caudate nucleus and globus pallidus).

Signs and symptoms	Structures involved
Contralateral hemiplegia/ hemiparesis (lower limb > upper limb)	Motor cortex
Contralateral sensory loss/ impairment (lower limb > upper limb)	Somatosensory cortex
Urinary incontinence	Superior frontal gyrus (bilateral)
Contralateral grasp reflex	Frontal lobe
Akinetic mutism, whispering, apathy	Frontal lobe (bilateral)
Apraxia of left limbs	Corpus callosum
Tactile agnosia	Corpus callosum
Spastic paresis of lower limb	Bilateral motor leg area

Posterior cerebral artery (PCA)

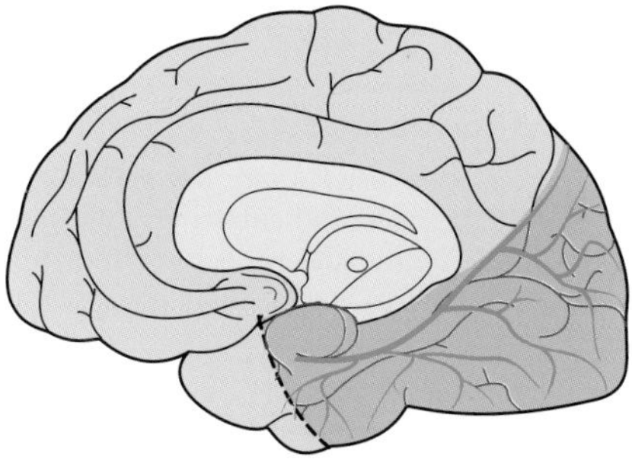

Figure 3.12 Posterior cerebral artery.

The posterior cerebral artery arises from the basilar artery. It supplies the occipital and temporal lobes, midbrain, choroid plexus, thalamus, subthalamic nucleus, optic radiation, corpus callosum and cranial nerves III and IV. The posterior communicating arteries connect the posterior cerebral arteries to the middle cerebral arteries anteriorly.

Signs and symptoms	Structures involved
Thalamic syndrome: hemisensory loss, chorea or hemiballism, spontaneous pain and dysaesthesias	Posterior nucleus of thalamus
Weber's syndrome: oculomotor paralysis and contralateral hemiplegia	Cranial nerve III and cerebral peduncle
Contralateral hemiballism	Subthalamic nucleus
Contralateral homonymous hemianopia	Primary visual cortex or optic radiation
Bilateral homonymous hemianopia, visual hallucinations	Bilateral occipital lobe
Alexia, colour anomia, impaired memory	Dominant corpus callosum (occipital lobe)
Memory defect, amnesia	Bilateral inferomedial portions of temporal lobe
Prosopagnosia	Calcarine sulcus and lingual gyrus (non-dominant occipital lobe)

Vertebral and basilar arteries

The vertebral arteries arise from the subclavian arteries at the root of the neck and enter the skull through the foramen magnum. Within the skull they fuse to form the basilar artery. They supply the medulla, pons, midbrain and cerebellum.

Signs and symptoms	Structures involved
Lateral medullary syndrome:	
– vertigo, vomiting, nystagmus	Vestibular nuclei
– ipsilateral limb ataxia	Spinocerebellar tract
– ipsilateral loss of facial pain and thermal sensation	Cranial nerve V
– ipsilateral Horner's syndrome	Descending sympathetic tract

Signs and symptoms	Structures involved
– ipsilateral dysphagia, hoarseness, vocal cord paralysis and reduced gag reflex – contralateral loss of pain and thermal sensation in trunk and limbs	Cranial nerves IX and X Lateral spinothalamic tract
Ipsilateral tongue paralysis and hemiatrophy	Cranial nerve XII
Contralateral impaired tactile sensation and proprioception	Medial lemniscus
Diplopia, lateral and vertical gaze palsies, pupillary abnormalities	Cranial nerve VI, medial longitudinal fasciculus
Bulbar palsy, tetraplegia, changes in consciousness	Bilateral corticospinal tracts
Pseudobulbar palsy, emotional instability	Bilateral supranuclear fibres, cranial nerves IX–XII
Locked-in syndrome	Bilateral medulla or pons
Coma, death	Brainstem

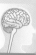

Signs and symptoms of injury to the lobes of the brain (adapted from Lindsay & Bone 2004, with permission)

Frontal lobe

Function	Signs of impairment
Precentral gyrus (motor cortex) Contralateral movement: face, arm, leg, trunk	Contralateral hemiparesis/hemiplegia
Broca's area (dominant hemisphere) Expressive centre for speech	Broca's dysphasia (dominant)

Function	Signs of impairment
Supplementary motor area Contralateral head and eye turning	Paralysis of contralateral head and eye movement
Prefrontal areas 'Personality', initiative	Disinhibition, poor judgement, akinesia, indifference, emotional lability, gait disturbance, incontinence, primitive reflexes, e.g. grasp
Paracentral lobule Cortical inhibition of bladder and bowel voiding	Incontinence of urine and faeces

Parietal lobe

Function	Signs of impairment
Postcentral gyrus (sensory cortex) Posture, touch and passive movement	Hemisensory loss/disturbance: postural, passive movement, localization of light touch, two-point discrimination, astereognosis, sensory inattention
Supramarginal and angular gyri *Dominant hemisphere (part of Wernicke's language area)*: integration of auditory and visual aspects of comprehension	Wernicke's dysphasia
Non-dominant hemisphere: body image, awareness of external environment, ability to construct shapes, etc.	Left-sided inattention, denies hemiparesis Anosognosia, dressing apraxia, geographical agnosia, constructional apraxia
Dominant parietal lobe Calculation, using numbers	Finger agnosia, acalculia, agraphia, confusion between right and left
Optic radiation Visual pathways	Homonymous quadrantanopia

Temporal lobe

Function	Signs of impairment
Superior temporal gyrus (auditory cortex) Hearing of language (dominant hemisphere), hearing of sounds, rhythm and music (non-dominant)	Cortical deafness, difficulty hearing speech – associated with Wernicke's dysphasia (dominant), amusia (non-dominant), auditory hallucinations
Middle and inferior temporal gyri Learning and memory	Disturbance of memory and learning
Limbic lobe Smell, emotional/affective behaviour	Olfactory hallucination, aggressive or antisocial behaviour, inability to establish new memories
Optic radiation Visual pathways	Upper homonymous quadrantanopia

Occipital lobe

Function	Signs of impairment
Calcarine sulcus	
Primary visual/striate cortex: Relay of visual information to parastriate cortex	Cortical blindness (bilateral involvement), homonymous hemianopia with or without macular involvement
Association visual/parastriate cortex: Relay of visual information to parietal, temporal and frontal lobes	Cortical blindness without awareness (striate and parastriate involvement), inability to direct gaze associated with agnosia (bilateral parieto-occipital lesions), prosopagnosia (bilateral occipito-temporal lesions)

Signs and symptoms of haemorrhage to other areas of the brain

Putamen

Function	Signs of impairment
Part of basal ganglia Involved in selective movement	Contralateral hemiplegia/hemiparesis, contralateral hemisensory loss, hemianopia (posterior segment), contralateral gaze palsy (posterior segment), Wernicke-type dysphasia (posterior segment, left side), anosognosia (posterior segment, right side), apathy, motor impersistence, temporary unilateral neglect (anterior segment), coma/death (large lesion)

Thalamus

Function	Signs of impairment
Thalamus Receives motor and sensory inputs and transmits them to the cerebral cortex	Contralateral hemiparesis/hemiplegia, contralateral hemisensory loss, impaired consciousness, ocular disturbances (varied), dysphasia (dominant), contralateral neglect (non-dominant)

Pons

Function	Signs of impairment
Part of brainstem Contains descending motor pathways, ascending sensory pathways and cranial nerve nuclei V–VIII	Coma/death (large bilateral lesions), locked-in syndrome (bilateral), tetraplegia (bilateral), lateral gaze palsy towards affected side, contralateral hemiplegia, contralateral hemisensory loss, ipsilateral facial weakness/sensory loss

Cerebellum

Function	Signs of impairment
Anterior lobe (spinocerebellum) Muscle tone, posture and gait control	Hypotonia, postural reflex abnormalities
Posterior lobe (neocerebellum) Coordination of skilled movements	Ipsilateral ataxia: dysmetria, dysdiadochokinesia, intention tremor, rebound phenomenon, dyssynergia, dysarthria
Flocculonodular lobe (vestibulocerebellum) Eye movements and balance	Disturbance of balance, unsteadiness of gait and stance, truncal ataxia, nystagmus, ocular disturbances

Cranial nerves

The cranial nerves form part of the peripheral nervous system and originate from the brain. Each nerve is named according to its function or appearance and is numbered using Roman numerals from I to XII. The numbers roughly correspond to their position as they descend from just above the brainstem (I and II), through the midbrain (III and IV), pons (V to VII) and medulla (VIII to XII).

Name	Function	Test	Abnormal signs
Olfactory (I)	Smell	Identify a familiar odour, e.g. coffee, orange, tobacco, with one nostril at a time	Partial or total loss of smell Altered or increased sense of smell
Optic (II)	Sight	Visual acuity: read with one eye covered Peripheral vision: detect objects or movement from the corner of the eye with the other eye covered	Visual fields defects, loss of visual acuity, colour-blind
Oculomotor (III)	Movement of eyelid and eyeball, constriction of pupil, lens accommodation	Follow the examiner's finger, which moves up and down and side to side, keeping the head in mid-position	Squint, ptosis, diplopia, pupil dilation
Trochlear (IV)	Movement of eyeball upwards	As for oculomotor	Diplopia, squint
Trigeminal (V)	Mastication, sensation for eye, face, sinuses and teeth	Test fascial sensation Clench teeth (the examiner palpates the masseter and temporalis muscles)	Trigeminal neuralgia, loss of mastication and sensation in eye, face, sinuses and teeth

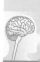

Abducens (VI)	Movement of eyeball into abduction, controls gaze	As for oculomotor	Gaze palsy
Facial (VII)	Facial movements, sensation and taste for anterior two-thirds of tongue, secretion of saliva and tears	Test ability to move the face, e.g. close eyes tightly, wrinkle brow, whistle, smile, show teeth	Bell's palsy, loss of taste and ability to close eyes
Vestibulocochlear (VIII)	Hearing, balance	Examiner rubs index finger and thumb together noisily beside one ear and silently beside the other. Patient identifies the noisy side	Tinnitus, deafness, vertigo, ataxia, nystagmus
Glossopharyngeal (IX)	Sensation and taste for posterior third of tongue, swallow, salivation, regulation of blood pressure	Swallow Evoke the gag reflex by touching the back of the throat with a tongue depressor	Loss of tongue sensation and taste, reduced salivation, dysphagia
Vagus (X)	Motor and sensation for heart, lungs, digestive tract and diaphragm, secretion of digestive fluids, taste, swallow, hiccups	As for glossopharyngeal	Vocal cord paralysis, dysphagia, loss of sensation from internal organs

Name	Function	Test	Abnormal signs
Accessory (XI)	Motor to soft palate, larynx, pharynx, trapezius and sternocleidomastoid	Rotate neck to one side and resist flexion, i.e. contract sternocleidomastoid. Shrug shoulders against resistance	Paralysis of innervated muscles
Hypoglossal (XII)	Tongue control and strap muscles of neck	Stick out the tongue. Push tongue into the left and right side of the cheek	Dysphagia, dysarthria, difficulty masticating

Key features of upper and lower motor neurone lesions

	Upper motor neurone	Lower motor neurone
Muscle tone	Increased	Decreased
Clonus	Present	Absent
Muscle fasciculation	Absent	Present
Tendon reflexes	Increased	Depressed or absent
Plantar response	Extensor (Babinski's sign)	Flexor (normal)
Distribution	Extensor weakness in upper limb and flexor weakness in lower limb Whole limb(s) involved	Weakness of muscle groups innervated by affected spinal segment/root, plexus or peripheral nerve

Upper motor neurone

Origin: cerebral cortex
Terminates: cranial nerve nuclei or spinal cord anterior horn

Lower motor neurone

Origin: cranial nerve motor nuclei or spinal cord anterior horn
Terminates: skeletal muscle motor unit

Functional implications of spinal cord injury

Level	Motor control	Personal independence	Equipment	Mobility
C1–C2	Swallow, talk, chew, blow (cough absent)	Type, turn pages, use telephone and computer	Hoist, respirator, mouthstick, reclining powered wheelchair using breath/chin control	Wheelchair
C3	Neck control, weak shoulder elevation	As above	Hoist, respirator, mouth/head stick, wheelchair as above	Wheelchair
C4	Respiration, neck control, shoulder shrug	Feed possible	Mouth/head stick, hoist, mobile arm supports, wheelchair as above	Wheelchair
C5	Shoulder external rotation, protraction, elbow flexion, supination	Feed, groom, roll in bed, weight shift, push wheelchair on flat, use brake	Adapted feeding/grooming equipment and hand splints, mobile arm supports, powered wheelchair with hand controls or lightweight manual with grips	Wheelchair
C6	Shoulder, elbow flexion, wrist extension, pronation. Weak elbow extension, wrist flexion and thumb control	Tenodesis grip, drink, write, personal ADL, transfers, dress upper body, light domestic chores, push wheelchair on slope	Adapted equipment and splints, transfer board, hand-controlled car, lightweight manual wheelchair, powered for short distances	Bed mobility, bed to chair transfers, wheelchair, car

C7	Elbow extension, finger flexion and extension, limited wrist flexion	Dress lower body, personal and skin care, showering, all transfers, pick up from floor, wheelchair sports	Bath board, shower chair, hand-controlled car, wheelchair as above	All transfers, wheelchair, car
C8	Wrist flexion, hand control	Bladder and bowel care	Grab rails, standing frame, non-adapted wheelchair	Stand in frame
T1–T5	Top half of intercostals and long back muscles	Trunk support, improved balance, assisted cough, negotiate kerbs with wheelchair, routine domestic chores	Bilateral knee–ankle orthoses with spinal attachment, standing frame/table	Full wheelchair independence, transfer floor to chair, mobilize with assistance for short distances
T6–T12	Abdominals	Good balance, weak to normal cough, improved stamina	Bilateral knee–ankle orthoses, crutches or frame	Mobilize independently indoors, transfer chair to crutches
L1–L2	Hip flexion		Calipers	Stairs, transfer floor to crutches

Level	Motor control	Personal independence	Equipment	Mobility
L3–L5	Knee extension, weak knee flexion, dorsiflexion and eversion		Ankle–foot orthoses, crutches/ sticks	
S1–S2	Hip extension	Improved standing balance		Normal gait without aids
S2–S4	Bladder, bowel and sexual function			

Glossary of neurological terms

Acalculia inability to calculate

Agnosia inability to interpret sensations such as sounds (auditory agnosia), three-dimensional objects by touch (tactile agnosia) or symbols and letters (visual agnosia)

Agraphia inability to write

Akinesia loss of movement

Alexia inability to read

Amnesia total or partial loss of memory

Amusia impaired recognition of music

Anomia inability to name objects

Anosmia loss of ability to smell

Anosognosia denial of ownership or the existence of a hemiplegic limb

Aphasia inability to generate and understand language whether verbal or written

Astereognosis inability to recognize objects by touch alone, despite intact sensation

Ataxia shaky and uncoordinated voluntary movements that may be associated with cerebellar or posterior column disease

Athetosis involuntary writhing movements affecting face, tongue and hands

Bradykinesia slowness of movement

Chorea irregular, jerky, involuntary movement

Clonus more than three rhythmic contractions of the plantarflexors in response to sudden passive dorsiflexion

Diplopia double vision

Dysaesthesia perverted response to sensory stimuli producing abnormal and sometimes unpleasant sensation

Dysarthria	difficulty articulating speech
Dysdiadochokinesia	clumsiness in performing rapidly alternating movements
Dysmetria	under- or overshooting while reaching towards a target
Dysphagia	difficulty or inability to swallow
Dysphasia	difficulty understanding language (receptive dysphasia) or generating language (expressive dysphasia)
Dysphonia	difficulty in producing the voice
Dyspraxia	inability to make skilled movements despite intact power, sensation and coordination
Dyssynergia	clumsy, uncoordinated movements
Dystonia	abnormal postural movements caused by co-contraction of agonists and antagonists, usually at an extreme of flexion or extension
Graphanaesthesia	inability to recognize numbers or letters traced onto the skin with a blunt object
Hemianopia	loss of half the normal visual field
Hemiballismus	sudden, involuntary violent flinging movements of an entire limb, usually unilateral
Hemiparesis	weakness affecting one side of the body
Hemiplegia	paralysis affecting one side of the body
Homonymous	affecting the same side, i.e. homonymous diplopia
Hyperacusis	increased sensitivity to sound
Hyperreflexia	increased reflexes
Hypertonia	increase in normal muscle tone
Hypertrophy	abnormal increase in tissue size
Kinaesthesia	perception of body position and movement
Miosis	pupil constriction
Nystagmus	involuntary movements of the eye

Paraesthesia	tingling sensation often described as 'pins and needles'
Paraphasia	insertion of inappropriate or incorrect words in person's speech
Paraplegia	paralysis of both legs
Paresis	muscle weakness
Photophobia	intolerance to light
Prosopagnosia	inability to recognize faces
Ptosis	drooping of the upper eyelid
Quadrantanopia	loss of quarter the normal visual field
Quadriplegia	paralysis of all four limbs
Stereognosis	ability to identify common objects by touch alone
Tetraplegia	another term for quadriplegia

Neurological tests

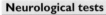

Finger–nose test

Hold your finger about an arm's length from the patient. Ask the patient to touch your finger with their index finger and then touch their nose, repeating the movement back and forth. Patients may demonstrate past pointing (missing your finger) or intention tremor.

Indicates: possible cerebellar dysfunction.

Heel–shin test

With the patient lying down, ask them to place one heel on the opposite knee and then run the heel down the tibial shaft towards the ankle and back again. Patients may demonstrate intention tremor, an inability to keep the heel on the shin or uncoordinated movements.

Indicates: possible cerebellar dysfunction.

Hoffman reflex

Flick the distal phalanx of the patient's third or fourth finger. Look for any reflex flexion of the patient's thumb.

Indicates: possible upper motor neurone lesion.

Joint position sense

Test the most distal joint of the limb, i.e. distal phalanx of the index finger or interphalangeal joint of the hallux. With the patient's eyes open, demonstrate the movement. To test, get the patient to close their eyes. Hold the joint to be tested at the sides between two fingers and move it up and down. Ask the patient to identify the direction of movement, ensuring that you are not moving more proximal joints or brushing against the neighbouring toes or fingers. If there is impairment, test more proximal joints.

Indicates: loss of proprioception.

Light touch

Use a wisp of cotton wool. With the patient's eyes open, demonstrate what you are going to do. To test, get the patient to close their eyes. Stroke the patient's skin with the cotton wool at random points, asking them to indicate every time they feel the touch.

Indicates: altered touch sensation.

Pin prick

Use a disposable neurological pin which has a sharp end and a blunt end. With the patient's eyes open, demonstrate what you are going to do. To test, get the patient to close their eyes. Test various areas of the limb randomly using sharp and blunt stimuli and get the patient to tell you which sensation they feel.

Indicates: altered pain sensation.

Plantar reflex (Babinski)

Apply a firm pressure along the lateral aspect of the sole of the foot and across the base of the toes, observing the big toe. If the big toe flexes, the response is normal. If the big toe extends and the other toes spread it indicates a positive Babinski's sign.

Indicates: A positive Babinski's sign signifies a possible upper motor neurone lesion.

Rapidly alternating movement

Ask the patient to hold out one hand palm up and then alternately slap it with the palmar and then dorsal aspect of the fingers of the other hand. Where there is a loss of rhythm and fluency it is referred to as dysdiadochokinesia. For the lower limbs get the patient to tap first one foot on the floor and then the other.

Indicates: possible cerebellar dysfunction.

Romberg's test

Patient stands with feet together and eyes open. Ask the patient to close their eyes (ensuring that you can support them if they fall). Note any excessive postural sway or loss of balance.

Indicates: proprioceptive or vestibular deficit if they fall only when they close their eyes.

Temperature

A quick test involves using a cold object such as a tuning fork and asking the patient to describe the sensation when applied to various parts of the body. For more formal testing, two test tubes are filled with cold and warm water and patients are asked to distinguish between the two sensations.

Indicates: altered temperature sensation.

Two-point discrimination

Requires a two-point discriminator, a device similar to a pair of blunted compasses. With the patient's eyes open, demonstrate what you are going to do. Get the patient to close their eyes. Alternately touch the patient with either one prong or two. Reduce the distance between the prongs until the patient can no longer discriminate between being touched by one prong or two prongs. Varies according to skin thickness but normal young patients can distinguish a separation of approximately 5 mm in the index finger and approximately 4 cm in the legs. Compare left to right.

Indicates: impaired sensory function.

Vibration sense

Use a 128 Hz tuning fork. Ask the patient to close their eyes. Place the tuning fork on a bony prominence or on the fingertips or toes. The patient should report feeling the vibration and not simply the contact of the tuning fork. If in doubt, apply the tuning fork and then stop it vibrating suddenly by pinching it between your fingers and see if the patient can correctly identify when it stops vibrating.

Indicates: altered vibration sense.

Modified Ashworth scale

Grade	Description
0	No increase in muscle tone
1	Slight increase in muscle tone, manifested by a catch and release or by minimal resistance at the end of the range of motion (ROM) when the affected part(s) is moved in flexion or extension
1+	Slight increase in muscle tone, manifested by a catch, followed by minimal resistance throughout the remainder (less than half) of the ROM
2	More marked increase in muscle tone through most of the ROM, but affected part(s) easily moved
3	Considerable increase in muscle tone passive, passive movement difficult
4	Affected part(s) rigid in flexion or extension

Neurological assessment

Patients present with a variety of conditions, and assessments need to be adapted to suit their needs. This section provides a basic framework for the subjective and objective neurological assessment of a patient.

Database

History of present condition
Past medical history
Drug history
Results of specific investigations (X-rays, CT scans, blood tests, etc.)

Subjective examination

Social situation
- family support
- accommodation
- employment
- leisure activities
- social service support

Normal daily routine
Indoor and outdoor mobility
Continence
Vision
Hearing
Swallowing
Fatigue
Pain
Other ongoing treatment
Past physiotherapy and response to treatment
Perceptions of own problems/main concern
Expectations of treatment

Objective examination

Posture and balance

Alignment
Neglect
Sitting balance
Standing balance
- Romberg's test

Voluntary movement

Range of movement
Strength

Coordination
- finger–nose test
- heel–shin test
- rapidly alternating movement

Endurance

Involuntary movement

Tremor
Clonus
Chorea
Associated reactions

Tone

Decreased/flaccid
Increased
- spasticity (clasp-knife)
- rigidity (cogwheel or lead-pipe)

Reflexes

Deep tendon reflexes
- biceps (C5/6)
- triceps (C7/8)
- knee (L3/4)
- ankle (S1/2)

Plantar reflex
Hoffman's reflex

Muscle and joint range

Passive range of movement

Sensory

Light touch
Pin prick
Two-point discrimination
Vibration sense
Joint position sense
Temperature
Vision and hearing

Functional activities

Bed mobility
Sitting balance
Transfers

Upper limb function
Mobility
Stairs

Gait

Pattern
Distance
Velocity
Use of walking aids
Orthoses
Assistance from others

Exercise tolerance/fatigue

Cognitive status

Attention
Orientation
Memory

Emotional state

References and further reading

Bromley I 2006 Tetraplegia and paraplegia: a guide for physiotherapists, 6th edn. Churchill Livingstone, Edinburgh

Davies P M 2000 Steps to follow: the comprehensive treatment of patients with hemiplegia, 2nd edn. Springer Verlag, Berlin

Douglas G, Nicol F, Robertson C 2005 Macleod's clinical examination, 11th edn. Churchill Livingstone, Edinburgh

Fitzgerald M J T, Gruener G, Mtui E 2006 Clinical neuroanatomy and neuroscience, 5th edn. Saunders, Edinburgh

Fowler T J, Scadding J W 2003 Clinical neurology, 3rd edn. Arnold, London

Fuller G 2008 Neurological examination made easy, 4th edn. Churchill Livingstone, Edinburgh

Hughes M, Miller T, Briar C 2007 Crash course: nervous system, 3rd edn. Mosby, Edinburgh

Lindsay K W, Bone I 2004 Neurology and neurosurgery illustrated, 4th edn. Churchill Livingstone, Edinburgh

Ropper A H, Brown R J 2005 Adams and Victor's principles of neurology, 8th edn. McGraw-Hill, New York

Stokes M 2004 Physical management in neurological rehabilitation, 2nd edn. Mosby, London

Respiratory

Respiratory anatomy illustrations **198**

Respiratory volumes and capacities **201**

Chest X-rays **203**

Auscultation **206**

Percussion note **208**

Interpreting blood gas values **208**

Respiratory failure **210**

Nasal cannula **211**

Sputum analysis **211**

Modes of mechanical ventilation **212**

Cardiorespiratory monitoring **215**

ECGs **218**

Biochemical and haematological studies **225**

Treatment techniques **232**

Tracheostomies **237**

Respiratory assessment **240**

References and further reading **242**

Respiratory anatomy illustrations

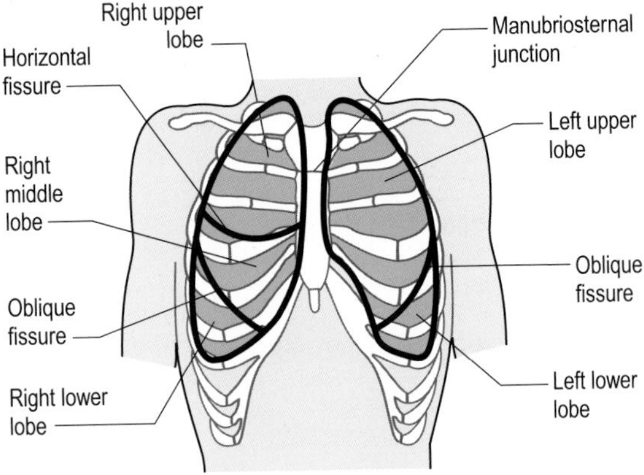
Right upper lobe
Horizontal fissure
Manubriosternal junction
Left upper lobe
Right middle lobe
Oblique fissure
Oblique fissure
Right lower lobe
Left lower lobe

Figure 4.1 Lung markings – anterior view.

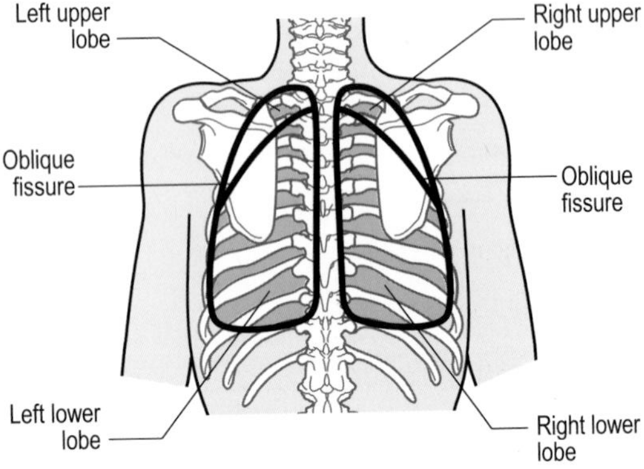
Left upper lobe
Right upper lobe
Oblique fissure
Oblique fissure
Left lower lobe
Right lower lobe

Figure 4.2 Lung markings – posterior view.

Useful lung markings*	
Apex	Anterior – 2.5 cm above clavicles Posterior – T1
Lower borders	Anterior – sixth rib Posterior – T10/11 Mid-axilla – eighth rib
Tracheal bifurcation	Anterior – manubriosternal junction Posterior – T4
Right horizontal fissure	Anterior – fourth rib (above the nipple)
Oblique fissures	Anterior – sixth rib (below the nipple) Posterior – T2/3
Left diaphragm	Anterior – sixth rib Posterior – T10 Mid-axilla – eighth rib
Right diaphragm	Anterior – fifth rib Posterior – T9 Mid-axilla – eighth rib

*These lung markings are approximate and can vary between individuals.

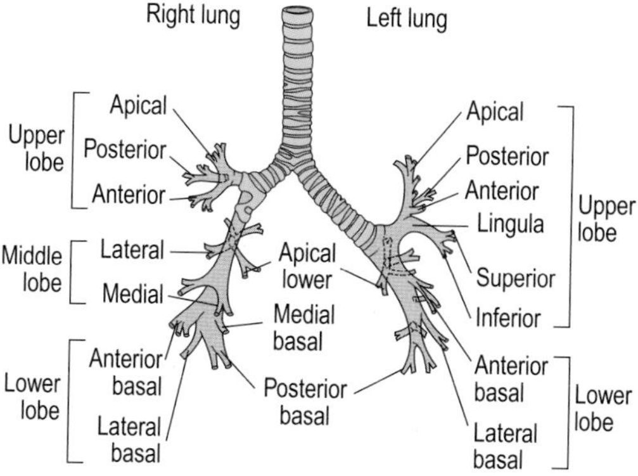
Right lung
Left lung
Upper lobe
Apical
Posterior
Anterior
Middle lobe
Lateral
Medial
Lower lobe
Anterior basal
Lateral basal
Apical lower
Medial basal
Posterior basal
Apical
Posterior
Anterior
Lingula
Superior
Inferior
Upper lobe
Anterior basal
Lateral basal
Lower lobe

Figure 4.3 Anterior view of bronchial tree.

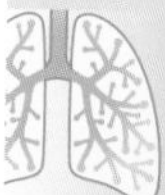

SECTION 4

RESPIRATORY

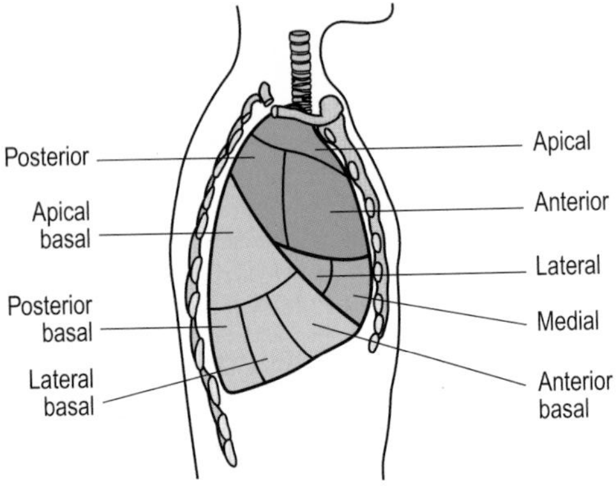
Posterior
Apical basal
Posterior basal
Lateral basal
Apical
Anterior
Lateral
Medial
Anterior basal

Figure 4.4 Bronchopulmonary segments – right lateral view.

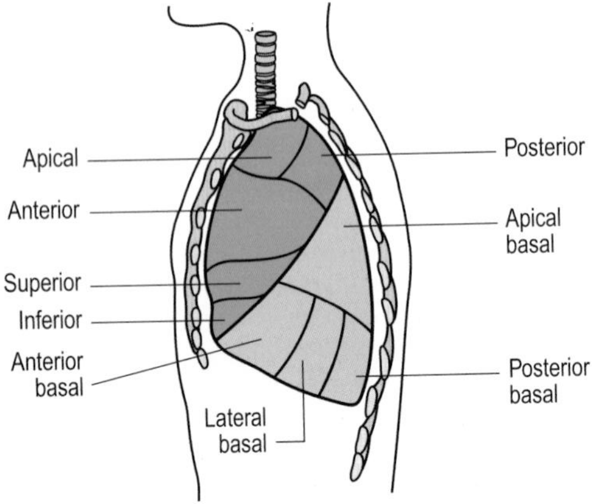
Apical
Anterior
Superior
Inferior
Anterior basal
Lateral basal
Posterior
Apical basal
Posterior basal

Figure 4.5 Bronchopulmonary segments – left lateral view.

Respiratory volumes and capacities

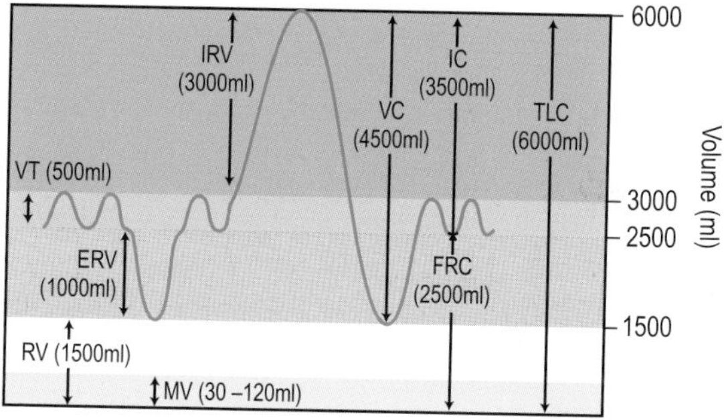

IRV
(3000ml)
VC
(4500ml)
IC
(3500ml)
TLC
(6000ml)
VT (500ml)
ERV
(1000ml)
FRC
(2500ml)
RV (1500ml)
MV (30 –120ml)
6000
3000
2500
1500
Volume (ml)

Figure 4.6 Respiratory volumes and capacities. Average volumes in healthy adult male.

Lung volumes

V_T (tidal volume)

Volume of air inhaled or exhaled during a single normal breath
Value: 500 mL

IRV (inspiratory reserve volume)

Maximum amount of air that can be inspired on top of a normal tidal inspiration
Value: 3000 mL

ERV (expiratory reserve volume)

Maximum amount of air that can be exhaled following a normal tidal expiration
Value: 1000 mL

RV (residual volume)

Volume of air remaining in the lungs after a maximal expiration
Value: 1500 mL

MV (minimal volume)
The amount of air that would remain if the lungs collapsed
Value: 30–120 mL

Lung capacities

A capacity is the combination of two or more lung volumes

TLC (total lung capacity)
Total volume of your lungs at the end of maximal inspiration

$$TLC = V_T + IRV + ERV + RV$$

Value: 6000 mL

VC (vital capacity)
Maximum amount of air that can be inspired and expired in a single breath

$$VC = V_T + IRV + ERV$$

Value: 4500 mL

IC (inspiratory capacity)
The maximum volume of air that can be inspired after a normal tidal expiration

$$IC = V_T + IRV$$

Value: 3500 mL

FRC (functional residual capacity)
Volume of air remaining in the lungs at the end of a normal tidal expiration

$$FRC = ERV + RV$$

Value: 2500 mL

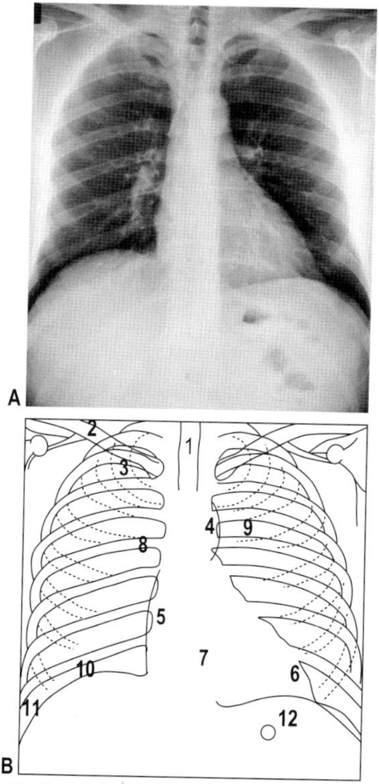
A
B
1
2
3
4
5
6
7
8
9
10
11
12

1 Air in the trachea
2 Clavicle
3 1st rib
4 Aortic arch
5 Right atrium
6 Left ventricle
7 Right ventricle
8 Right hilum
9 Left hilum
10 Right hemidiaphragm
11 Costophrenic angle
12 Gastric bubble

Figure 4.7 A Normal PA chest X-ray (from Pryor & Prasad 2008); **B** structures normally visible on X-ray.

Analysing chest X-rays

Adopt a systematic approach when analysing X-rays. You should check the following:

Patient's details

- Name, date and time of X-ray

Is it anteroposterior (AP) or posteroanterior (PA)? Supine or erect?

- AP X-rays are taken using a mobile machine with the patient in supine. The heart appears larger and the scapulae are visible.
- PA X-rays are taken in the radiology department with the patient standing erect. The quality is generally better and the scapulae are out of the way.

Is the patient positioned symmetrically?

- The medial ends of the clavicle should be equidistant from the adjacent vertebral body. If the patient is rotated the position of the heart, spine and rib cage may appear distorted.

Degree of inspiration

- On full inspiration the sixth or seventh rib should intersect the midpoint of the right hemidiaphragm anteriorly or the ninth rib posteriorly.

Exposure

- If the film appears too dark it is overpenetrated (overexposed).
- If the film appears too light it is underpenetrated (underexposed).
  Think of toast: dark is overdone and white is underdone.
- The spinous processes of the cervical and upper thoracic vertebra should be visible, as should the outline of the mid-thoracic vertebral bodies.

Extrathoracic soft tissues

- Surgical emphysema is often seen in the supraclavicular areas, around the armpit and the lateral chest wall.

- The lateral wall of the chest may be obscured by breast shadows.

Invasive medical equipment

- Note the position and presence of any tubes, cannulas, electrodes, etc.
- The tip of the endotracheal tube should lie about 2 cm above the carina.

Bony structures

- Check for fractures, deformities and osteoporosis.

Intercostal spaces

- Small intercostal spaces and steeply sloping ribs indicate reduced lung volume.
- Large intercostal spaces and horizontal ribs indicate hyperinflation.

Trachea

- Lies centrally with the lower third inclining slightly to the right.
- Deviation of the trachea indicates mediastinal shift. It shifts towards collapse and away from tumours, pleural effusions and pneumothoraces.
- Bifurcation into the left and right bronchi is normally seen. The right bronchus follows the line of the trachea whereas the left bronchus branches off at a more acute angle.

Hila

- Made up of the pulmonary vessels and lymph nodes.
- The left and right hilum should be roughly equal in size, though the left hilum appears slightly higher than the right. Their silhouette should be sharp.

Heart

- On a PA film the diameter of the heart is usually less than half the total diameter of the thorax. In the majority of cases, one-third of the cardiac shadow lies on the right and two-thirds on the left, which should be sharply defined. The density of both sides should be equal. The heart may appear bigger on an AP film or if the patient is rotated.

Diaphragm

- The right side of the diaphragm is about 2 cm higher than the left because the right lobe of the liver is situated directly underneath it. Both hemidiaphragms should be dome shaped and sharply defined.
- The costophrenic angle is where the diaphragm meets the ribs.
- The cardiophrenic angle is where the diaphragm meets the heart.

Auscultation

Auscultation should be conducted in a systematic manner, comparing the same area on the left and right side while visualizing the underlying lung structures. Ideally patients should be sitting upright and be asked to breathe through the mouth to reduce nose turbulence.

Breath sounds

Normal

More prominent at the top of the lungs and centrally, with the volume decreasing towards the bases and periphery. Expiration is shorter and quieter than inspiration and follows inspiration without a pause.

Abnormal (bronchial breathing)

Similar to the breath sounds heard when listening over the trachea. They are typically loud and harsh and can be heard throughout inspiration and expiration. Expiration is longer than inspiration and there is a pause between the two. They occur if air is replaced by solid tissue, which transmits sound more clearly. Caused by consolidation, areas of collapse with adjacent open bronchus, pleural effusion, tumour.

Diminished

Breath sounds will be reduced if air entry is compromised by either an obstruction or a decrease in airflow. Caused by pneumothorax, pleural effusion, emphysema, collapse with occluded bronchus, atelectasis, inability to breathe deeply, obesity.

Added sounds

Crackles

Heard when airways that have been narrowed or closed, usually by secretions, are suddenly forced open on inspiration. Usually classified as fine (originating from small, distal airways), coarse (from large, proximal airways), localized or widespread. They can be further defined as being early or late, depending on when they are heard on inspiration or expiration.

Early inspiratory – reopening of large airways (e.g. bronchiectasis and bronchitis)
Late inspiratory – reopening of alveoli and peripheral airways (e.g. pulmonary oedema, pulmonary fibrosis, pneumonia, atelectasis)
Early expiratory – secretions in large airways
Late expiratory – secretions in peripheral airways

Wheeze

Caused by air being forced through narrowed or compressed airways. Described as either high or low pitched and monophonic (single note) or polyphonic (where several airways may be obstructed). Airway narrowing can be caused by bronchospasm, mucosal oedema or sputum retention. An expiratory wheeze with prolonged expiration is usually indicative of bronchospasm, while a low-pitched wheeze throughout inspiration and expiration is normally caused by secretions.

Pleural rub

If the pleural surfaces are inflamed or infected they become rough and rub together, creating a creaking or grating sound. Heard equally during inspiration and expiration.

Voice sounds

In normal lung tissue, voice sounds are indistinct and unintelligible. When there is consolidation, sound is transmitted more clearly and loudly and speech can be distinguished. Voice sounds can be diminished in the presence of emphysema, pneumothorax and pleural effusion. They can be heard through a stethoscope (vocal resonance) or felt by hand (vocal fremitus). To test voice sounds patients can be asked to say or whisper '99' repeatedly.

Percussion note

Elicited by placing the middle finger of one hand firmly in the space between the ribs and tapping the distal phalanx sharply with the middle finger of the other hand.

The pitch of the note is determined by whether the lungs contain air, solid or fluid and will either sound normal, resonant, dull or stony dull.

Resonant = normal
Hyper-resonant = emphysema (bullae) or pneumothorax
Dull = consolidation, areas of collapse, pleural effusion

Interpreting blood gas values

Arterial blood analysis	Reference ranges in adults
pH	7.35–7.45 pH
PaO_2	10.7–13.3 kPa (80–100 mmHg)
$PaCO_2$	4.7–6.0 kPa (35–45 mmHg)
HCO_3^-	22–26 mmol/L
Base excess	−2 to +2

Assessing acid–base disorders

Assessing acid–base disorders involves examining the pH, $PaCO_2$ and HCO_3^-:

- pH – a low pH (<7.4) indicates a tendency towards acidosis, a high pH (>7.4) indicates a tendency towards alkalosis.
- $PaCO_2$ – an increase in $PaCO_2$ leads to acidosis, a decrease to alkalosis.
- HCO_3^- – an increase in HCO_3^- leads to alkalosis, a decrease to acidosis.

Assessment

1. Establish whether the patient's pH is acidotic, alkalotic or normal.
2. If the pH is acidotic establish whether this is due to:
   - increased $PaCO_2$ – indicating respiratory acidosis
   - decreased HCO_3^- – indicating metabolic acidosis.
3. If the pH is alkalotic establish whether this is due to:
   - decreased $PaCO_2$ – indicating respiratory alkalosis
   - increased HCO_3^- – indicating metabolic alkalosis.
4. If the pH is within normal range the original abnormality can be identified by comparing the pH to the $PaCO_2$ and the HCO_3^-. If the pH is below 7.4 (tending towards acid) then the component that correlates with acidosis (increased $PaCO_2$ or decreased HCO_3^-) is the cause and the other is the compensation. Likewise, if the pH is above 7.4 (tending towards alkaline) the component that correlates with alkalosis (decreased $PaCO_2$ or increased HCO_3^-) is the cause and the other is the compensation.

Simple acid–base disorders

	pH	$PaCO_2$	HCO_3^-
Respiratory acidosis			
Uncompensated	↓	↑	N
Compensated	N	↑	↑
Respiratory alkalosis			
Uncompensated	↑	↓	N
Compensated	N	↓	↓
Metabolic acidosis			
Uncompensated	↓	N	↓
Compensated	N	↓	↓
Metabolic alkalosis			
Uncompensated	↑	N	↑
Compensated	N	↑	↑

↓ = decreased; ↑ = increased; N = normal.

Base excess

Allows assessment of the metabolic component of acid–base disturbances and therefore the degree of renal compensation that has occurred. A base deficit (less than −2) indicates a metabolic acidosis and a base excess (greater than +2) correlates with metabolic alkalosis.

Respiratory failure

Broadly defined as an inability of the respiratory system to maintain blood gas values within normal ranges. There are two types:

Type I (hypoxaemic respiratory failure)

A decreased PaO_2 (hypoxaemia) with a normal or slightly reduced $PaCO_2$ due to inadequate gas exchange. Causes include pneumonia, emphysema, fibrosing alveolitis, severe asthma and adult respiratory distress syndrome.

Defined as $PaO_2 < 8$ kPa (60 mmHg).

Type II (ventilatory failure)

A decreased PaO_2 with an increased $PaCO_2$ (hypercapnia) caused by hypoventilation. Causes include neuromuscular disorders (e.g. muscular dystrophy, Guillain–Barré), lung diseases (e.g. asthma, COPD), drug-related respiratory drive depression and injuries to the chest wall.

Defined as $PaO_2 < 8$ kPa (60 mmHg), $PaCO_2 > 6.7$ kPa (50 mmHg).

Arterial blood gas classification of respiratory failure

	pH	$PaCO_2$	HCO_3^-
Acute	↓	↑	N
Chronic	N	↑	↑
Acute on chronic	↓	↑	↑

↓ = decreased; ↑ = increased; N = normal.

Nasal cannula

The following values are approximate as the patient's flow rates, ability to breathe through the nose, type of cannula and build-up of nasal mucus may all affect the amount of oxygen received. As a general rule the FiO_2 is raised by 3–4% for each litre of oxygen.

To convert litres of O_2 to FiO_2
RA ≈ 21% FiO_2
1 L/min ≈ 24% FiO_2
2 L/min ≈ 28% FiO_2
3 L/min ≈ 32% FiO_2
4 L/min ≈ 36% FiO_2
5 L/min ≈ 40% FiO_2
6 L/min ≈ 44% FiO_2

RA = room air.

$>$ 6 L/min has little effect on FiO_2 and may lead to irritation and drying of the nasal mucosa.

Sputum analysis (Middleton & Middleton 2008, with permission)

	Description	**Causes**
Saliva	Clear watery fluid	
Mucoid	Opalescent or white	Chronic bronchitis without infection, asthma
Muco-purulent	Slightly discoloured, but not frank pus	Bronchiectasis, cystic fibrosis, pneumonia

Purulent	Thick, viscous: – yellow – dark green/brown – rusty – redcurrant jelly	 *Haemophilus* *Pseudomonas* *Pneumococcus, Mycoplasma* *Klebsiella*
Frothy	Pink or white	Pulmonary oedema
Haemoptysis	Ranging from blood specks to frank blood, old blood (dark brown)	Infection (tuberculosis, bronchiectasis), infarction, carcinoma, vasculitis, trauma, also coagulation disorders, cardiac disease
Black	Black specks in mucoid secretions	Smoke inhalation (fires, tobacco, heroin), coal dust

Modes of mechanical ventilation

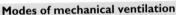

Controlled mechanical ventilation (CMV)

Delivers a preset number of breaths to the patient at a preset tidal volume, pressure and flow rate. The ventilator performs all the work of breathing – the patient cannot trigger the machine or breathe spontaneously. Patients on CMV are sedated and paralysed.

Assist/control ventilation (ACV)

Spontaneously breathing patients trigger a breath and the ventilator delivers gas at a preset tidal volume or preset pressure. The ventilator will initiate a breath automatically should the patient fail to trigger within a preset time.

Intermittent mandatory ventilation (IMV)

Delivers a preset number of breaths at a preset tidal volume and flow rate but allows the patient to take spontaneous breaths between machine-delivered breaths.

Synchronized intermittent mandatory ventilation (SIMV)

Synchronizes breaths from the ventilator with the patient's spontaneous breaths. If the patient fails to take a spontaneous breath within a set time the ventilator delivers a mandatory breath at either a preset tidal volume (SIMV/volume cycled) or preset inspiratory pressure (SIMV/pressure cycled).

Pressure support (PS)

Patients breathe spontaneously, triggering the ventilator to deliver a set level of positive pressure to assist air entry and reduce the work of breathing. The patient controls the tidal volume, respiratory rate and flow rate. Pressure support can be added to SIMV to compensate for the resistance from the endotracheal tube, making it easier for the patient to breathe.

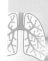

High-frequency ventilation

This mode of ventilation does not try to imitate normal physiological breathing. Instead it delivers low tidal volumes at high respiratory rates. This results in lower airway pressures, thereby reducing the risk of complications associated with barotrauma. There are three types:

- *High-frequency positive pressure ventilation*: delivers small tidal volumes at high respiratory rates (60–100 breaths/min).
- *High-frequency oscillation ventilation*: oscillates small bursts of gas to and fro at high rates (up to 3000 cycles/min).
- *High-frequency jet ventilation*: delivers a short, rapid, high-pressure jet to the airways through a small-bore cannula (100–600 cycles/min).

Continuous positive airway pressure (CPAP)

A high flow of gas delivered continuously throughout inspiration and expiration during spontaneous breathing. The alveoli and smaller airways are splinted open, increasing lung volume at the end of expiration (i.e. the functional residual capacity), thereby reversing atelectasis and improving gas exchange. It also increases lung compliance and decreases the work of breathing.

Bilevel positive airway pressure (BiPAP)

Similar to CPAP, positive airway pressure is delivered throughout inspiration and expiration during spontaneous breathing but the level of positive airway pressure alters between inspiration and expiration. A higher level is delivered during inspiration and a lower level during expiration. The alteration between pressure levels is synchronized with the patient's breathing. This is usually by means of a trigger that is sensitive to changes in flow (triggered or spontaneous mode) but the ventilator can also deliver breaths should the patient fail to inhale spontaneously (timed/spontaneous mode or assist-control mode).

Non-invasive ventilation (NIV)

NIV is the provision of ventilatory support without intubation, usually via a mask or similar device, to the upper airway. Positive pressure ventilation is the most common form, though negative pressure ventilation is used in some situations. Positive pressure devices may be pressure, volume or time controlled and the following modes may be used: controlled mechanical ventilation, assist/control ventilation, pressure support ventilation (assisted spontaneous breathing), CPAP, BiPAP and proportional assist ventilation.

Contraindications to NIV (British Thoracic Society 2002, with permission)

- Facial trauma/burns
- Recent facial, upper airway or upper gastrointestinal tract surgery*
- Fixed obstruction of the upper airway
- Inability to protect airway*
- Life-threatening hypoxaemia*
- Haemodynamic instability*
- Severe co-morbidity*
- Impaired consciousness*
- Confusion/agitation*

- Vomiting
- Bowel obstruction*
- Copious respiratory secretions*
- Focal consolidation on chest radiograph*
- Undrained pneumothorax*

*NIV may be used, despite the presence of these contraindications, if it is to be the 'ceiling' of treatment.

Cardiorespiratory monitoring

Arterial blood pressure (ABP)

Measured via an intra-arterial cannula which allows continuous monitoring of the patient's blood pressure and also provides an access for arterial blood sampling and blood gas analysis.

Normal value: 95/60–140/90 mmHg in adults (increases gradually with age)
Hypertension: >145/95 mmHg
Hypotension: <90/60 mmHg

Cardiac output (CO)

Amount of blood pumped into the aorta each minute.

$$CO = HR \times SV$$

Normal value: 4–8 L/min

Cardiac index (CI)

Cardiac output related to body size. Body surface area is calculated by using the patient's weight and height and a nomogram. Allows reliable comparison between patients of different sizes.

$$CI = CO \div \text{ body surface area}$$

Normal value: 2.5–4 L/min/m^2

Central venous pressure (CVP)

Measured via a central venous cannula inserted into the internal or external jugular vein or subclavian vein with the tip resting close to the right atrium within the superior vena cava. Provides information on circulating blood volume, the effectiveness of the heart to pump that volume, vascular tone and venous return.

Normal value: 3–15 cmH_2O

Cerebral perfusion pressure (CPP)

Pressure required to ensure adequate blood supply to the brain.

$$CPP = MAP - ICP$$

Normal value: >70 mmHg

Ejection fraction (EF)

The stroke volume (SV) as a percentage of the total volume of the ventricle prior to systolic contraction, i.e. end-diastolic volume (EDV).

$$EF = SV \div EDV$$

Normal value: 65–75%

Heart rate (HR)

The number of times the heart contracts in a minute.

Normal value: 50–100 beats/min
Tachycardia: >100 beats/min at rest
Bradycardia: <50 beats/min at rest

Intracranial pressure (ICP)

Pressure exerted by the brain tissue, cerebrospinal fluid and blood volume within the rigid skull and meninges. Neurological insults such as space-occupying lesions, cerebral oedema, hydrocephalus, cerebral haemorrhage, hypoxia and infection cause this pressure to rise, resulting in a decreased blood supply to the brain. When treating patients with raised ICP, minimize handling and ensure that the head is maintained in midline and raised 15–30° from supine. A marked degree of hip flexion should be avoided to ensure optimal circulation and prevent potential increase in ICP.

Normal value: 0–10 mmHg

Mean arterial pressure (MAP)

Measures the average pressure of blood being pushed through the circulatory system. It relates to cardiac output and systemic vascular resistance and reflects tissue perfusion pressure.

$$\text{MAP} = (\text{diastolic BP} \times 2) + (\text{systolic BP}) \div 3$$

Normal value: 80–100 mmHg
$<$ 60 mmHg indicates inadequate circulation to the vital organs

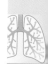

Oxygen saturation (SpO_2)

Arterial oxygen saturation is measured using non-invasive pulse oximetry.

Normal value: 95–98%

Pulmonary artery pressure (PAP)

A pulmonary artery balloon catheter (Swan–Ganz) is inserted via the CVP catheter route and floated into the pulmonary artery via the right ventricle. The PAP measures pressures of the blood in the vena cava, right atrium and right ventricle and provides a measure of the ability of the right side of the heart to push blood through the lungs and to the left side of the heart.

Normal value: 15–25/8–15 mmHg
Mean value: 10–20 mmHg

Pulmonary artery wedge pressure (PAWP)

Similar to PAP but the Swan–Ganz catheter is moved further along until it wedges in a small pulmonary artery. The balloon tip is inflated to occlude the artery in order to allow measurement of the pressure in the pulmonary capillaries in front of it and the left atrium. PAWP is also known as pulmonary capillary wedge pressure (PCWP).

Normal value: 6–12 mmHg

Respiratory rate (RR)

Number of breaths taken in a minute.

Normal value: 12–16 breaths/min
Tachypnoea: >20 breaths/min
Bradypnoea: <10 breaths/min

Stroke volume (SV)

The amount of blood ejected from the ventricles during each systolic contraction. Affected by preload (amount of tension on the ventricular wall before it contracts), afterload (resistance that the ventricle must work against when it contracts) and contractility (force of contraction generated by the myocardium).

$$SV = (CO \times 1000) \div HR$$

Normal value: 60–130 mL/beat

Systemic vascular resistance (SVR)

Evaluates the vascular component of afterload in the left ventricle. Vasocontriction will increase systemic vascular resistance while vasodilation will decrease it.

$$SVR = (MAP - CVP \div CO) \times 79.9$$

Normal value: 800–1400 dyn $\cdot$ s $\cdot$ cm^{-5}

ECGs

ECGs detect the sequence of electrical events that occur during the contraction (depolarization) and relaxation (repolarization) cycle of the heart. Depolarization is initiated by the sinoatrial (SA) node, the heart's natural pacemaker, which transmits the electrical stimulus to the atrioventricular (AV) node. From here the impulse is conducted through the bundle

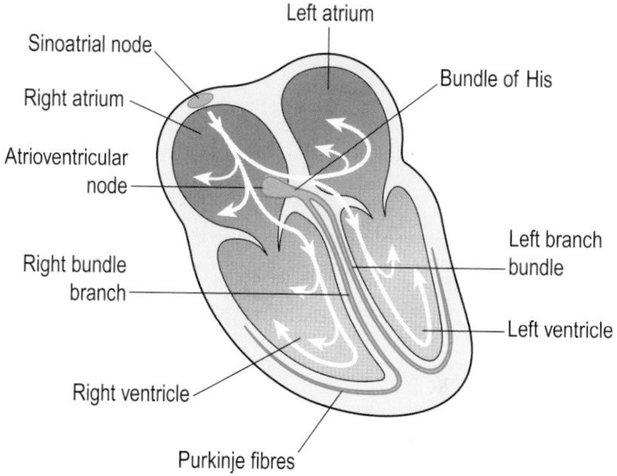
Left atrium
Sinoatrial node
Bundle of His
Right atrium
Atrioventricular node
Left branch bundle
Right bundle branch
Left ventricle
Right ventricle
Purkinje fibres

Figure 4.8 Conduction system of the heart.

of His and along the bundle branches to the Purkinje fibres, causing the heart to contract.

The atrioventricular (AV) node can also function as a pacemaker when there is a dysfunction of the SA node, e.g. failure to generate an impulse (sinus arrest), when the impulse generated is too slow (sinus bradycardia) or when the impulse is not conducted to the AV node (SA block, AV block).

ECGs are recorded on graphed paper that travels at 25 mm/s. It is divided into large squares of 5 mm width, which represents 0.2 s horizontally. Each square is then divided into five squares of 1 mm width (i.e. 0.04 s horizontally). Electrical activity is measured in millivolts (mV). A 1 mV signal moves the recording stylus vertically 1 cm (i.e. two large squares).

An ECG complex consists of five waveforms labelled with the letters P, Q, R, S and T, which represent the electrical events that occur in one cardiac cycle.

The P wave represents the activation of the atria (atrial depolarization).

- P amplitude: <2.5 mm
- P duration: 0.06–0.12 s

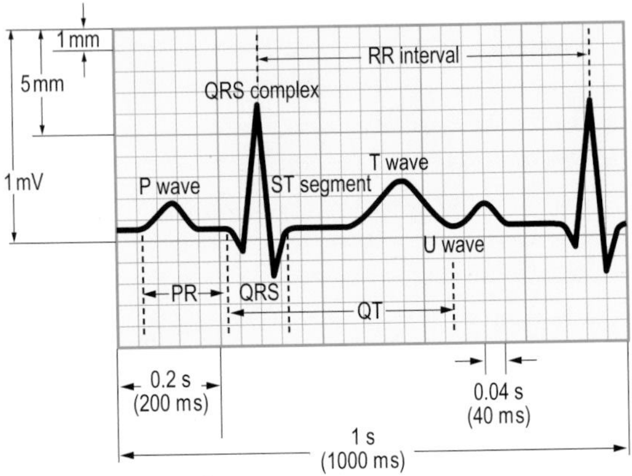
1 mm
5 mm
1 mV
RR interval
QRS complex
T wave
P wave
ST segment
U wave
PR
QRS
QT
0.2 s
(200 ms)
0.04 s
(40 ms)
1 s
(1000 ms)
Paper speed = 25 mm/s

Figure 4.9 Normal ECG.

The PR interval represents the time between the onset of atrial depolarization and the onset of ventricular depolarization, i.e. the time taken for the impulse to travel from the SA node through the AV node and the His–Purkinje system.

- PR duration: 0.12–0.20 s

The QRS complex represents the activation of the ventricles (ventricular depolarization).

- QRS amplitude: 5–30 mm
- QRS duration: 0.06–0.10 s

The ST segment represents the end of ventricular depolarization and the beginning of ventricular repolarization.

The T wave represents ventricular repolarization.

- T amplitude: $<$10 mm (approximately more than one-eighth but less than two-thirds of corresponding R wave)

The QT interval represents the total time for ventricular depolarization and repolarization.

- QT duration: 0.35–0.45 s

The U wave represents repolarization of the His–Purkinje system and is not always present on an ECG.

Examples of ECGs

Normal sinus rhythm

- Regular rhythms and rates (60–100 beats/min)
- Has a P wave, QRS complex and T wave; all similar in size and shape

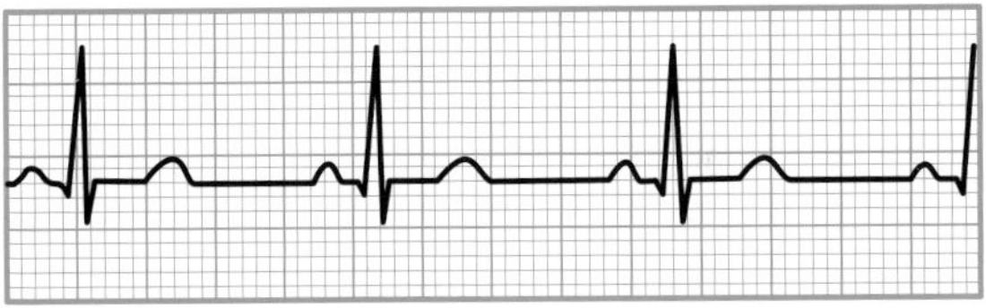

Figure 4.10 Sinus rhythm.

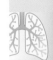

Sinus bradycardia

Defined as a sinus rhythm with a resting heart rate of less than 60 beats/min.

- Heart rate <60 beats/min
- Regular sinus rhythm

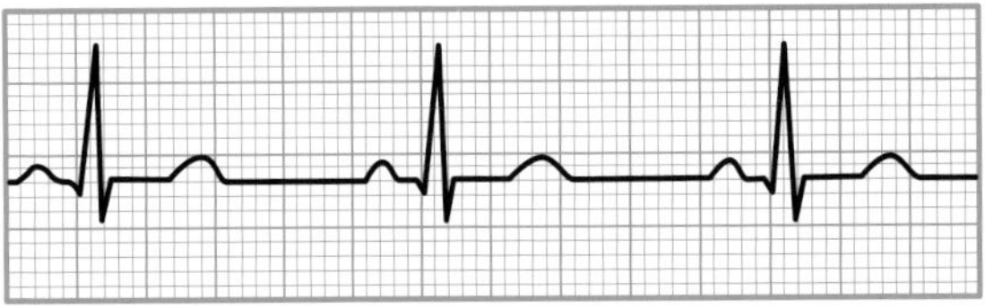

Figure 4.11 Sinus bradycardia.

Causes include cardiomyopathy, acute myocardial infarction, drugs (e.g. β-blockers, digoxin, amiodarone), obstructive jaundice, raised intracranial pressure, sick sinus syndrome, hypothermia, hypothyroidism, electrolyte abnormalities.

Can be a normal finding in extremely fit individuals and during sleep.

Sinus tachycardia

Defined as a sinus rhythm with a resting heart rate of more than 100 beats/min.

- Heart rate >100 beats/min
- Regular sinus rhythm

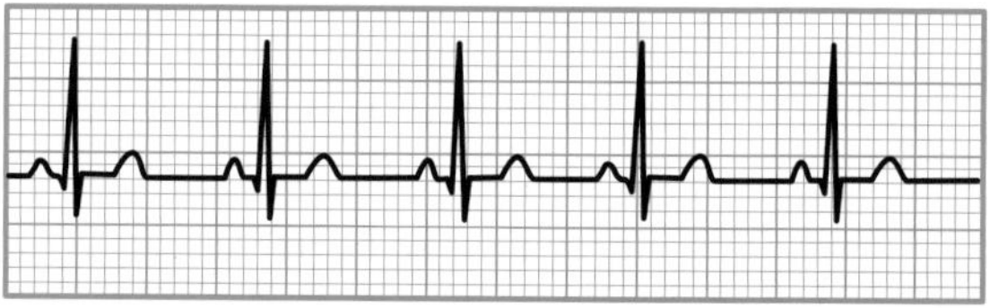

Figure 4.12 Sinus tachycardia.

Causes include sepsis, fever, anaemia, pulmonary embolism, hypovolaemia, hypoxia, hyperthyroidism, phaeochromocytoma, drugs (e.g. salbutamol, alcohol, caffeine).

Can occur as a response to increased demand for blood flow, e.g. exercise or in high emotional states, e.g. fear, anxiety, pain.

Atrial fibrillation

Where rapid, unsynchronized electrical activity is generated in the atrial tissue, causing the atria to quiver. Transmission of the impulses to the ventricles via the AV node is variable and unpredictable, leading to an irregular heartbeat.

- Absent P wave replaced by fine baseline oscillations (atrial impulses fire at a frequency of 350–600 beats/min)
- Irregular ventricular complexes; RR interval irregular
- Ventricular rate varies between 100 and 180 beats/min but can be slower

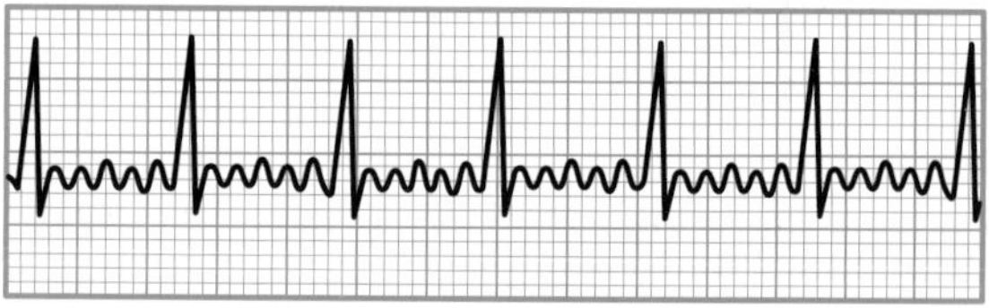

Figure 4.13 Atrial fibrillation.

Causes include hypertension, coronary artery disease, mitral valve disease, post-cardiac surgery, sick sinus syndrome, pneumonia, pulmonary embolism, hyperthyroidism, alcohol misuse, chronic pulmonary disease.

Ventricular ectopics or premature ventricular contractions (PVCs)

Early beats (ectopics) usually caused by electrical irritability in the ventricular conduction system or myocardium. Can occur in normal individuals and be asymptomatic. However, can indicate impending fatal arrhythmias in patients with heart disease. Can occur singly, in clusters of two or more or in repeating patterns such as bigeminy (every other beat) or trigeminy (every third beat).

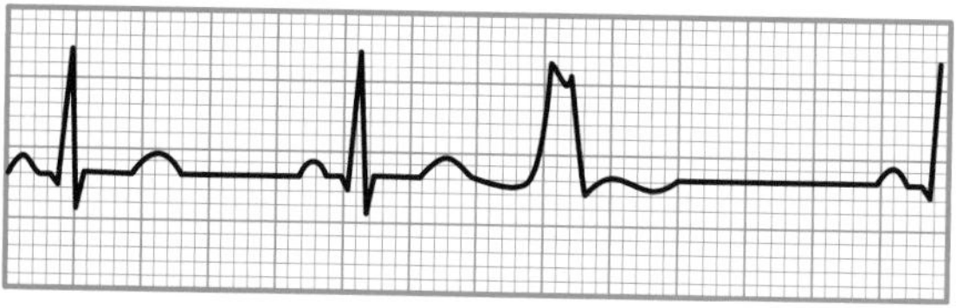

Figure 4.14 Ventricular ectopics and PVCs.

- Irregular rhythm during PVC; however, underlying rhythm and rate is usually regular, i.e. sinus
- P wave absent, QRS complex wide and early, T wave in opposite direction from QRS complex during PVC

Causes include acute myocardial infarction, valvular heart disease, electrolyte disturbances, metabolic acidosis, medications including digoxin and tricyclic antidepressants, drugs such as cocaine, amphetamines and alcohol, anaesthetics and stress.

Ventricular tachycardia

Defined as three or more heartbeats of ventricular origin at a rate exceeding 100 beats/minute. May occur in short bursts of less than 30 seconds and may terminate spontaneously with few or no symptoms (non-sustained). Episodes lasting more than 30 seconds (sustained) lead to rapid deterioration and ventricular fibrillation that requires immediate treatment to prevent death.

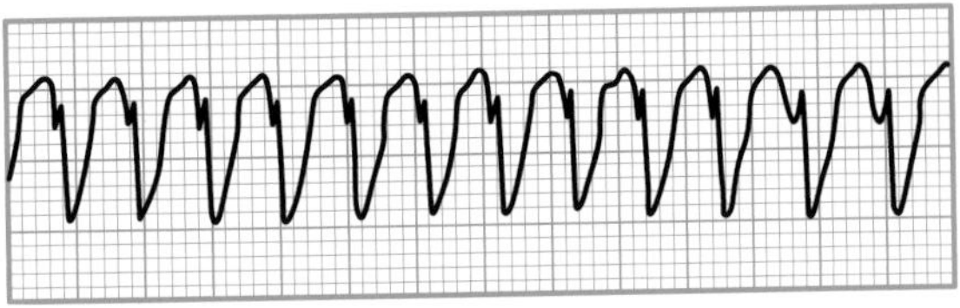

Figure 4.15 Ventricular tachycardia.

- Ventricular rate 100–200 beats/min
- Ventricular rhythm is usually regular
- QRS complex is wide, P wave is absent

Causes include acute myocardial infarction, myocardial ischaemia, cardiomyopathy, mitral valve prolapse, electrolyte imbalance, drugs (digoxin, anti-arrhythmics), myocarditis.

Ventricular fibrillation

Rapid, ineffective contractions of the ventricles caused by chaotic electrical impulses resulting in no cardiac output. Unless treated immediately, it is fatal.

Ventricular fibrillation is the most commonly identified arrhythmia in cardiac arrest patients and the primary cause of sudden cardiac death (SCD).

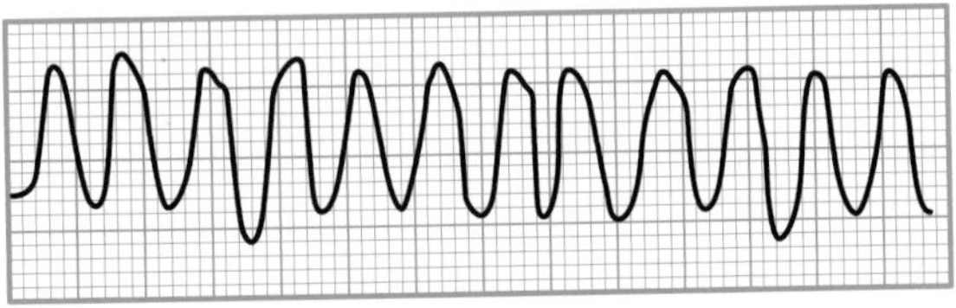

Figure 4.16 Ventricular fibrillation.

No recognizable pattern: irregular, chaotic, immeasurable.

Biochemical and haematological studies

Blood serum studies

Test	Function	Interpretation
Albumin 36–47 g/L	Most abundant plasma protein. Maintains osmotic pressure of the blood. Transports blood constituents such as fatty acids, hormones, enzymes, drugs and other substances	*Increased*: relative increase with haemoconcentration, where there is severe loss of body water *Decreased*: malnutrition, malabsorption, severe liver disease, renal disease, gastrointestinal conditions causing excessive loss, thyrotoxicosis, chemotherapy, Cushing's disease
Bilirubin 2–17 mmol/L	Pigment produced by the breakdown of haem	*Increased*: hepatitis, biliary tract obstruction, haemolysis, haematoma *Decreased*: iron deficiency, anaemia
C-reactive protein $<$7 mg/L	Protein produced in the acute inflammatory phase of injury. Index for monitoring disease activity	*Increased*: pyrexia, all inflammatory conditions (e.g. rheumatoid arthritis, pneumococcal pneumonia), trauma, during late pregnancy

Test	Function	Interpretation
Calcium 2.1–2.6 mmol/L	Nerve impulse transmission, bone and teeth formation, skeletal and myocardial muscle contraction, activation of enzymes, blood coagulation, cell division and repair, membrane structure and absorption of vitamin B_{12}	*Increased (hypercalcaemia)*: hyperparathyroidism, malignancy, Paget's disease, osteoporosis, immobilization, renal failure *Decreased (hypocalcaemia)*: hypoparathyroidism, vitamin D deficiency, acute pancreatitis, low blood albumin, low blood magnesium, large transfusion of citrated blood, increased urine excretion, respiratory acidosis
Creatine kinase *Men*: 30–200 U/L *Women*: 30–150 U/L	Enzyme found in heart, brain and skeletal muscle. Increased when one of these areas is stressed or damaged. Testing for a specific creatine kinase isoenzyme indicates area of damage (e.g. raised CK-MB indicates damage to heart)	*Increased*: heart (myocardial infarction, myocarditis, open heart surgery), brain (brain cancer, trauma, seizure) and skeletal muscle damage (intramuscular injections, trauma, surgery, strenuous exercise, muscular dystrophy)
Creatinine 55–150 mmol/L	End-product of normal muscle metabolism	*Increased*: renal failure, urinary obstruction, muscle disease *Decreased*: pregnancy, muscle wasting
Glucose 3.6–5.8 mmol/L	Metabolized in the cells to produce energy	*Increased*: diabetes mellitus, Cushing's disease, patients on steroid therapy *Decreased*: severe liver disease, adrenocortical insufficiency, drug toxicity, digestive diseases

Lactate dehydrogenase 230–460 U/L	Enzyme that converts pyruvic acid into lactate. High levels found in myocardial and skeletal muscle, the liver, lungs, kidneys and red blood cells	*Increased*: tissue damage due to myocardial infarction, liver disease, renal disease, cellular damage in trauma, hypothyroidism, muscular diseases
Magnesium 0.7–1.0 mmol/L	Neuromuscular transmission, cofactor in activation of many enzyme systems for cellular metabolism (e.g. phosphorylation of glucose, production and functioning of ATP), regulation of protein synthesis	*Increased (hypermagnesaemia)*: renal failure, adrenal insufficiency, excessive oral or parenteral intake of magnesium, severe hydration *Decreased (hypomagnesaemia)*: excessive loss from GIT (diarrhoea, nasogastric suction, pancreatitis), decreased gut absorption, renal disease, long-term use of certain drugs (e.g. diuretics, digoxin), chronic alcoholism, increased aldosterone secretion, polyuria
Phosphate 0.8–1.4 mmol/L	Bone formation, formation of high energy compounds (e.g. ATP), nucleic acid synthesis, enzyme activation	*Increased (hyperphosphataemia)*: renal failure, hypoparathyroidism, chemotherapy, excessive phosphorus intake *Decreased (hypophosphataemia)*: hyperparathyroidism, chronic alcoholism, diabetes, respiratory alkalosis, excessive glucose ingestion, hypoalimentation, chronic use of antacids

Test	Function	Interpretation
Potassium 3.6–5.0 mmol/L	Nerve impulse transmission, contractility of myocardial, skeletal and smooth muscle	*Increased (hyperkalaemia)*: renal failure, increased intake of potassium, metabolic acidosis, tissue trauma (e.g. burns and infection), potassium-sparing diuretics, adrenal insufficiency *Decreased (hypokalaemia)*: potassium-wasting diuretics, vomiting, diarrhoea, metabolic alkalosis, excess aldosterone secretion, polyuria, profuse sweating
Sodium 136–145 mmol/L	Regulates body's water balance, maintains acid–base balance and electrical nerve potentials	*Increased (hypernatraemia)*: excessive fluid loss or salt intake, water deprivation, diabetes insipidus, excess aldosterone secretion, diarrhoea *Decreased (hyponatraemia)*: kidney disease, excessive water intake, adrenal insufficiency, diarrhoea, profuse sweating, diuretics, congestive heart failure, inappropriate secretion of ADH
Urea 2.5–6.5 mmol/L	Waste product of metabolism	*Increased*: renal failure, decreased renal perfusion because of heart disease, shock *Decreased*: high carbohydrate/low protein diets, late pregnancy, malabsorption, severe liver damage

Haematological studies (data from Matassarin-Jacobs 1997, with permission of W B Saunders)

Test	Assesses	Interpretation
Red blood cell count (RBC) *Men:* 4.5–6.5 $\times 10^{12}$/L *Women:* 3.8–5.3 $\times 10^{12}$/L	Blood loss, anaemia, polycythaemia (increase in Hb concentration of the blood)	*Increased*: polycythaemia vera, dehydration, cardiac and pulmonary disorders characterized by cyanosis, acute poisoning *Decreased*: leukaemia, anaemia, fluid overload, haemorrhage
White blood cell count (WBC) 4.0–11.0 $\times 10^9$/L	Detects infection or inflammation. Monitors response to radiation and chemotherapy	*Increased*: leukaemia, tissue necrosis, infection *Decreased*: bone marrow suppression
White blood cell differential *Neutrophils:* 1.5–7.0 $\times 10^9$/L *Eosinophils:* 0.0–0.4 $\times 10^9$/L *Lymphocytes:* 1.2–3.5 $\times 10^9$/L *Monocytes:* 0.2–1.0 $\times 10^9$/L *Basophils:* 0.0–0.2 $\times 10^9$/L	Evaluates body's ability to resist infection. Detects and classifies leukaemia	*Increased:* Neutrophil – bacterial infection, non-infective acute inflammation, tissue damage Eosinophil – allergic reaction, parasitic worm infections Lymphocyte – viral infection, chronic bacterial infection Monocyte – chronic bacterial infections, malignancies Basophil – myeloproliferative disorders

Test	Assesses	Interpretation
Packed cell volume (PCV)/haematocrit (Hct) *Men:* 0.40–0.54 L/L *Women:* 0.35–0.47 L/L	Blood loss and fluid balance	*Increased*: polycythaemia, dehydration *Decreased*: anaemia, acute blood loss, haemodilution
Haemoglobin (Hb) *Men:* 130–180 g/L *Women:* 115–165 g/L	Anaemia and polycythaemia	*Increased*: polycythaemia, dehydration *Decreased*: anaemia, recent haemorrhage, fluid overload
Platelets (Plt) 150–400 × 10^9/L	Severity of thrombocytopenia	*Increased*: polycythaemia vera, splenectomy, malignancy *Decreased*: anaemias, infiltrative bone marrow disease, haemolytic disorders, disseminated intravascular coagulopathy, idiopathic thrombocytopenic purpura, viral infections, AIDS, splenomegaly, with radiation or chemotherapy
Prothrombin time (PT) 12–16 s	Measures extrinsic clotting time of blood plasma and clotting factor deficiencies	*Increased*: bile duct obstruction, liver disease, disseminated intravascular coagulation, malabsorption of nutrients from GIT, vitamin K deficiency, warfarin therapy, factor I (fibrinogen), II (prothrombin), V, VII, X deficiency

Activated partial thromboplastin time (APTT) 30–40 s	Measures intrinsic clotting time of blood plasma and clotting factor deficiencies	*Increased*: liver disease, disseminated intravascular coagulation, factor XI, VIII (haemophilia A) and IX (haemophilia B) deficiency, hypofibrinogenaemia, malabsorption from GIT, heparin or warfarin therapy
International normalized ratio (INR) 0.89–1.10	Standardized measure of clotting time derived from the PT. An INR of 1 is assigned to the time it takes for normal blood to clot	*Increased*: indicates excessive bleeding tendencies *Decreased*: indicates increased risk of thrombosis
Erythrocyte sedimentation rate (ESR) *Men*: 3–15 mm/h *Women*: 1–10 mm/h	The rate at which red blood cells settle in a tube of blood over 1 hour. A non-specific test that screens for significant inflammatory, infectious or malignant disease	*Increased*: autoimmune disease, malignancy, acute post-trauma, severe infection (mainly bacterial), myocardial infarction *Decreased*: heart failure, sickle cell anaemia, steroid treatment

Values vary from laboratory to laboratory, depending on testing methods used. These reference ranges should be used as a guide only. All reference ranges apply to adults only; they may differ in children.

Treatment techniques

Positioning

Positioning the patient optimizes cardiovascular and cardiopulmonary function and thus oxygen transport. Correct positioning of the patient can maximize lung volume, lung compliance and the ventilation/perfusion ratio. It can also reduce the work of breathing and aid secretion removal and cough. This may involve positioning adult patients in side lying with the 'good' lung (dependent) facing down and the 'bad' lung (non-dependent) facing uppermost. Always monitor the patient after positioning.

Precautions when placing 'bad' lung up
Recent pneumonectomy
• Large pleural effusion
• Bronchopleural fistula
• Presence of a large tumour in a main stem bronchus

Note: Positioning small children and infants to maximize ventilation/perfusion – rather than for postural drainage and removal of secretions – requires a different approach from that used with adults. In children with unilateral lung disease the good lung should be positioned uppermost to improve oxygenation.

Postural drainage

Positioning the patient according to the anatomy of the bronchial tree in order to use gravity to assist drainage of secretions.

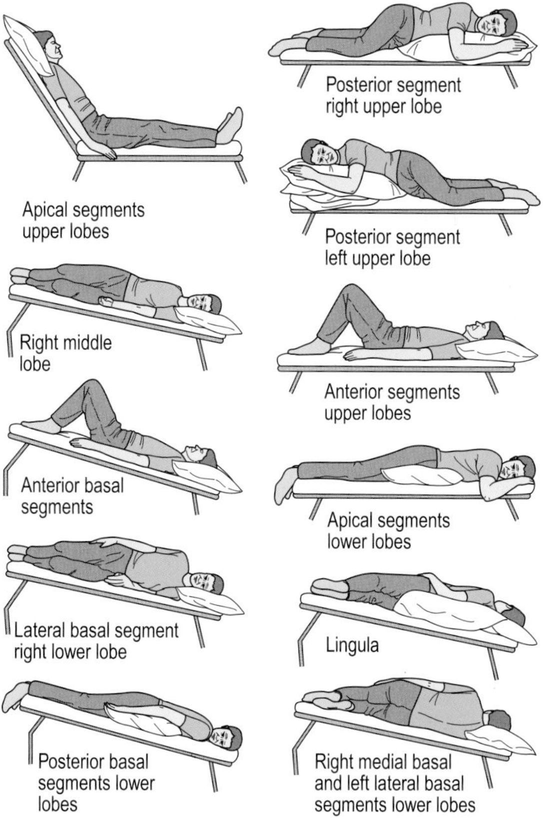
Apical segments
upper lobes
Posterior segment
right upper lobe
Posterior segment
left upper lobe
Right middle
lobe
Anterior segments
upper lobes
Anterior basal
segments
Apical segments
lower lobes
Lateral basal segment
right lower lobe
Lingula
Posterior basal
segments lower
lobes
Right medial basal
and left lateral basal
segments lower lobes

Figure 4.17 Postural drainage positions.

Contraindications and precautions for head-down position (Harden 2004, with permission)

Contraindications

- Hypertension
- Severe dyspnoea

- Recent surgery
- Severe haemoptysis
- Nose bleeds
- Advanced pregnancy
- Hiatus hernia
- Cardiac failure
- Cerebral oedema
- Aortic aneurysm
- Head or neck trauma/surgery

Precautions

- Diaphragmatic paralysis/weakness
- Mechanical ventilation

Manual chest clearance techniques

These can be used while the patient is in a postural drainage position to aid the clearance of secretions. Manual techniques include percussion, vibrations and shaking.

	Contraindications	Precautions
Percussion	Directly over rib fracture Directly over surgical incision or graft	Profound hypoxaemia Bronchospasm Pain
	Frank haemoptysis Severe osteoporosis	Osteoporosis Bony metastases Near chest drains
Vibrations	Directly over rib fracture Directly over surgical incision Severe bronchospasm	Long-term oral steroids Osteoporosis Near chest drains
Shaking	Directly over rib fracture Directly over surgical incision	Long-term oral steroids Osteoporosis Bony metastases Near chest drains Severe bronchospasm

From Harden 2004, with permission.

Active cycle of breathing technique (ACBT)

This consists of three different breathing techniques, namely breathing control (normal tidal breaths), thoracic expansion exercises (deep inspiratory breaths, usually combined with a 3 s end-inspiratory hold) and forced expiration technique (forced expirations following a breath in that can be performed at different lung volumes), that are repeated in cycles in order to mobilize and clear bronchial secretions. These can be used in different combinations according to the patient's needs and in conjunction with other treatment techniques.

Contraindications

- None if technique(s) adapted to suit the patient's condition

Precautions

- Bronchospasm

Airway suction

The removal of bronchial secretions through a suction catheter inserted via the nose (nasopharyngeal/NP) or mouth (oropharyngeal), or via a tracheostomy or endotracheal tube using vacuum pressure (usually in the range 8.0–20 kPa/60–150 mmHg).

Contraindications

- CSF leak/basal skull fracture (applies to nasopharyngeal approach only)
- Stridor
- Severe bronchospasm
- Pulmonary oedema

Precautions

- Clotting disorders
- Recent oesophagectomy, lung transplant or pneumonectomy

Adverse effects

- Tracheobronchial trauma
- Bronchospasm
- Atelectasis

- Pneumothorax
- Hypoxia
- Cardiac arrhythmias
- Raised ICP

Manual hyperinflation

The use of a rebreathing bag to manually inflate the lungs in order to increase lung volume, aid the removal of secretions and assess or improve lung compliance. The peak airway pressure being delivered should not exceed 40 cmH_2O.

Contraindications

- Undrained pneumothorax
- Bullae
- Surgical emphysema
- Cardiovascular instability
- Patients at risk of barotrauma, e.g. emphysema, fibrosis
- Recent pneumonectomy/lobectomy (first 10 days)
- Severe bronchospasm (if peak airway pressure >40 cmH_2O)
- Unexplained haemoptysis
- Acute head injury

Adverse effects

- Barotrauma
- Haemodynamic compromise – reduced or increased blood pressure
- Cardiac arrhythmia
- Reduced oxygen saturation
- Raised intracranial pressure
- Reduced respiratory drive
- Bronchospasm

Considerations when treating patients with raised ICP
Minimize suction
Minimize manual techniques
Minimize manual hyperinflation (maintain hypocapnia)
Consider sedation/inotropic support if ICP increased or unstable
Monitor CPP: should be >70 mmHg

Intermittent positive pressure breathing (IPPB)

Assisted breathing using positive airway pressure to deliver gas throughout inspiration until a preset pressure is reached. Inspiration is triggered when the patient inhales and expiration is passive.

Effects

- Increases tidal volume
- Reduces work of breathing
- Assists clearance of bronchial secretions
- Improves alveolar ventilation

Contraindications

IPPB should not normally be used when any of the following conditions are present. If in doubt, medical advice should be sought.

- Undrained pneumothorax
- Facial fractures
- Acute head injury
- Large bullae
- Lung abscess
- Severe haemoptysis
- Vomiting
- Tumour or obstruction in proximal airways
- Surgical emphysema
- Recent lung and oesophageal surgery

Tracheostomies

A tracheostomy is an opening in the anterior wall of the trachea to facilitate ventilation. It is sited below the level of the vocal cords.

Indications

- Provide and maintain a patent airway when the upper airways are obstructed.
- Provide access for the removal of tracheobronchial secretions.

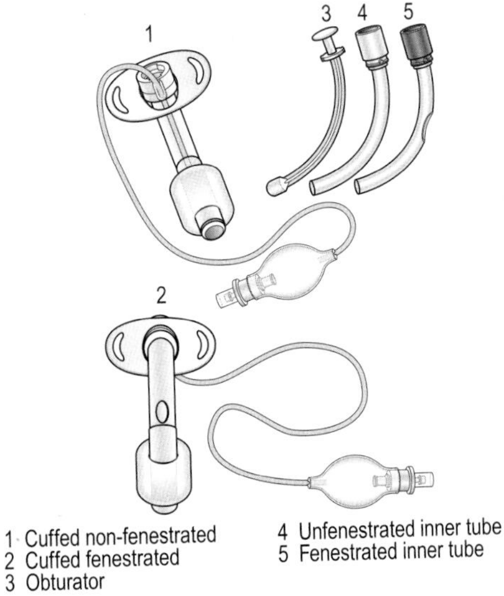
1
2
3
4
5
1 Cuffed non-fenestrated
2 Cuffed fenestrated
3 Obturator
4 Unfenestrated inner tube
5 Fenestrated inner tube

Figure 4.18 Different types of tracheostomy tubes.

- Prevent aspiration of oral and gastric secretions in patients unable to protect their own airway.
- Used in patients who need longer-term ventilation.

Types of tube

Metal or plastic

- Metal tubes are used by long-term tracheostomy patients as they are more durable. They are made of either stainless steel or sterling silver and do not have connections for respiratory equipment, e.g. a resuscitation bag. On some tubes an adaptor can be attached.
- Plastic tubes are cheaper and therefore more disposable.

Cuffed or uncuffed

- Cuffed tubes have an air-filled sac at their distal end. When inflated a cuffed tube provides a seal between the trachea and the tube. It protects the airway against aspiration and allows positive pressure ventilation. Patients cannot speak when the cuff is inflated, unless the tube is fenestrated.

- Uncuffed tubes are used for paediatric patients as the air space around the tube can be sealed without the need for a cuff. Also used when the cuff is no longer required for ventilation, when there is no risk of aspiration, or in patients on long-term ventilation.

Fenestrated

- Fenestrated tubes enable air to pass through the tube and over the vocal cords, allowing speech. They can also be used as part of the weaning process by allowing patients to breathe through the tube and use their upper airway.

Single or double lumen

- Single lumen tubes consist of a single cannula. Used for invasive ventilation. They are for short-term use only as they carry the risk of becoming blocked by secretions and obstructing the airway.
- Double lumen tubes consist of an inner and outer cannula. The inner cannula is removable and can be cleaned to prevent the accumulation of secretions. To allow speech the inner tube and outer tube need to be fenestrated. However, during suctioning the inner tube must be replaced with an unfenestrated tube to prevent the catheter passing through the fenestration. It must also be in place if the patient is put on positive pressure ventilation in order to maintain pressure.

Mini tracheostomy

- A small tracheostomy that is primarily indicated for sputum retention as it allows regular suctioning. Talking and swallowing are unaffected.

Complications

- Haemorrhage
- Pneumothorax
- Tracheal tube misplacement

- End of tube blocked if pressed against carina or tracheal wall
- Surgical emphysema
- Secretions occluding tube
- Herniation of cuff causing tube blockage
- Stenosis of trachea due to granulation
- Tracheo-oesophageal fistula
- Infection of tracheostomy site
- Tracheal irritation, ulceration and necrosis caused by overinflated cuff or excessive tube movement

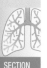

Respiratory assessment

Patients present with a variety of conditions, and assessments need to be adapted to suit their needs. This section provides a basic framework for the subjective and objective respiratory assessment of a patient.

Database

- History of present condition
- Past medical history
- Drug history
- Family history
- Social history
  - support at home
  - home environment
  - occupation and hobbies
  - smoking

Subjective examination

- Patient's main concern
- Symptoms
  - shortness of breath
  - cough (productive or non-productive)
  - pain
  - wheeze
- Functional ability/exercise tolerance

Objective examination

X-rays and other diagnostic imaging (e.g. MRI, CT)

Charts

- Blood pressure
- Heart rate
- Temperature
- Oxygen requirement
- Oxygen saturation
- Respiratory rate
- Weight
- Peak flow
- Spirometry
- Fluid balance
- Urine output
- Medications

+ ITU/HDU charts

- Mode of ventilation
- FiO_2
- Heart rhythm
- Pressure support/volume control
- Airway pressure
- Tidal volume
- I : E ratio
- PEEP
- MAP
- CVP
- GCS
- ABGs
- Blood chemistry

Observation

- General appearance
- Position
- Oxygen therapy
- Humidification
- Lines and drains
- Presence of wheeze or cough

- Sputum
  - colour
  - volume
  - viscosity
- Quality of voice
- Ability to talk in full sentences
- Skin colour
- Jugular venous pressure
- Oedema
- Clubbing
- Flapping tremor
- Chest
  - shape
  - breathing pattern
  - work of breathing
  - chest wall movement
  - respiratory rate

Palpation

- Chest excursion
- Skin hydration
- Trachea
- Percussion note

Auscultation

- Breath sounds
- Added sounds
- Voice sounds

Functional ability

Exercise tolerance

References and further reading

British Thoracic Society Standards of Care Committee, 2002 Guidelines on non-invasive ventilation in acute respiratory failure. Thorax 57: 192–211

Chung E K 2001 Pocket guide to ECG diagnosis, 2nd edn. Blackwell Science, Cambridge, MA

Hampton J R 2003 ECG made easy, 6th edn. Churchill Livingstone, Edinburgh
Harden B 2004 Emergency physiotherapy. Churchill Livingstone, Edinburgh
Hillegass E A, Sadowsky H S 2001 Essentials of cardiopulmonary physical therapy, 2nd edn. W B Saunders, Philadelphia
Hough A 2001 Physiotherapy in respiratory care: an evidence-based approach to respiratory and cardiac management, 3rd edn. Nelson Thornes, Cheltenham
Irwin S, Tecklin J S 2004 Cardiopulmonary physical therapy: a guide to practice, 4th edn. Mosby, St Louis
Jones M, Moffatt F 2002 Cardiopulmonary physiotherapy. BIOS, Oxford
McGhee M 2003 A guide to laboratory investigations, 4th edn. Radcliffe Medical Press Ltd, Abingdon
Martini F H 2006 Fundamentals of anatomy and physiology, 7th edn. Pearson Benjamin Cummings, London
Matassarin-Jacobs E 1997 Assessment of clients with haematological disorders. In: Black J M, Matassarin-Jacobs E (eds) Medical-surgical nursing: clinical management for continuity of care, 5th edn. W B Saunders, Philadelphia
Middleton S, Middleton P G 2008 Assessment and investigation of patient's problems. In: Pryor J A, Prasad S A Physiotherapy for respiratory and cardiac problems, 4th edn. Churchill Livingstone, Edinburgh, p. 1–20
Paz J C, West M P 2002 Acute care handbook for physical therapists, 2nd edn. Butterworth-Heinemann, Boston
Pryor J A, Prasad S A 2008 Physiotherapy for respiratory and cardiac problems, 4th edn. Churchill Livingstone, Edinburgh
Richards A, Edwards S 2008 A nurse's survival guide to the ward, 2nd edn. Churchill Livingstone, Edinburgh
Smith M, Ball V 1998 Cardiovascular/respiratory physiotherapy. Mosby, London
Springhouse 2007 ECG interpretation made incredibly easy, 4th edn. Lippincott, Williams & Wilkins, Philadelphia
Stillwell S B 2006 Mosby's critical care nursing reference, 4th edn. Mosby, St Louis
Ward J, Ward J, Leach R M, Weiner C M 2006 The respiratory system at a glance, 2nd edn. Blackwell, Oxford
Whiteley S M, Bodenham A, Bellamy M C 2004 Churchill's pocketbook of intensive care, 2nd edn. Churchill Livingstone, Edinburgh
Wilkins R L, Sheldon R L, Krider S J 2006 Clinical assessment in respiratory care, 5th edn. Mosby, St Louis

Pathology

Alphabetical listing of pathologies **246**

Diagnostic imaging **281**

Electrodiagnostic tests **283**

SECTION 5

Acute respiratory distress syndrome (ARDS)

ARDS can be caused by a wide variety of factors including pneumonia, sepsis, smoke inhalation, aspiration, major trauma and burns. As a result, the body launches an inflammatory response that affects the alveolar epithelium and pulmonary capillaries. In ARDS the alveolar walls break down and the pulmonary capillaries become more permeable allowing plasma and blood to leak into the interstitial and alveolar spaces, while at the same time the capillaries become blocked with cellular debris and fibrin. The lungs become heavy, stiff and waterlogged and the alveoli collapse. This leads to ventilation/perfusion mismatch and hypoxaemia and patients normally require mechanical ventilatory support to achieve adequate gas exchange. Symptoms usually develop within 24–48 hours after the original injury or illness but can develop 5–10 days later.

Adhesive capsulitis

A condition that affects the glenohumeral joint synovial capsule and is characterized by a significant restriction of active and passive shoulder movement.

The aetiology is unknown but it has been linked to diabetes, heart disease, shoulder trauma or surgery, inflammatory disease, cervical disease and hyperthyroidism. The condition usually affects the middle-aged, particularly women. It normally follows three distinct phases, each lasting approximately 6–9 months (although this can be extremely variable):

Phase 1: increasing pain accompanied by increasing stiffness
Phase 2: decreasing pain with the stiffness remaining
Phase 3: decreasing stiffness and gradual return to normal function

Also known as frozen shoulder.

AIDS (acquired immunodeficiency syndrome)

Caused by infection with the human immunodeficiency virus (HIV), which destroys a subgroup of lymphocytes and monocytes, resulting in suppression of the immune system. The virus enters the host cell and causes a mutation of its DNA so that the host cell becomes an infective agent (known as the provirus). Signs and symptoms include fever, malaise, painful throat, swollen lymph nodes and aching muscles in the initial period following infection. After a variable period of latency (1–15 years) weight loss, night sweats, long-lasting fever and diarrhoea occur as AIDS itself develops, which eventually progresses to the acquisition of major opportunistic infections and cancers such as pneumonia or Kaposi's sarcoma (a malignant skin tumour appearing as purple to dark brown plaques). Antiretroviral drugs are used to prolong the lives of infected individuals although there is no cure or vaccine for the disease.

Alzheimer's disease

A form of dementia that is characterized by slow, progressive mental deterioration. Symptoms may start with mild forgetfulness, difficulty remembering names and faces or recent events and progress to memory failure, disorientation, speech disturbances, motor impairment and aggressive behaviour. It is the most common form of dementia and is distinguished by the presence of neuritic plaques (primarily in the hippocampus and parietal lobes), and neurofibrillary tangles (mainly affecting the pyramidal cells of the cortex). Definitive diagnosis is post-mortem.

Ankylosing spondylitis

A chronic inflammatory disease of synovial joints, involving the capsule and its attached ligaments and tendons. The spinal and sacroiliac joints are primarily affected, resulting in pain, stiffness, fatigue, loss of movement and function. Bone gradually forms in the outer layers of the annulus fibrosus and the anterior longitudinal ligament and, as the disease progresses, the vertebrae fuse together. 'Bamboo spine' is the term commonly used to describe its appearance on X-ray. The disease is more common in young males.

Asthma

A chronic inflammatory disease of the airways that makes them hyper-responsive to a wide range of stimuli including allergens, pollution, infection, exercise and stress. As a result the airways narrow, leading to coughing, wheezing, chest tightness and difficulty breathing. These symptoms can range from mild to severe; and may even result in death.

Baker's cyst

Distension of the popliteal bursa, which may be accompanied by herniation of the synovial membrane of the knee-joint capsule forming a fluid-filled sac at the back of the knee. Associated with rheumatoid arthritis and osteoarthritis.

Bell's palsy

An acute, lower motor neurone paralysis of the face, usually unilateral, related to inflammation and swelling of the facial nerve (VII) within the facial canal or at the stylomastoid foramen. Symptoms include inability to close the eye on the affected side, hyperacusis and impairment of taste. Good recovery is common.

Boutonnière deformity

A flexion deformity of the proximal interphalangeal joint combined with a hyperextension deformity of the distal interphalangeal joint. Caused by a rupture of the central slip of the extensor tendon at its insertion into the base of the middle phalanx. This causes the proximal phalanx to push upwards through the lateral slips. The most common causes are rheumatoid arthritis and direct trauma.

Broca's dysphasia

A lesion of Broca's area, on the inferior frontal cortex, causing non-fluent, hesitant speech that is characterized by poor grammar and reduced word output while meaning is preserved. Persistent repetition of a word or phrase (perseveration) can occur and writing may be impaired but comprehension remains relatively intact. Broca's area is near the motor cortex for the face and arm and so may be associated with weakness in these areas.

Bronchiectasis

Dilatation and destruction of the bronchi as a result of recurrent inflammation or infection. It may be present from birth (congenital bronchiectasis) or acquired as a result of another disorder (acquired bronchiectasis). Causes of infection include impaired mucociliary clearance due to congenital disorders such as primary ciliary dyskinesia or cystic fibrosis as well as bronchial obstruction and impaired inflammatory response, either acquired after a severe episode of inflammation or secondary to immunodeficiency. The inability of the airways to clear secretions in the bronchi leads to a vicious circle of infection, damage and obstruction of the bronchi. Clinical features include: productive cough, episodic fever, pleuritic pain and night sweats. Patients may develop pneumothorax, respiratory and heart failure, emphysema and haemoptysis.

Bronchiolitis

A common respiratory problem affecting young infants. Caused by inflammation of the bronchioles due to infection by the human respiratory syncytial virus (RSV). Commonly occurs in winter. Signs and symptoms are similar to those of the common cold and include runny or blocked nose, temperature, difficulty feeding, a dry cough, dyspnoea and wheeze. In severe cases, hypoxia, cyanosis, tachypnoea and a refusal to eat may develop and hospitalization is necessary.

Bronchitis

An inflammation of the bronchi. Acute bronchitis is commonly associated with viral respiratory infections, i.e. the common cold or influenza, causing a productive cough, fever and wheezing. Chronic bronchitis is defined as a cough productive of sputum for 3 months a year for more than 2 consecutive years. It is characterized by inflammation of the airways leading to permanent fibrotic changes, excessive mucus production and thickening of the bronchial wall. This results in sputum retention and narrowing and obstruction of the airways.

In severe cases irreversible narrowing of the airways leads to dyspnoea, cyanosis, hypoxia, hypercapnia and heart failure. These patients are often described as 'blue bloaters'.

Brown-Séquard syndrome

A neurological condition that occurs when there is damage to one half of the spinal cord. Below the lesion there is motor loss on the same side and loss of pain and temperature on the opposite side.

Bulbar palsy

A bilateral or unilateral lower motor neurone lesion that affects the nerves supplying the bulbar muscles of the head and neck. Causes paralysis or weakness of the muscles of the jaw, face, palate, pharynx and larynx leading to impaired swallow, cough, gag reflex and speech.

Bursitis

Inflammation of the bursa caused by mechanical irritation or infection. Bursas that are commonly affected include the prepatellar, olecranon (can be associated with gout), subacromial, trochanteric, semimembranosus and the 'bunion' associated with hallux valgus. May or may not be painful.

Carpal tunnel syndrome

Compression of the median nerve as it passes beneath the flexor retinaculum, caused by inflammation due to joint disease, trauma, repetitive injury or during menopause. Characterized by pain, numbness, tingling or burning sensation in the distribution of the median nerve, i.e. the radial three and a half fingers and nail beds and the associated area of the palm. Symptoms are often worse at night. Patients also complain of clumsiness performing fine movements of the hand, particularly in the early morning.

Cerebral palsy

An umbrella term for a variety of posture and movement disorders arising from permanent brain damage incurred before, during, or immediately after birth. The disorder is most frequently associated with premature births and is often complicated by other neurological problems including epilepsy, visual, hearing and sensory impairments, communication and feeding difficulties, cognitive and behavioural problems. Common causes include intrauterine infection, intrauterine cerebrovascular insult, birth asphyxia, postnatal meningitis and postnatal cerebrovascular insult. The most common disability is a spastic paralysis, which can be associated with choreoathetosis (irregular, repetitive, writhing and jerky movements).

Charcot–Marie–Tooth disease

A progressive hereditary disorder of the peripheral nerves that is characterized by gradual progressive distal weakness and wasting, mainly affecting the peroneal muscle in the leg. Early symptoms include difficulty running and foot deformities. The disease is slowly progressive and in the late stages the arm muscles can also be involved. Also known as hereditary motor sensory neuropathy (HMSN).

Chondromalacia patellae

Refers to degeneration of the patellar cartilage causing pain around or under the patella. Common among teenagers and young adults, especially girls, it is linked to structural changes and muscle imbalance associated with periods of rapid growth. This leads to excessive and uneven pressure on patellar cartilage. May also result from an acute injury to the patella.

Chronic fatigue syndrome

A condition where patients complain of long-term, persistent fatigue along with other symptoms such as muscle pain, joint pains, disturbed sleep, poor concentration, headaches, sore throat and tender lymph nodes in the armpit and neck, though patients will not necessarily have all of them. Diagnosis is based on symptoms and tests that rule out other causes. No single cause of the disease has been established.

Chronic obstructive pulmonary disease (COPD)

An umbrella term for respiratory disorders that lead to obstruction of the airways. COPD is associated mainly with emphysema and chronic bronchitis but also includes chronic asthma. Risk factors include smoking, recurrent infection, pollution and genetics. Symptoms include cough, dyspnoea, excessive mucus production and chest tightness. Patients may also develop oedema and heart failure.

Claw toe

A flexion deformity of both the proximal interphalangeal and the distal interphalangeal joints combined with an extension deformity of the metatarsophalangeal joint.

Coccydynia

Pain around the coccyx. Often due to trauma, such as a fall onto the buttocks, or childbirth; however, the cause is often unknown.

Compartment syndrome

Soft tissue ischaemia caused by increased pressure in a fascial compartment of a limb. This increased pressure can have a number of causes but the main ones are swelling following major trauma, a cast being applied too tightly over an injured limb, or repetitive strain injury. Signs and symptoms are pain, pale/plum colour, absent pulse, paraesthesia and loss of active movement. If left untreated, it leads to necrosis of nerve and muscle in the affected compartment, which is known as Volkmann's ischaemic contracture.

Complex regional pain syndrome (CRPS)

An umbrella term for a number of conditions, usually affecting the distal extremities, whose common features include unremitting severe pain (often described as burning) and autonomic changes in the affected region such as swelling, tenderness, restriction of movement, increased skin temperature, sweating, discoloration of the skin (usually blue or dusky red) and osteoporosis. CRPS is subdivided into two groups:

Group II – conditions where there has been an injury to a major peripheral nerve (e.g. sciatic nerve). Also referred to as causalgia ('hot pain').

Group I – conditions where minor or major trauma has occurred but there is no identifiable nerve injury, e.g. after Colles' fractures. Also referred to as reflex sympathetic dystrophy and Sudeck's atrophy.

Conversion disorder

A psychological disorder in which conflict or stress is 'converted' into physical symptoms such as blindness, deafness, loss of sensation, gait abnormalities, paralysis and seizures, for which no underlying cause can be found.

Coxa vara

Any condition that affects the angle between the femoral neck and shaft so that it is less than the normal 120–135°. It can be either congenital (present at birth), developmental (manifests clinically during early childhood and progresses with growth) or acquired (mal-united and non-united fractures, a slipped upper femoral epiphysis, Perthes' disease and bone 'softening', e.g. osteomalacia, Paget's disease).

Cubital tunnel syndrome

Compression of the ulnar nerve as it passes through the cubital tunnel (between the medial epicondyle and the olecranon). Symptoms include pain, weakness and dysaesthesia along the medial aspect of the elbow, forearm and hand.

Cystic fibrosis

A progressive genetic disorder of the mucus-secreting glands of the lungs, pancreas, mouth, gastrointestinal tract and sweat glands. Chloride ion secretion is reduced and sodium ion absorption is accelerated across the cell membrane, resulting in the production of abnormally viscous mucus. This thickened mucus lines the intestine and lung leading to malabsorption, malnutrition and poor growth as well as recurrent respiratory infections that eventually lead to chronic lung disease. The increased concentration of sodium in sweat upsets the mineral balance in the blood and causes abnormal heart rhythms. Other complications include male infertility, diabetes mellitus, liver disease and vasculitis. The disease is eventually fatal.

De Quervain's syndrome

See 'Tenovaginitis'.

Developmental dysplasia of the hip

Used to describe a spectrum of disorders causing hip dislocation either at birth or soon afterwards. The acetabulum is abnormally shallow so that the femoral head is easily displaced. Females and the left hip are more commonly affected.

Diabetes insipidus

A condition that leads to frequent excretion of large amounts of diluted urine. The symptoms of excessive thirst and urination are similar to diabetes mellitus but the two conditions are unrelated. Urine excretion is governed by antidiuretic hormone (ADH), which is made in the hypothalamus and stored in the pituitary gland. Diabetes insipidus is caused by damage to the pituitary gland or by insensitivity of the kidneys to ADH. This leads to the body losing its ability to maintain fluid balance.

Diabetes mellitus

A chronic condition caused by the body's inability to produce or effectively use the hormone insulin to regulate the transfer of glucose from the blood into the cells. This leads to higher than normal levels of blood sugar. If not corrected this can lead to coma, kidney failure and ultimately, death. In the long term, high levels of glucose can damage blood vessels, nerves and organs leading to cardiovascular disease, chronic renal failure, retinal damage and poor wound healing.

There are two types of diabetes:

Type I – little or no insulin is produced. Requires lifelong treatment with insulin injections, diet control and lifestyle adaptations.

Type II – the body produces inadequate amounts of insulin or is unable to utilize insulin effectively. Mainly occurs in people over the age of 40 and is linked to obesity.

Diffuse idiopathic skeletal hyperostosis (DISH)

A condition that is characterized by widespread calcification and ossification of ligaments, tendons and joint capsule insertions. Mainly affects the spine with calcification of the anterior longitudinal ligament, which radiologically gives the appearance of candle wax dripping down the spine. Other joints may be affected with ossification of ligament and tendon insertions. Radiographically distinguishable from spondyloarthropathies and degenerative disc disease in that underlying bone and disc height are preserved and the facet joints are unaffected. It mainly affects men over 50 and is most cases it is asymptomatic, though some patients complain of stiffness and mild pain. The cause is unknown. Also known as Forestier's disease.

Dupuytren's contracture

Thickening and shortening of the palmar aponeurosis together with flexion contracture of one or more fingers. The cause is unknown.

Ehlers–Danlos syndrome (EDS)

A hereditary disorder of connective tissue that represents a collection of disorders (types I–X) characterized by a combination of joint hypermobility and hyperextensible (stretchy) skin. EDS types I and II are associated with mutations of collagen and feature high degrees of hypermobility, which may materialize in deformity or excessive dislocation. Type III, however, is associated with greater skin extensibility resulting in more obvious scarring or striae in the skin (in the thigh or lumbar region). The poorest prognosis is associated with EDS type IV, which results from a mutation in procollagen. Although rare, it commonly causes death through arterial rupture.

Emphysema

The walls of the terminal bronchioles and alveoli are destroyed by inflammation and lose their elasticity. This causes excessive airway collapse on expiration which traps air in the enlarged alveolar sacs. This irreversible airways obstruction leads to symptoms of dyspnoea, productive cough, wheeze, recurrent respiratory infection, hyperinflated chest and weight loss. These patients are often described as 'pink puffers' who may hyperventilate, typically overusing their accessory respiratory muscles, and breathe with pursed lips in order to maintain airway pressure to decrease the amount of airway collapse.

Empyema

A collection of pus in the pleural cavity following nearby lung infection. Can cause a build-up of pressure in the lung which causes pain and shortness of breath.

Enteropathic arthritis

This form of chronic inflammatory arthritis is associated with ulcerative colitis or Crohn's disease, which are types of inflammatory bowel disease (IBD). It affects around a fifth of IBD sufferers and it mainly affects the peripheral joints such as the knees, ankles and elbows.

Fibromyalgia/fibrositis

A non-articular rheumatological disorder associated with widespread myofascial and joint pain and pain and tenderness in at least 11 of 18 trigger points. Other problems associated with fibromyalgia include fatigue, disturbed sleep, depression, anxiety and morning stiffness. The cause and pathogenesis of fibromyalgia is unknown, but it can either develop on its own or together with other conditions such as rheumatoid arthritis or systemic lupus erythematosus.

Forestier's disease

See 'Diffuse idiopathic skeletal hyperostosis'.

Freiberg's disease

Degenerative aseptic necrosis of the metatarsal head, usually the second metatarsal head, which mainly affects athletic females aged 10–15 years.

Ganglion

An abnormal but harmless cystic swelling that often develops over a tendon sheath or joint capsule, especially on the back of the wrist.

Golfer's elbow (medial epicondylitis)

Tendinopathy of the common origin of the forearm flexors causing pain and tenderness at the medial aspect of the elbow and down the forearm.

Gout

Characterized by attacks of acute joint inflammation secondary to hyperuricaemia (raised serum uric acid) where monosodium urate or uric acid crystals are deposited into the joint cavity. The disease usually affects middle-aged men and mainly affects the big toe. If the disease progresses, urates may be deposited in the kidney (stones) or the soft tissues (tophi), especially the ears. Further joint destruction can occur.

Guillain–Barré syndrome (GBS)

An acute inflammatory polyneuropathy that usually occurs 1–4 weeks after fever associated with viral infection or following immunization. Thought to be an autoimmune disorder, it leads to segmental demyelination of spinal roots and axons, denervation atrophy of muscle and inflammatory infiltration of the brain, liver, kidneys and lungs. Clinical features include loss of sensation in hands and feet, symmetrical progressive ascending motor weakness, paralysis, muscle wasting, diminished reflexes, pain and autonomic disturbances. In severe cases, the respiratory and bulbar systems are affected and ventilation/tracheostomy may be required. Recovery is common.

Haemothorax

Blood in the pleural cavity. Commonly due to chest trauma but also found in patients with lung and pleural cancer and in those who have undergone thoracic or heart surgery.

Hallux valgus

A lateral deviation of the great toe at the metatarsophalangeal joint. The metatarsal head becomes prominent (bunion) and, along with the overlying bursa, may become inflamed.

Hammer toe

An extension deformity of the metatarsophalangeal joint, combined with a flexion deformity of the proximal interphalangeal joint. The second toe is the most commonly affected.

Hereditary disorders of connective tissue

See 'Joint hypermobility syndrome', 'Marfan syndrome', 'Ehlers–Danlos syndrome', 'Osteogenesis imperfecta'.

Herpes zoster

See 'Shingles'.

Horner's syndrome

A group of symptoms caused by a lesion of the sympathetic pathways in the hypothalamus, brainstem, spinal cord, C8–T2 ventral spinal roots, superior cervical ganglion or internal carotid sheath. It causes ipsilateral pupil constriction, drooping of the upper eyelid and loss of facial sweating on the affected side of the face.

Huntingdon's disease

A hereditary disease caused by a defect in chromosome 4 that can be inherited from either parent. Onset is insidious and occurs between 35 and 50 years of age. Symptoms include sudden, involuntary movements (chorea) accompanied by behavioural changes and progressive dementia.

Hyperparathyroidism

Overactivity of the parathyroid glands leads to excessive secretion of parathyroid hormone (PTH), which regulates levels of calcium and phosphorus. Overproduction of PTH causes excessive extraction of calcium from the bones and leads to hypercalcaemia. Symptoms include fatigue, memory loss, renal stones and osteoporosis.

Hyperthyroidism

Occurs when the thyroid gland produces too much thyroxine, a hormone that regulates metabolism. This increase in metabolism causes most body functions to accelerate and symptoms may include tachycardia, palpitations, hand tremors, nervousness, shortness of breath, irritability, anxiety, insomnia, fatigue, increased bowel movements, muscle weakness, heat intolerance, weight loss despite an increase in appetite, thinning of skin and fine brittle hair. Also known as overactive thyroid or thyrotoxicosis.

Hyperventilation syndrome

Breathing in excess of metabolic requirements, which causes low arterial carbon dioxide levels, leading to alkalosis and changes in potassium and calcium ion distribution. As a result, neuromuscular excitability and vasoconstriction occur. Clinical features include light-headedness, dizziness, chest pain, palpitations, breathlessness, tachycardia, anxiety, paraesthesia and tetanic cramps.

Hypothyroidism

Occurs when the thyroid gland does not produce enough thyroxine, a hormone that regulates metabolism. This decrease in metabolism causes most body functions to slow down and symptoms may include tiredness, weight gain, dry skin and hair, cold intolerance, hoarse voice, memory loss, muscle cramps, constipation and depression. Also known as underactive thyroid.

Interstitial lung disease

An umbrella term for a wide range of respiratory disorders characterized by inflammation and, eventually, fibrosis of the lung connective tissue. The bronchioles, alveoli and vasculature may all be affected, causing the lungs to stiffen and decrease in size. Examples of interstitial lung disease include fibrosing alveolitis, asbestosis, pneumoconiosis, bird fancier's or farmer's lung, systemic lupus erythematosus, scleroderma, rheumatoid disease, cryptogenic pulmonary fibrosis and sarcoidosis.

Joint hypermobility syndrome (JHS)

Hypermobility describes a condition in which joint movement is in excess of normal range. In some cases this poses no problem to the individual but in others it makes joints more susceptible to soft tissue injury and internal derangement, arthritis, arthralgias and myalgias. Joint hypermobility with associated symptoms is termed joint hypermobility syndrome (JHS). The clinical features and number of joints affected are highly variable and features may include a history of dislocation/subluxation/sprains, tendinitis, proprioceptive deficit, skin hyperextensibility, striae atrophicae, autonomic dysfunction and prolapse (mitral, rectal, uterine). JHS is said to overlap with the hereditary disorders of connective tissue, which include Marfan syndrome, Ehlers–Danlos syndrome and osteogenesis imperfecta.

Jones fracture

A stress fracture of the proximal fifth metatarsal. The fracture occurs within 1.5 cm distal to the tuberosity of the metatarsal.

Köhler's disease

A condition where the navicular bone undergoes avascular necrosis. The cause is unclear but it mainly affects boys around the age of 5 years.

Locked-in syndrome

A rare neurological disorder characterized by total paralysis of all voluntary muscles except those controlling eye movement and some facial movements. May be caused by traumatic brain injury, vascular disease, demyelinating diseases or overdose. Patients are unable to speak or move but sight, hearing and cognition are normal. Prognosis for recovery is poor with most patients not regaining function.

Lung abscess

A pus-filled necrotic cavity within the lung parenchyma caused by infection.

Mallet toe/finger

A flexion deformity of the distal interphalangeal joint due to damage to the extensor tendon at its insertion into the distal phalanx. The result is an inability to extend the distal phalanx.

March fracture

A stress fracture of the metatarsal. Usually affects the second or third metatarsal but it can affect the fourth and fifth. Initially the fracture may not be visible on X-ray but abundant callus is seen on later X-rays.

Marfan syndrome (MFS)

A hereditary disorder of connective tissue that is thought to result from a mutation in the fibrillin gene. Patients present with a distinct collection of features known as the marfanoid habitus which include a tall, slender body, an elongated head and long extremities (fingers, toes, hands, arms and legs), pectus excavatum, pectus carinatum, scoliosis, myopia and dislocation of the ocular lens. MFS also carries an increased risk of aortic aneurysm.

Meningitis

An acute inflammation of the meninges due to infection by bacteria or viruses. Age groups most at risk are the under-5s, especially infants under 1 year, and adolescents between 15 and 19 years of age. The most common causes of bacterial meningitis in young children are *Neisseria meningitidis* (meningococcal meningitis) and *Haemophilus influenzae.* The classic triad of clinical features is fever, headache and neck stiffness. Skin rash and septic shock may occur where septicaemia has developed as a result of widespread meningococcal infection. Other signs in adults include confusion and photophobia. Onset of symptoms may be gradual or sudden; however, deterioration is rapid, often requiring intensive supportive therapy.

Morton's metatarsalgia

A fibrous thickening of the digital nerve as it travels between the metatarsals. Can be caused by irritation, trauma or compression. Usually occurs between the third and fourth toes. Symptoms include burning, numbness, paraesthesia and pain in the ball of the foot. Also known as plantar neuroma and plantar digital neuritis.

Motor neurone disease

A group of progressive degenerative diseases of the motor system occurring in middle to late adult life, causing weakness, wasting and eventual paralysis of muscles. It primarily affects the anterior horn cells of the spinal cord, the motor nuclei of the brainstem and the corticospinal tracts. There are three distinct types:

Progressive muscle atrophy

Starts early in life, typically before 50 years of age. Affects the cervical region leading to atrophy of the muscles of the hand. Involvement spreads to the arms and shoulder girdle and may extend to the legs.

Amyotrophic lateral sclerosis

There are upper motor neurone changes as well as lower motor neurone changes. Characterized by weakness and atrophy in the hands, forearms and legs but may also spread to the body and face.

Progressive bulbar palsy

Caused by damage to the motor nuclei in the bulbar region in the brainstem which results in wasting and paralysis of muscles of the mouth, jaw, larynx and pharynx. General features include pain and spasms, dyspnoea, dysphagia, dysarthria and sore eyes.

Multiple sclerosis

A chronic, progressive disease characterized by multiple demyelinating lesions (plaques) throughout the central nervous system. It predominantly affects young adults in temperate latitudes and is more prevalent in women. The disease is usually characterized by recurrent relapses (attacks) followed by remissions, although some patients follow a chronic, progressive course. The plaques interfere with normal nerve impulses along the nerve fibre, and the site of the lesions and the degree of inflammation at each site leads to a variety of neurological signs and symptoms. Common symptoms include visual disturbances, ataxia, sensory and motor disturbance, bulbar dysfunction, fatigue, bladder and bowel symptoms, cognitive and emotional disturbances, pain and spasm.

Muscular dystrophy

A group of genetically determined progressive muscle wasting diseases in which the affected muscle fibres degenerate and are replaced by fat and connective tissue. Duchenne muscular dystrophy is the most common form, affecting boys before the age of 4 years. Clinical features include difficulty walking, pseudohypertrophy of proximal muscles, postural problems, diminished reflexes and difficulty standing from squatting (Gower's sign).

Myalgic encephalomyelitis

See 'Chronic fatigue syndrome'.

Myasthenia gravis

A disorder of the neuromuscular junction caused by an impaired ability of the neurotransmitter acetylcholine to induce muscular contraction, most likely due to an autoimmune destruction of the postsynaptic receptors for acetylcholine. It predominantly affects adolescents and young adults (mainly women) and is characterized by abnormal weakness and fatiguing of some or all muscle groups to the point of temporary paralysis. Onset of symptoms is usually gradual and includes drooping of the upper eyelid, double vision, dysarthria and weakness of other facial muscles.

Myositis ossificans

Growth of bone in the soft tissues near a joint that occurs after fracture or severe soft tissue trauma, particularly around the elbow. Also occurs in a congenital progressive form, usually leading to early death during adolescence.

Osgood–Schlatter disease

Seen mainly in teenage boys, it affects the tibial tubercle. Vigorous physical activity can cause the patellar tendon to pull at its attachment to the tibial tuberosity, resulting in detachment of small cartilage fragments.

Osteoarthritis

A chronic disease of articular cartilage, associated with secondary changes in the underlying bone, causing joint inflammation and degeneration. Primarily affects the large, weight-bearing joints such as the knee and hip, resulting in pain, loss of movement and loss of normal function.

Osteochrondritis

An umbrella term for a variety of conditions where there is compression, fragmentation or separation of a piece of bone, e.g. Osgood–Schlatter, osteochrondritis dissecans, Perthes', Scheuermann's, Sever's, Sinding–Larsen–Johansson disease.

Osteochrondritis dissecans

Seen mainly in adolescent boys, it is a gradual localized separation of a fragment of bone and cartilage into a joint. The medial femoral condyle and the capitulum of the humerus are the most common sites. The loose body can enter the joint space, resulting in pain, swelling and reduced movement.

Osteogenesis imperfecta

A hereditary disorder of connective tissue caused by an abnormal synthesis of type I collagen. As a result, bone is susceptible to fracture and deformity and connective tissue may also be affected. There are several different forms, which vary in appearance and severity. In its mildest form, features may include a history of fractures (which mainly occur before puberty), lax joints, low muscle tone, tinted sclera ranging from nearly white to dark blue or grey and adult-onset deafness. Those with a more severe form of the disease suffer short stature, progressive bone deformity and frequent fractures. Some types of the disease can be fatal in the perinatal period. Also known as brittle bone disease.

Osteomalacia

Softening of the bone caused by a deficiency in vitamin D from poor nutrition, lack of sunshine or problems absorbing or metabolizing vitamin D. A lack of vitamin D leads to incomplete calcification of the bones so that they become weak and easily fractured. This is particularly noticeable in the long bones, which become bowed. In children, the condition is called rickets.

Osteomyelitis

An inflammation of the bone and bone marrow due to infection. The most common causes are infection of an open fracture or postoperatively after bone or joint surgery. The infection is often spread from another part of the body to the bone via the blood.

Osteoporosis

A reduction in bone density which results from the body being unable to form enough new bone or when too much calcium and phosphate is reabsorbed back into the body from existing bones. This leads to thin, weak, brittle bones that are susceptible to fracture. Osteoporosis is common in postmenopausal women where a loss of ovarian function results in a reduction in oestrogen production. It can also be caused by prolonged disuse and non-weight-bearing, endocrine disorders such as Cushing's disease, and steroid therapy.

Paget's disease

Characterized by an excessive amount of bone breakdown associated with abnormal bone formation causing the bones to become enlarged, deformed and weak. Normal architecture of the trabeculae is affected, making the bones brittle. Paget's disease is usually confined to individual bones although more than one bone can be affected. Also known as osteitis deformans. The cause remains unknown.

Parkinson's disease

A degenerative disease of the substantia nigra that reduces the amount of dopamine in the basal ganglia. Depletion of dopamine levels affects the ability of the basal ganglia to control movement, posture and coordination and leads to the characteristic symptoms of rigidity, slowness of voluntary movement, poor postural reflexes and resting tremor. Parkinson's has a gradual, insidious onset and affects mainly those aged between 50 and 65 years. Early symptoms of Parkinson's include aches and stiffness, difficulty with fine manipulative movements, slowness of walking, resting tremor of head, hands (pill rolling) and feet, while later symptoms may include shuffling gait, difficulties with speech, a mask-like appearance and depression.

Pellegrini–Stieda syndrome

Local calcification of the femoral attachment of the medial collateral ligament (MCL), usually following direct trauma or a sprain/tear of the MCL. Signs and symptoms include chronic pain and tenderness, difficulty extending and twisting the knee, marked restriction of knee range of movement and a tender lump over the proximal portion of the knee.

Perthes' disease

Seen mainly in young boys, it affects the upper femoral epiphysis, which becomes ischaemic and necrotic. The tissues of the femoral head become soft and fragmented but eventually reform over a period of several years. However, the reformed head is flatter and larger than the original, which can lead to deformity, shortening and secondary osteoarthritis. The cause is unknown.

Piriformis syndrome

Irritation of the sciatic nerve by the piriformis muscle. Swelling of the muscle through injury or overuse causes it to compress on the sciatic nerve, resulting in deep buttock pain and pain along the posterior thigh and calf.

Plantar fasciitis

An inflammatory or degenerative condition affecting the plantar fascia. Pain is usually felt along the medial aspect of the calcaneal tuberosity where the plantar aponeurosis inserts and may extend down the proximal plantar fascia.

Pleural effusion

A collection of excess fluid in the pleural cavity which can be caused by a number of mechanisms:

- increased hydrostatic pressure, e.g. congestive heart failure
- decreased plasma-oncotic pressure, e.g. cirrhosis of the liver, malnutrition
- increased capillary permeability, e.g. inflammation of the pleura
- impaired lymphatic absorption, e.g. malignancy
- communication with peritoneal space and fluid, e.g. ascites.

The fluid can either be clear/straw-coloured and have a low protein content (known as a transudate), indicating a disturbance of the normal pressure in the lung, or it can be cloudy and have a high protein content (known as an exudate), indicating infection, inflammation or malignancy.

Pleurisy

Inflammation of the pleura causing severe pain as a result of friction between their adjoining surfaces. Pain is focused at the site of the inflammation and is increased with deep inspiration and coughing. Most commonly associated with pneumonia but also tuberculosis, rheumatic diseases and chest trauma.

Pneumonia

An inflammation of the lung tissue, mostly caused by bacterial or viral infection but also by fungi or aspiration of gastric contents. Pneumonia can be divided into two types:

- Community-acquired pneumonia: most commonly caused by the bacterium *Streptococcus pneumoniae*
- Hospital-acquired pneumonia: tends to be more serious as patients are often immunocompromised and they may be infected by bacteria resistant to antibiotics.

The most common infective agents are bacteria such as *Pseudomonas*, *Klebsiella* and *Escherichia coli*. Clinical features include cough, pleuritic pain, fever, fatigue and, after a few days, purulent and/or blood-stained sputum.

Pneumothorax

A collection of air in the pleural cavity following a lesion in the lung or trauma to the chest, which causes the lung to collapse. Clinical features include acute pain, dyspnoea and decreased movement of the chest wall on the affected side. They are classified by how they are caused and divided into three types:

Spontaneous pneumothorax

Caused by rupture of an emphysematous bulla, in association with diseases such as asthma, cystic fibrosis, pneumonia or COPD. It can also develop in people with no underlying lung disease and frequently affects tall, thin young men, especially smokers.

Traumatic pneumothorax

Caused by traumatic injury to the chest, e.g. perforation of lung tissue by fractured ribs or stab wound, or during medical procedures such as insertion of central venous lines, lung biopsies or mechanical ventilation.

Tension pneumothorax

Produced when pressure within the pleural cavity increases as a result of a tear in the visceral pleura acting as a one-way valve, allowing air to enter on inspiration but preventing it from escaping on expiration. In severe cases it can cause a mediastinal shift, impairing venous return, leading to respiratory and cardiac arrest. Clinical features include increased respiratory distress, cyanosis, hypotension, tachycardia and tracheal deviation.

Poliomyelitis

Poliomyelitis is a highly contagious infectious disease caused by one of three types of poliovirus. The extent of the disease varies, with some people experiencing no or mild symptoms, while others develop the paralytic form of the disease. It can strike at any age, but affects mainly children under the age of 3 years. The poliovirus destroys motor neurones in the anterior horn. The muscles of the legs are affected more often than those of the arm but the paralysis can spread to the muscles of the thorax and abdomen. In the most severe form (bulbar polio), the motor neurones of the brainstem are attacked, reducing breathing capacity and causing difficulty in swallowing and speaking. Without respiratory support, bulbar polio can result in death.

Polyarteritis nodosa

A vasculitic syndrome where small and medium-sized arteries are attacked by rogue immune cells causing inflammation and necrosis. Tissue supplied by the affected arteries, most commonly the skin, heart, kidneys and nervous system, is damaged by the impaired blood supply. Common manifestations are fever, renal failure, hypertension, neuritis, skin lesions, weight loss and muscle and joint pain.

Polymyalgia rheumatica

A vasculitic syndrome associated with fever and generalized pain and stiffness, especially in the shoulder and pelvic girdle areas. Symptoms usually begin abruptly and it mainly affects women over 50. Severe cases can suffer loss of vision, stroke and migraines due to involvement of the cranial arteries.

Polymyositis

An autoimmune, inflammatory muscle disease of unknown aetiology causing progressive weakness of skeletal muscle. The muscles of the shoulder girdle, hip and pelvis are most commonly affected, although, less commonly, the distal musculature or swallowing can be affected. The muscles can ache and be tender to touch. The disease sometimes occurs with a skin rash over the upper body and is known as dermatomyositis.

Post polio syndrome

A recurrence or progression of neuromuscular symptoms that appears in people who have recovered from acute paralytic poliomyelitis, usually 15–40 years after the original illness. Symptoms include progressive muscle weakness, severe fatigue and pain in muscles and joints.

Primary ciliary dyskinesia

A genetic condition affecting the cilia causing abnormal ciliary activity and consequently, poor mucociliary clearance. Can be associated with situs inversus (the location of internal organs on the opposite side of the body), and where the two conditions exist together this is known as Kartagener's syndrome. Sperm can also be affected as they share a similar structure to cilia, leading to infertility in males. Clinical features include recurrent ear, sinus and chest infections, which can eventually lead to bronchiectasis.

Pseudobulbar palsy

An upper motor neurone lesion that affects the corticomotoneuronal pathways and results in weakness and spasticity of the oral and pharyngeal musculature. Leads to slurring of speech and dysphagia. Patients also exhibit emotional incontinence. They are unable to control their emotional expression and may laugh or cry without apparent reason.

Psoriatic arthritis

A chronic autoimmune and heritable disorder associated with psoriasis. Only a minority of psoriasis sufferers are affected and it can either precede or follow the onset of the skin disease. Males and females are affected equally and it can sometimes be indistinguishable from rheumatoid arthritis. It can affect any joint, though the most common pattern is for one large joint to be infected along with a number of small joints in the fingers or toes.

Pulmonary embolus

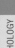

A blockage in the pulmonary arterial circulation most commonly caused by blood clots from the veins in the pelvis or the legs. This causes a ventilation/perfusion imbalance and leads to arterial hypoxaemia. Risk factors include prolonged bed rest or prolonged sitting (e.g. long flights), oral contraception, surgery, pregnancy, malignancy and fractures of the femur.

Pulmonary oedema

Accumulation of fluid in the lungs. Usually caused by left ventricular failure whereby a back pressure builds up in the pulmonary veins eventually causing fluid to be pushed from the veins into the alveoli. Pulmonary oedema can also be caused by myocardial infarction, damage to mitral or aortic valves, direct lung injury, severe infection, poisoning or fluid overload. Symptoms include shortness of breath, wheezing, sweating, tachycardia and coughing up white or pink-tinged frothy secretions.

Raynaud's phenomenon

A vasospastic disorder affecting the arterioles of the hands and feet, usually triggered by cold weather or emotional stress. The affected digits first turn pale and cold (ischaemia), then blue (cyanosis) and then bright red (reperfusion). The condition can either be primary, with no known cause, or secondary to an underlying disease such as systemic lupus erythematosus, polymyositis, rheumatoid arthritis and scleroderma.

Reactive arthritis

A chronic inflammatory disease that is caused by gastrointestinal or genitourinary infections. The syndrome is classically composed of arthritis (usually involving the lower limb), urethritis and conjunctivitis; although not all three symptoms occur in all affected individuals. It mainly affects males aged 20–40.

Reiter's syndrome

See 'Reactive arthritis'.

Rheumatoid arthritis

Thought to be an autoimmune disease involving the synovium, often affecting several joints at the same time. The joints are affected symmetrically and eventually there is destruction of articular cartilage, capsule, ligaments and tendons, leading to deformity. Clinical features include stiffness, pain, swelling, heat, loss of movement and function. Other manifestations of the disease include subcutaneous nodules, osteoporosis, vasculitis, muscle weakness, fatigue and anaemia. The disease is more common in young to middle-aged women.

Sarcoidosis

An autoimmune disease that is characterized by the formation of nodules or lumps (granulomas) in one or more organs of the body. It mainly affects the lungs, eyes, skin, and lymph glands and may change how the organ functions. Patients commonly present with dyspnoea, persistent dry cough, skin rashes, or eye inflammation. They may also complain of being unwell or fatigued, and suffer fever and weight loss. In some cases the patients are asymptomatic. The cause is unknown.

Scheuermann's disease

Seen mainly in adolescent boys, it is a growth disturbance of the thoracic vertebral bodies, resulting in degeneration of the intervertebral disc into the vertebral endplate. Can lead to a thoracic kyphosis of varying severity.

Septic arthritis

An infection in the joint caused by bacteria (e.g. *Staphylococcus aureus*) or, rarely, by a virus or fungus. Patients present with pain, swelling, erythema, restricted movement and fever. In most cases it only affects one joint. Risk factors include recent joint trauma, surgery or replacement, intravenous drug abuse, immunosuppressants, bacterial infection and existing joint conditions, e.g. rheumatoid arthritis. Early diagnosis is essential as delay can result in joint destruction. Also known as pyogenic arthritis and infective arthritis.

Seronegative spondyloarthropathies

A group of inflammatory joint disorders that include ankylosing spondylitis, psoriatic arthritis and Reiter's syndrome. They all share notable characteristics: the spine is usually affected, though other large joints are occasionally implicated; there is a strong link to human leukocyte antigen HLA-B27;

there is an absence of rheumatoid factor in the blood; males are predominantly affected; enthesopathy (inflammation of the ligaments and tendon where they attach to bone) commonly occurs, and onset is usually before the age of 40.

Sever's disease

A painful inflammation of the calcaneal apophysis that mainly affects growing, active children between the ages of 9 and 14. The pull of the Achilles tendon at its insertion causes traction of the apophysis, resulting in localized pain and tenderness of the heel. It is exacerbated by sport and activities like running and jumping.

Shingles

An infection of a sensory nerve and the area of skin that it supplies by the varicella/zoster virus (chickenpox). Following chickenpox infection the virus remains dormant in a sensory nerve ganglion but can be reactivated later in life. Characterized by pain, paraesthesia and the appearance of a rash along the dermatomal distribution of the affected nerve. Mainly occurs in the trunk although the face and other parts of the body can be affected. Occurs predominantly in the middle-aged and older population as well as the immunocompromised. Also known as herpes zoster.

Sinding–Larsen–Johansson disease

Seen mainly in adolescent boys, it affects the inferior pole of the patella. Most commonly occurs in running and jumping sports, which cause the patellar tendon to pull at its attachment at the inferior patellar pole. Results in fragmentation of the inferior patella and/or calcification in the proximal patellar tendon.

Sjögren's syndrome

An autoimmune disorder in which the body's immune system attacks the moisture-producing glands, such as the salivary and tear glands. This produces the primary features of dry eyes and dry mouth. It can be primary or secondary to other autoimmune diseases such as rheumatoid arthritis, systemic sclerosis, systemic lupus erythematosus and polymyositis. Ninety per cent of those affected are women.

Sleep apnoea

A cessation of breathing for more than 10 seconds caused by recurrent collapse of the upper airway leading to disturbed sleep. This may occur as a result of loss of muscle tone in the pharynx as the patient relaxes during sleep (obstructive sleep apnoea) and is usually associated with obesity or enlarged tonsils or adenoids. It may also be caused by abnormal central nervous system control of breathing (central sleep apnoea) or occur as a result of a restrictive disorder of the chest wall, e.g. scoliosis or ankylosing spondylitis, where normal use of accessory respiratory muscles is inhibited during sleep. Pulmonary hypertension, respiratory and/or heart failure may develop in severe cases.

Spina bifida

A developmental defect that occurs in early pregnancy in which there is incomplete closure of the neural tube. The posterior part of the affected vertebrae does not fuse, leaving a gap or split. There are three main types:

Spina bifida occulta

A mild form in which there is no damage to the meninges or spinal cord. The defect is covered with skin that may be dimpled, pigmented or hairy. In the vast majority of cases it presents with no symptoms. However, in some cases the spinal cord may become tethered against the vertebrae, with possible impairment of mobility or bladder control.

Spina bifida cystica

When a blister-like sac or cyst balloons out through the opening in the vertebrae.

There are two forms:

Meningocele: the spinal cord and nerves remain in the spinal canal but the meninges and cerebrospinal fluid balloon out through the opening in the vertebrae, forming a sac. This is the least common form of spina bifida.

Myelomeningocele: the spinal cord and nerves are pushed out through the opening, along with the meninges and cerebrospinal fluid. The spinal cord at this level is damaged, leading to paralysis and loss of sensation below the affected segment. This is the most serious and more common form and is often associated with hydrocephalus.

Spinal muscular atrophies (SMA)

A group of inherited degenerative disorders of the anterior horn cell causing muscle atrophy. There are three main types, which are classified by age of onset: *SMA I (Werdnig–Hoffman disease)* is the most severe form with onset from preterm to 6 months. It causes weakness and hypotonia ('floppy' babies) leading to death within 3 years. *SMA II (intermediate type)* usually develops between 6 and 15 months of age. It has the same pathological features as SMA I but progresses more slowly. *SMA III (Wohlfart–Kugelberg–Welander disease)* has a late onset, between 1 year and adolescence, leading to progressive, proximal limb weakness.

Spinal stenosis

Narrowing of the spinal canal, nerve root canals or intervertebral foramina. May be caused by a number of factors, including loss of disc height, osteophytes, facet hypertrophy, disc prolapse and hypertrophic ligamentum flavum.

Compression of the nerve root may lead to radiating leg or arm pain, numbness and paraesthesia in the affected dermatome, muscle weakness, neurogenic claudication and low back pain. In severe cases the spinal cord may be compromised.

Spondylolisthesis

A spontaneous forward displacement of one vertebral body upon the segment below it (usually L5/S1). Displacement may be severe, causing compression of the cauda equina, requiring urgent surgical intervention. Spondylolisthesis is classified according to its cause:

I Dysplastic – congenital
II Isthmic – fatigue fracture of the pars interarticularis due to overuse

III Degenerative – osteoarthritis
IV Traumatic – acute fracture
V Pathological – weakening of the pars interarticularis by a tumour, osteoporosis, tuberculosis or Paget's disease

In rare cases the displacement may be backwards, known as a retrolisthesis.

Spondylolysis

A defect in the pars interarticularis of the lumbar vertebrae (usually L5), often the result of a fatigue fracture. It can be unilateral or bilateral and may or may not progress to spondylolisthesis.

Spondylosis

Degeneration and narrowing of the intervertebral discs leading to the formation of osteophytes at the joint margin and arthritic changes of the facet joints. The lowest three cervical joints are most commonly affected, causing neck pain and stiffness, sometimes with radiation to the upper limbs, although the condition may remain symptomless. In some cases osteophytes may encroach sufficiently upon an intervertebral foramen to cause nerve root pressure signs, or, more rarely, the spinal canal to cause dysfunction in all four limbs and possibly the bladder. The vertebral artery can also be involved.

Stroke/cerebrovascular accident (CVA)

An illness in which part of the brain is suddenly severely damaged or destroyed as a consequence of an interruption to the flow of blood in the brain. This interruption may be caused by a blood clot (ischaemic stroke) or by a ruptured blood vessel (haemorrhagic stroke), either within the brain (intracerebral) or around the brain (subarachnoid). The most common symptoms of stroke are numbness, weakness or paralysis on one side of the body, contralateral to the side of the brain in which the cerebrovascular accident occurred. Other symptoms include dysphasia, dysphagia, dysarthria, dyspraxia, disturbance of vision and perception, inattention or unilateral neglect, and memory or attention problems. Where symptoms resolve within 24 hours, this is known as a transient ischaemic attack (TIA).

Swan neck deformity

A hyperextension deformity of the proximal interphalangeal joint combined with a flexion deformity of the distal interphalangeal joints and, sometimes, a flexion deformity of the metacarpophalangeal joints due to failure of the proximal interphalangeal joint's volar/palmar plate. Usually seen in rheumatoid arthritis.

Systemic lupus erythematosus (SLE)

A chronic, inflammatory autoimmune connective tissue disorder involving the skin, joints and internal organs. Clinical features and severity can vary widely depending on the area affected but may include butterfly rash on face, polyarthritis, vasculitis, Raynaud's phenomenon, anaemia, hypertension, neurological disorders, renal disease, pleurisy and alopecia. Of those affected by the disease, around 90% are women.

Systemic sclerosis (scleroderma)

An autoimmune connective tissue disorder that causes an increase in collagen metabolism. Excessive collagen deposits cause damage to microscopic blood vessels in the skin (scleroderma) and other organs (systemic sclerosis), leading to fibrosis and degeneration. Any organ can be affected and its effects can be localized or diffuse, as well as progressive. Middle-aged women are most commonly affected. Clinical features include oedema of hands and feet, contractures and finger deformities, alteration of facial features and dry, shiny, tight skin.

Talipes calcaneovalgus

A common deformity of the foot and ankle, usually postural, where the foot is dorsiflexed and everted, and is resistant to plantarflexion. Common in breech births and often associated with developmental dysplasia of the hip.

Talipes equinovarus

A common deformity of the foot and ankle, often congenital, where the foot is plantarflexed, adducted and supinated. This deformity can either be fixed (structural talipes) or passively corrected (positional talipes). Males are more commonly affected. Also known as club foot.

Tarsal tunnel syndrome

Compression of the posterior tibial nerve or its branches as it passes through the tarsal tunnel (behind the medial malleolus). Symptoms include pain, dysaesthesia and weakness in the medial and plantar aspects of the foot and ankle. Can be confused with plantar fasciitis.

Tennis elbow (lateral epicondylitis)

Tendinopathy of the common origin of the forearm extensors causing pain and tenderness at the lateral aspect of the elbow and down the forearm.

Tenosynovitis

Inflammation of the synovial lining of a tendon sheath caused by mechanical irritation or infection, often associated with overuse and repetitive movements. A similar inflammatory process can affect the paratenon of those tendons without synovial sheaths (peritendinitis).

Tenovaginitis

Inflammatory thickening of the fibrous tendon sheath, sometimes leading to the formation of nodules, usually caused by repeated minor injury. Characterized by restricted movement of the tendon and pain. Common sites to be affected are the flexor sheaths in the fingers or thumb ('trigger' finger) and the sheaths of the extensor pollicis brevis and abductor pollicis longus tendons (de Quervain's syndrome).

Thoracic outlet syndrome

An umbrella term for a group of conditions that result from compression of the neurovascular bundle in the cervicoaxillary canal. Common sites of compression are the costoclavicular space (between the first rib and the clavicle) and the triangle between the anterior scalene, middle scalene and first rib. Causes include muscle shortening and spasm, poor posture, stretching of the lower trunk of the brachial plexus, traumatic structural changes, or, more rarely, congenital anatomical abnormalities such as an enlarged C7 transverse process, cervical rib or clavicular bony abnormality. Clinical features include paraesthesia, pain, subjective weakness, oedema, pallor, discoloration or venous engorgement involving the neck and affected shoulder and upper limb.

Torticollis

Refers to the position of the neck in a number of conditions (rotated and tilted to one side). From the Latin *torti* meaning twisted and *collis* meaning neck.

Congenital torticollis

Caused by injury, and possible contracture, of the sternocleidomastoid by birth trauma or malpositioning in the womb. Seen in babies and young children.

Acquired torticollis

Acute torticollis (wry neck) is caused by spasm of the neck muscles (usually trapezius and sternocleidomastoid) that often results from a poor sleeping position. Usually resolves within a few days. *Spasmodic torticollis* is a focal dystonia caused by disease of the central nervous system which leads to prolonged and involuntary muscle contraction.

Transverse myelitis

A demyelinating disorder of the spinal cord where inflammation spreads more or less completely across the tissue of the spinal cord, resulting in a loss of its normal function to transmit nerve impulses up and down. Paralysis and numbness affect the legs and trunk below the level of diseased tissue. Causes include spinal cord injury, immune reaction, atherosclerotic vascular disease and viral infection, e.g. smallpox, measles or chickenpox. Some patients progress to multiple sclerosis. Recovery varies.

Trigeminal neuralgia

A condition that is characterized by brief attacks of severe, sharp, stabbing facial pain in the territory of one or more divisions of the trigeminal nerve (cranial nerve V). It can be caused by degeneration of the nerve or compression on it (e.g. by a tumour), though often the cause is unknown. Attacks can last for several days or weeks after which the patient may be pain-free for months.

Trigger finger

See 'Tenovaginitis'.

Tuberculosis

A chronic infectious disease caused by *Mycobacterium tuberculosis* that is spread via the circulatory system or the lymph nodes. Any tissue can be infected but the lungs are the most common site as the route of infection is most often by inhalation, although it can also be by ingestion. Other sites of infection include lymph nodes, bones, gastrointestinal tract, kidneys, skin and meninges. The disease is characterized by the development of granulomas in the infected tissues. The initial lesion that develops on first exposure to the disease is referred to as the primary complex. The primary lesion can be asymptomatic and heal itself with no further complications. However, the disease can be reactivated, especially following infection, inadequate immunity and malnutrition, and is known as post-primary tuberculosis. Clinical features include cough, haemoptysis, weight loss, fatigue, fever and night sweats.

Wernicke's dysphasia

A lesion of Wernicke's area (posterolateral left temporal and inferior parietal language region of the left cortex) causing fluent but nonsensical speech. Writing and comprehension are greatly impaired. The patient is unaware of the language problem.

Diagnostic imaging

Plain radiography (X-rays)

An image formed by exposure to short wavelengths of electromagnetic radiation (X-rays) that pass through the body and hit a photographic receptor (radiographic plate or film) placed behind the patient's body. The X-rays pass through soft tissue such as muscle, skin and organs and turn the plate black while hard tissue such as bone blocks the X-rays leaving the film white. Useful for detecting fractures, dislocations and many bony abnormalities including degenerative joint disease, spondylolisthesis, infections, tumours, avascular necrosis and metabolic bone diseases. Two views in planes at right angles to each other, usually anteroposterior and lateral, are usually required in order to adequately examine a region.

Can be used in conjunction with the instillation of iodinated contrast material into various structures of the body. These block the X-rays and help visualize the structure:

Angiography (blood vessels): cerebral aneurysms, vascular malformations and occluded or stenosed arteries and veins
Arthrography (joints): internal derangements of joints
Discography (intervertebral disc space): disc pathology
Myelography (thecal sac): compressive lesions of the spinal cord and cauda equina.
Tenography (tendon sheath): tendon pathology and ligament ruptures

Computed tomography (CT)

Involves scanning part of the body from several angles by rotating a thin X-ray beam and detector around it. The data from the X-rays is then compared and reconstructed by computer to produce a cross-sectional image, which can be manipulated to emphasize bony or soft tissue structures. Provides good detail of bony structures, especially cortical bone, and is particularly useful for complex fractures and dislocations as well as for osteochondral lesions, stress fractures, loose bodies and certain spinal pathologies such as stenosis and disc herniation. It can also be used for diagnosing aneurysms, brain tumours and brain damage and detecting tumours and abscesses throughout the body. As with plain film radiography, it can also be used in conjunction with the administration of iodinated contrast material into various body structures to image the brain, neck, chest, abdomen and pelvis.

Magnetic resonance imaging (MRI)

A cross-sectional image is formed by placing the body in a powerful magnetic field and using radiofrequency pulses to excite hydrogen nuclei within tissue cells. The signals emitted by the nuclei are measured and reconstructed by computer to create an image of soft tissue and bone. Different pulse sequences are used to accentuate different characteristics of tissue. T1-weighted images show good anatomical detail with fluid being dark and fat being bright. T2-weighted images are better at identifying soft tissue pathology but anatomical detail is less clear. Fluid appears bright.

MRI provides superior soft tissue contrast in multiple imaging planes and is used to examine the central nervous, musculoskeletal and cardiovascular systems. MRI has no known adverse physiological effects. It is often used with gadolinium, an intravenous contrast agent, to improve diagnostic accuracy (T1-weighted). Patients with a cardiac pacemaker, brain aneurysm clip or other metallic implants with the exception of those attached to bone, i.e. prosthetic joints, cannot undergo MRI.

Radionuclide scanning

Involves the administration of a radioactive label (radioisotope) along with a biologically active substance that is readily taken up by the tissue being examined, e.g. iodine for the thyroid gland. The radioisotope emits a particular type of radiation that can be picked up by gamma ray cameras or detectors as it travels through the body. Highly active cells in the target organ will take up more of the radionuclide and emit more gamma rays resulting in 'hot spots'. Is used to identify areas of abnormal pathology. Bone scans detect areas of increased activity and can pick up metastatic disease, infection (osteomyelitis) and fractures. It can also be used to investigate kidney, liver and spleen function, coronary blood flow, thyroid activity and to detect pulmonary emboli in the lungs.

Dual-energy X-ray absorptiometry (DEXA) scanning

The most commonly used technique to measure bone mineral density. Two low-dose photon (X-ray) beams of different energies are transmitted through the bone being examined and are measured by a detector on the other side of the patient. The denser the bone, the fewer the X-rays that reach the detector. Used to diagnose and grade osteoporosis and assess the risk of a particular bone becoming fractured. The World Health Organization has defined bone mass according to the DEXA scan's T-scores, which are standard deviation (SD) measurements referenced to the young adult mean.

Normal: not more than 1 standard deviation below the average value

Osteopenia: more than 1 but less than 2.5 standard deviations below the average value

Osteoporosis: more than 2.5 standard deviations below the average value

Ultrasound

Involves high-frequency sound waves being directed into the body via a transducer, which are then reflected back from different tissue interfaces and converted into a real-time image. Can be used to examine a broad range of soft tissue structures (abdomen, peripheral musculoskeletal system, fetus in pregnancy, thyroid, eyes, neck, prostate and blood flow (Doppler)). However, it cannot penetrate bone or deep structures.

Electrodiagnostic tests

Electroencephalography (EEG)

A technique that records the electrical activity of the brain via electrodes attached to the scalp. Used in the diagnosis of epilepsy, coma and certain forms of encephalitis.

Evoked potentials (EP)

A technique that studies nerve conduction of specific sensory pathways within the brain by measuring the time taken for the brain to respond to a stimulus. The stimulus may either be visual (e.g. flashed light, which measures conduction in the occipital pathways), auditory (e.g. click, which measures conduction in the auditory pathways) or somatosensory (e.g. electrical stimulation of a peripheral nerve, which measures conduction in the parietal cortex). Used for detecting multiple sclerosis, brainstem and cerebellopontine angle lesions (e.g. acoustic neuroma), various cerebral metabolic disorders in infants and children as well as lesions in the sensory pathways (e.g. brachial plexus injury and spinal cord tumour).

Nerve conduction studies

Measures conduction along a sensory or motor peripheral nerve following stimulation of that nerve from two different sites. The conduction velocity is calculated by dividing the distance between the two sites by the difference in conduction times between the two sites. Useful in the diagnosis of nerve entrapments (e.g. carpal tunnel syndrome), peripheral neuropathies, motor and sensory nerve damage and multifocal motor neuropathy.

Electromyography (EMG)

Involves the insertion of a needle electrode into muscle to record spontaneous and induced electrical activity within that particular muscle. Used in the diagnosis of a broad range of myopathies and neuropathies.

SECTION 6

Pharmacology

Drug classes **286**

A–Z of drugs **289**

Prescription abbreviations **316**

Further reading **316**

Drug classes

ACE inhibitors

Angiotensin-converting enzyme (ACE) inhibitors allow blood vessels to dilate by preventing the formation of angiotensin II, a powerful artery constrictor. Used in the treatment of heart failure, hypertension, diabetic nephropathy and post-myocardial infarction.

Analgesics

Used to relieve pain and can be divided into opioids and non-opioids.

Opioids block transmission of pain signals within the brain and spinal cord. They include morphine and pethidine and are used to treat moderate to severe pain arising from surgery, serious injury and terminal illness.

Non-opioids are less powerful and work by blocking the production of prostaglandins, thereby preventing stimulation of nerve endings at the site of pain. They include paracetamol and non-steroidal anti-inflammatory drugs such as aspirin.

Antibiotics

Used to treat bacterial disorders ranging from minor infections to deadly diseases. Antibiotics work by destroying the bacteria or preventing them from multiplying while the body's immune system works to clear the invading organism. There are different classes of antibiotic, which include penicillins (amoxicillin, ampicillin, benzylpenicillin), cephalosporins (cefaclor, cefotaxime, cefuroxime), macrolides (erythromycin), tetracyclines (oxytetracycline, tetracycline), aminoglycosides (gentamicin) and glycopeptides (vancomycin).

Antiemetics

Act by blocking signals to the vomiting centre in the brain which triggers the vomiting reflex. Used to prevent or treat vomiting and nausea caused by motion sickness, vertigo, digestive tract infection and to counteract the side-effects of some drugs.

Antiepileptics

Used to prevent or terminate epileptic seizures. There are several types of epilepsy, each treated by a specific antiepileptic medication. It is therefore essential to classify the type of seizure in order to treat it effectively and minimize side-effects.

Antiretrovirals

Specific antiviral drugs for the treatment of infection caused by the human immunodeficiency virus (HIV). There are two groups:

Reverse transcriptase inhibitors reduce the activity of the reverse transcriptase enzyme, which is vital for virus replication. They are divided according to their chemical structure into nucleoside and non-nucleoside inhibitors.

Protease inhibitors interfere with the protease enzyme.

To reduce the development of drug resistance the drugs are used in combination. Treatment is usually initiated with a combination of two nucleoside reverse transcriptase inhibitors (NRTI) plus a non-nucleoside reverse transcriptase inhibitor (NNRTI) or a protease inhibitor (often referred to as 'triple therapy'). Antiretrovirals are not a cure for HIV but they increase life expectancy considerably. However, they are toxic and treatment regimens have to be carefully balanced.

β-blockers

Prevent stimulation of the β-adrenoreceptors in the heart muscle (mainly β_1-receptors) and peripheral vasculature, bronchi, pancreas and liver (mainly β_2-receptors). Used to treat hypertension, angina, myocardial infarction, arrhythmias and thyrotoxicosis. Can also be used to alleviate some symptoms of anxiety. Since blocking β-adrenoreceptors in the lungs can lead to constriction of air passages, care needs to be taken when treating patients with asthma or COPD.

Benzodiazepines

Increase the inhibitory effect of gamma-aminobutyric acid (GABA), which depresses brain cell activity in the higher centres of the brain controlling consciousness. Used for anxiety, insomnia, convulsions, sedation for medical procedures and alcohol withdrawal.

Bronchodilators

Dilate the airways to assist breathing when constricted or congested with mucus. There are two main types:

Sympathomimetics (e.g. salbutamol) stimulate β_2-adrenoreceptors on the surface of bronchial smooth muscle cells causing the muscle to relax.

Anticholinergics (e.g. ipratropium bromide) act by blocking the neurotransmitters that trigger muscle contraction.

Both are used to treat asthma and other conditions associated with reversible airways obstruction such as COPD.

Calcium channel blockers

Interfere with the transport of calcium ions through the cell walls of cardiac and vascular smooth muscle. Reduce the contractility of the heart, depress the formation and conduction of impulses in the heart and cause peripheral vasodilation. Used to treat angina, hypertension and arrhythmias.

Corticosteroids

Reduce inflammation by inhibiting the formation of inflammatory mediators, e.g. prostaglandins. Used to control many inflammatory disorders thought to be caused by excessive or inappropriate activity of the immune system, e.g. asthma, rheumatoid arthritis, lupus, eczema, as well as inflammation caused by strain and damage to muscles and tendons. Also known as glucocorticoids.

Diuretics

Work on the kidneys to increase the amount of sodium and water excreted. There are different types of diuretic that work on the nephron:

Thiazides (bendroflumethiazide/bendrofluazide)
Loop (furosemide/frusemide, bumetanide)
Potassium-sparing (amiloride, spironolactone)
Osmotic (mannitol)
Carbonic anhydrase inhibitors (acetazolamide, dorzolamide)

Used to treat hypertension (thiazides), chronic heart failure and oedema (loop diuretics, thiazides or a combination of both), glaucoma (carbonic anhydrase inhibitors or osmotic), raised intracranial pressure (osmotic).

Inotropes

Work by increasing the contractility of the heart muscle. They can be divided into three groups:

Cardiac glycosides (e.g. digoxin) assist activity of heart muscle by increasing intracellular calcium storage in myocardial cells. Used for heart failure and supraventricular arrhythmias.

Sympathomimetics (e.g. dobutamine, dopamine) stimulate β_1-receptors on the heart which increase the rate and force of myocardial contraction. Provide inotropic support in infarction, cardiac surgery, cardiomyopathies, septic shock and cardiogenic shock.

Phosphodiesterase inhibitors (e.g. milrinone) inactivate cyclic AMP, which increases the force of myocardial contraction and relaxes vascular smooth muscle. Used to treat congestive heart failure.

Mucolytics

Reduce the viscosity of bronchopulmonary secretions by breaking down their molecular complexes. Used to treat excessive or thickened mucus secretions.

Non-steroidal anti-inflammatory drugs (NSAIDs)

Inhibit the production of prostaglandins, which are responsible for inflammation and pain following tissue damage. They are called non-steroidals to distinguish them from corticosteroids, which have a similar function. Used for inflammatory diseases, pain and pyrexia.

A–Z of drugs

Acetylcysteine (mucolytic)

Reduces the viscosity of secretions associated with impaired or abnormal mucus production. Administered with a

bronchodilator as it can cause bronchospasm and inhibit ciliary function. Also used as an antidote for paracetamol overdose.
Side-effects: bronchoconstriction, nausea and vomiting.

Aciclovir (antiviral)

Used against infections caused by herpes virus (herpes simplex and varicella zoster).
Side-effects are rare.

Adenosine (anti-arrhythmic)

Reverses supraventricular tachycardias to sinus rhythm.
Side-effects: chest pain, dyspnoea, nausea, bronchospasm, facial flush.

Adrenaline/epinephrine (sympathomimetic agent)

Used during cardiopulmonary resuscitation to stimulate heart activity and raise low blood pressure. Adrenaline (epinephrine) acts as a vasoconstrictor and is used to reduce bleeding and prolong the effects of local anaesthetic. It is also used to treat anaphylactic shock as it raises blood pressure and causes bronchodilation. Since it lowers pressure in the eye by decreasing production of aqueous humour it is used for glaucoma and eye surgery.
Side-effects: dry mouth, anxiety, restlessness, palpitations, tremor, headache, blurred vision, hypertension, tachycardias.

Alendronate (bisphosphonate)

Inhibits the release of calcium from bone by interfering with the activity of osteoclasts, thereby reducing the rate of bone turnover. Used in the prophylaxis and treatment of postmenopausal osteoporosis and corticosteroid-induced osteoporosis. Often used in conjunction with calcium tablets. Also used in the treatment of Paget's disease, hypercalcaemia of malignancy and in bone metastases in breast cancer.
Side-effects: oesophageal irritation and ulceration, gastrointestinal upset, increased bone pain in Paget's disease.

Alfentanil (opioid analgesic)

Fast-acting, it is used as a respiratory depressant in patients needing prolonged assisted ventilation. Also used as an analgesic during surgery and to enhance anaesthesia.

Side-effects: drowsiness, nausea, vomiting, constipation, dizziness, dry mouth.

Allopurinol (anti-gout)

A prophylactic for gout and uric acid kidney stones.
Side-effects: rash, itching, nausea.

Aminophylline (xanthine)

Acts as a bronchodilator and is used for reversible airways obstruction and intravenously for acute severe asthma.
Side-effects: tachycardias, palpitations, nausea, headache, insomnia, arrhythmias, convulsions.

Amiodarone (anti-arrhythmic)

Slows nerve impulses in the heart muscle. Used to treat ventricular and supraventricular tachycardias and prevent recurrent atrial and ventricular fibrillation.
Side-effects: photosensitivity, reversible corneal depositions, liver damage and thyroid disorders.

Amitriptyline (tricyclic antidepressant)

Used as a long-term treatment for depression, particularly when accompanied by anxiety or insomnia, owing to its sedative properties. In low doses it is also useful for the treatment of neuropathic pain. It is also sometimes used to treat nocturnal enuresis (bedwetting) in children.
Side-effects: drowsiness, sweating, dry mouth, blurred vision, dizziness, fainting, palpitations, gastrointestinal upset.

Amlodipine (calcium channel blocker)

Used to treat hypertension and angina. Can be used safely by asthmatics and non-insulin-dependent diabetics.
Side-effects: oedema, headache, dizziness, fatigue, sleep disturbances, palpitations, flushing, gastrointestinal upset.

Amoxicillin (penicillin antibiotic)

See antibiotics in 'Drug classes'.

Ampicillin (penicillin antibiotic)

See antibiotics in 'Drug classes'.

Aspirin (NSAID)

Used as an anti-inflammatory, as an analgesic and to reduce fever. It also inhibits thrombus formation and is used to reduce the risk of heart attacks and stroke.
Side-effects: gastric irritation leading to dyspepsia and bleeding, and wheezing in aspirin-sensitive asthmatics.

Atenolol (β-blocker)

Used to treat hypertension, angina and arrhythmias.
Side-effects: muscle ache, fatigue, dry eyes, bradycardia and atrioventricular (AV) block, hypotension, cold peripheries.

Atorvastatin (statin)

Lowers low-density lipoprotein (LDL) cholesterol and is prescribed for those who have not responded to diet and lifestyle modification to protect them from cardiovascular disease.
Side-effects: mild: gastrointestinal upset, headache, fatigue, rarely myositis.

Atracurium (non-depolarizing muscle relaxant)

Used as a muscle relaxant during surgery and to facilitate intermittent positive pressure breathing in intensive care unit.
Side-effects: skin rash, flushing, hypotension.

Atropine (antimuscarinic)

Relaxes smooth muscle by blocking the action of acetylcholine and is used to treat irritable bowel syndrome. Can be used to paralyse ciliary action and enlarge the pupils during eye examinations. Also used to reverse excessive bradycardia, in cardiopulmonary resuscitation and for patients who have been poisoned with organophosphorous anticholinesterase drugs.
Side-effects: blurred vision, dry mouth, thirst, constipation, flushing, dry skin.

Azathioprine (immunosuppressant)

Prevents rejection of transplanted organs by the immune system and in a number of autoimmune and collagen diseases (including rheumatoid arthritis, polymyositis, systemic lupus erythematosus).
Side-effects: nausea, vomiting, hair loss, loss of appetite, bone marrow suppression.

Baclofen (skeletal muscle relaxant)

Acts on the central nervous system to reduce chronic severe spasticity resulting from a number of disorders, including multiple sclerosis, spinal cord injury, brain injury, cerebral palsy or stroke.

Side-effects: drowsiness, nausea, urinary disturbances.

Beclometasone (corticosteroid)

Given by inhaler and used to control asthma in those who do not respond to bronchodilators alone. Also used in creams to treat inflammatory skin disorders and to relieve and prevent symptoms of vasomotor and allergic rhinitis.

Side-effects: cough, nasal discomfort/irritation, hoarse voice, sore throat, nosebleed (with inhalers/nasal spray).

Bendroflumethiazide/bendrofluazide (thiazide diuretic)

Used to treat hypertension, cardiac failure and resistant oedema. Also reduces urinary calcium excretion and so decreases rate of recurrence in patients with recurrent renal stones.

Side-effects: hypokalaemia, dehydration, postural hypotension, gout and hyperglycaemia.

Benzylpenicillin (penicillin antibiotic)

See antibiotics in 'Drug classes'.

Budesonide (corticosteroid)

Used as an inhaler in the prophylactic treatment of asthma and COPD. Also given systemically in a controlled-release form for Crohn's disease.

Side-effects: nasal irritation, cough, sore throat.

Calcitonin (salmon)/salcatonin (hormone)

Regulates bone turnover and is used to treat hypercalcaemia in Paget's disease of bone and metastatic cancer. Also given for prophylaxis and treatment of osteoporosis and for short-term pain relief following vertebral fracture or in metastatic disease.

Side-effects: gastrointestinal upset, flushing.

Captopril (ACE inhibitor)

Reduces peripheral vasoconstriction and is used to treat hypertension, congestive heart failure, post-myocardial infarction and diabetic nephropathy.

Side-effects: postural hypotension, persistent dry cough, rash, loss of taste, reduced kidney function.

Carbamazepine (anticonvulsant)

Used to reduce likelihood of generalized tonic-clonic seizures and partial seizures. Also used to relieve severe pain in trigeminal neuralgia and for prophylaxis of bipolar disorder.
Side-effects: drowsiness, ataxia, blurred vision, confusion, nausea, loss of appetite.

Cefaclor (cephalosporin antibiotic)

See antibiotics in 'Drug classes'.

Cefotaxime (cephalosporin antibiotic)

See antibiotics in 'Drug classes'.

Cefuroxime (cephalosporin antibiotic)

See antibiotics in 'Drug classes'.

Celecoxib (NSAID)

Used to relieve the symptoms of osteoarthritis and rheumatoid arthritis. Has a relatively selective action on the inflammatory response compared to other NSAIDs, causing fewer gastrointestinal disturbances. However, it also associated with a greater risk of adverse cardiovascular effects.
Side-effects: dizziness, fluid retention, hypertension, headache, itching, insomnia.

Chlorpromazine (antipsychotic)

Has a sedative effect and is used to control the symptoms of schizophrenia and to treat agitation without causing confusion and stupor. Also used to treat nausea and vomiting in terminally ill patients.
Side-effects: extrapyramidal symptoms (e.g. parkinsonian symptoms, dystonia, akathisia, tardive dyskinesia), hypotension, dry mouth, blurred vision, urinary retention, constipation, jaundice.

Ciclosporin (immunosuppressant)

Used to prevent rejection of organ and tissue transplantation. Also used to treat rheumatoid arthritis, and severe resistant psoriasis and dermatitis when other treatments have failed.

Side-effects: nephrotoxicity, hypertension, increased body hair, nausea, tremor, swelling of gums.

Cimetidine (anti-ulcer – H_2-receptor antagonist)

Decreases gastric acid production and is used to treat gastric and duodenal ulcers, and for gastro-oesophageal reflux disease.
Side-effects: none.

Ciprofloxacin (antibacterial)

Treats mainly Gram-negative infection and some Gram-positive infections. Used for chest, intestine and urinary tract infections and to treat gonorrhoea.
Side-effects: nausea, vomiting, abdominal pain, diarrhoea.

Clomipramine (tricyclic antidepressant)

Used for long-term treatment of depression, especially when associated with phobic and obsessional states.
Side-effects: drowsiness, sweating, dry mouth, blurred vision, dizziness, fainting, palpitations, gastrointestinal upset.

Clonidine (α_2-adrenoceptor agonist)

Acts centrally to reduce sympathetic activity and thereby reduces peripheral vascular reactivity. Used in the prophylaxis of migraine and in the treatment of menopausal flushing. Sometimes used to treat hypertension.
Side-effects: gastrointestinal upset, dry mouth, headache, dizziness, rash, sedation, nocturnal unrest, depression, bradycardia, fluid retention.

Codeine phosphate (opioid analgesic)

A mild opioid analgesic that is similar to, but weaker than, morphine. Used to treat mild to moderate pain and is often combined with a non-opioid analgesic such as paracetamol (to form co-codamol). Also used as a cough suppressant and for the short-term control of diarrhoea.
Side-effects: constipation.

Dexamethasone (corticosteroid)

Suppresses inflammatory and allergic disorders. Used to diagnose Cushing's disease. Used to treat cerebral oedema, congenital adrenal hyperplasia, nausea and vomiting associated with chemotherapy and various types of shock.

Side-effects: indigestion, acne, increased body hair, moon-face, hypertension, weight gain/oedema, impaired glucose tolerance, cataract, glaucoma, osteoporosis, peptic ulcer, candida.

Diazepam (benzodiazepine)

Has a wide range of uses. Most commonly used to reduce anxiety, relax muscles, promote sleep and in the treatment of alcohol withdrawal. Also used for febrile convulsions and status epilepticus.
Side-effects: daytime drowsiness, dizziness, unsteadiness, confusion in the elderly. Dependence develops with prolonged use.

Didanosine (ddI) (antiretroviral – NRTI)

Prevents the replication of HIV and therefore the progression of AIDS by blocking the action of the reverse transcriptase enzyme. Usually used in combination with other antiretroviral drugs.
Side-effects: pancreatitis, peripheral neuropathy, headache, insomnia, gastrointestinal upset, fatigue, breathlessness, cough, blood disorders, rash, liver damage.

Diclofenac (NSAID)

Used to relieve mild to moderate pain associated with inflammation such as rheumatoid arthritis, osteoarthritis and musculoskeletal disorders. Also used to treat acute gout and postoperative pain.
Side-effects: gastrointestinal disorders.

Digoxin (cardiac glycoside)

Used in heart failure to control breathlessness, tiredness and fluid retention. Also used to treat supraventricular arrhythmias, particularly atrial fibrillation.
Side-effects: anorexia, nausea, vomiting, diarrhoea, visual disturbances, headache, tiredness, palpitations.

Dihydrocodeine/DF118 (opioid analgesic)

Similar to, but weaker than, morphine and more potent than codeine. Used to relieve moderate acute and chronic pain and is often combined with a non-opioid analgesic such as paracetamol (to form co-dydramol).

Side-effects: drowsiness, nausea, vomiting, constipation, dizziness, dry mouth.

Diltiazem (calcium channel blocker)

Used to prevent and treat angina and to lower high blood pressure.
Side-effects: bradycardia, headache, nausea, dizziness, dry mouth, hypotension, ankle and leg swelling.

Dobutamine (inotropic sympathomimetic)

Provides inotropic support in acute severe heart failure, cardiac surgery, cardiomyopathies, septic shock and cardiogenic shock.
Common side-effect: tachycardias.

Donepezil (anticholinesterase)

Inhibits the breakdown of acetylcholine. Used to improve cognitive function in mild to moderate dementia due to Alzheimer's disease, although the underlying disease process is not altered.
Side-effects: gastrointestinal upset, fatigue, insomnia, muscle cramps.

Dopamine (inotropic sympathomimetic)

Used to treat cardiogenic shock after myocardial infarction, hypotension after cardiac surgery, acute severe heart failure and to start diuresis in chronic heart failure.
Side-effects: nausea, vomiting, peripheral vasoconstriction, hypotension, hypertension, tachycardia.

Dornase alfa (mucolytic)

A synthetic version of a naturally occurring human enzyme that breaks down the DNA content of sputum. Used by inhalation in cystic fibrosis to facilitate expectoration.
Side-effects: pharyngitis, laryngitis, chest pain.

Dosulepin/Dothiepin (tricyclic antidepressant)

Used for long-term treatment of depression, especially when associated with agitation, anxiety and insomnia.
Side-effects: drowsiness, sweating, dry mouth, blurred vision, dizziness, fainting, palpitations, gastrointestinal upset.

Doxapram (respiratory stimulant)

Used in hospital to treat acute exacerbations of COPD with type II respiratory failure when ventilation is unavailable or contraindicated.
Side-effects: tachycardia, hypertension, cerebral oedema, hyperthyroidism, dizziness, sweating, confusion, seizures, nausea, vomiting, perineal warmth.

Efavirenz (antiretroviral – NNRTI)

Used to treat HIV infection, specifically HIV type 1 (HIV-1) in combination with other antiretroviral drugs. Not effective for HIV-2.
Side-effects: gastrointestinal upset, rash, itching, anxiety, depression, sleep disturbances, dizziness, headache, impaired concentration.

Enalapril (ACE inhibitor)

Used in the treatment of hypertension, chronic heart failure and in the prevention of recurrent myocardial infarction following a heart attack.
Side-effects: postural hypotension, persistent dry cough, rash, loss of taste, reduced kidney function, dizziness, headache.

Epinephrine/adrenaline (sympathomimetic agent)

See 'Adrenaline'.

Erythromycin (macrolide antibiotic)

See antibiotics in 'Drug classes'.

Estradiol (oestrogen for hormone replacement therapy)

A naturally occurring female sex hormone used to treat menopausal and postmenopausal symptoms such as hot flushes, night sweats and vaginal atrophy. Can also be used for the prevention of osteoporosis in high-risk women with early menopause.
Side-effects: withdrawal bleeding, sodium and fluid retention, gastrointestinal upset, weight changes, breast enlargement, venous thromboembolism.

Etidronate (bisphosphonate)

Inhibits the release of calcium from bone by interfering with the activity of osteoclasts, thereby reducing the rate of bone

turnover. Used in the prophylaxis and treatment of postmenopausal osteoporosis and corticosteroid-induced osteoporosis. Often used in conjunction with calcium tablets. Also used in the treatment of Paget's disease, hypercalcaemia of malignancy and in bone metastases in breast cancer.
Side-effects: oesophageal irritation and ulceration, gastrointestinal upset, increased bone pain in Paget's disease.

Fentanyl (opioid analgesic)

Used to depress respiration in patients needing prolonged assisted ventilation. Also used as an analgesic during surgery and to enhance anaesthesia.
Side-effects: drowsiness, nausea, vomiting, constipation, dizziness, dry mouth.

Ferrous sulphate (iron salt)

Used to treat iron-deficiency anaemia.
Side-effects: nausea, epigastric pain, constipation or diarrhoea, darkening of faeces.

Flucloxacillin (penicillin antibiotic)

See antibiotics in 'Drug classes'.

Fluoxetine (selective serotonin re-uptake inhibitor)

More commonly known by its brand name, Prozac, it increases serotonin levels and is used to treat depressive illness, obsessive–compulsive disorder and bulimia nervosa.
Side-effects: headache, nervousness, insomnia, anxiety, nausea, diarrhoea, weight loss, sexual dysfunction.

Furosemide/frusemide (loop diuretic)

A powerful, fast-acting diuretic that is used in emergencies to reduce acute pulmonary oedema secondary to left ventricular failure. It also reduces oedema and dyspnoea associated with chronic heart failure and is used to treat oliguria secondary to acute renal failure.
Side-effects: postural hypotension, hypokalaemia, hyponatraemia, hyperuricaemia, gout, dizziness, nausea.

Gabapentin (anticonvulsant)

Used as an adjunct in the management of partial and general epileptic seizures, as well as for the treatment of neuropathic pain. Can also be used in trigeminal neuralgia.

Side-effects: drowsiness, dizziness, ataxia, nystagmus, tremor, diplopia, gastrointestinal upset, peripheral oedema, amnesia, paraesthesia.

Gentamicin (aminoglycoside antibiotic)

See antibiotics in 'Drug classes'.

Gliclazide (sulphonylurea)

Oral antidiabetic drug that lowers blood sugar and is used to treat type II diabetes mellitus.
Side-effects: hypoglycaemia, weight gain.

GTN/glyceryl trinitrate (organic nitrate)

A potent coronary and peripheral vasodilator that relieves angina and is used to treat heart failure.
Side-effects: headaches, dizziness, flushing, postural hypotension, tachycardias.

Haloperidol (antipsychotic)

Used to control violent and dangerously impulsive behaviour associated with psychotic disorders such as schizophrenia, mania and dementia. Also used to treat motor tics.
Side-effects: parkinsonism, acute dystonia, akathisia, drowsiness, postural hypotension.

Heparin (anticoagulant)

Prevents blood clots forming and is used to prevent and treat deep vein thrombosis and pulmonary embolism. Also used in the management of unstable angina, myocardial infarction and acute occlusion of peripheral arteries.
Side-effects: haemorrhage, thrombocytopenia.

Hydrocortisone (corticosteroid)

Given as replacement therapy for adrenocortical insufficiency. Suppresses a variety of inflammatory and allergic disorders, e.g. psoriasis, eczema, rheumatic disease, inflammatory bowel disease. Also used as an immunosuppressant following organ transplant and for treating shock.
Side-effects: indigestion, acne, increased body hair, moonface, hypertension, weight gain/oedema, impaired glucose tolerance, cataract, glaucoma, osteoporosis, peptic ulcer, candida.

Hyoscine (muscarinic antagonist)

Used to manage motion sickness, giddiness and nausea caused by disturbances of the inner ear and reduce intestinal spasm in irritable bowel syndrome. Used as a pre-medication to dry bronchial secretions before surgery.
Side-effects: sedation, dry mouth, blurred vision.

Ibuprofen (NSAID)

Used to reduce pain, stiffness and inflammation associated with conditions such as rheumatoid arthritis, osteoarthritis, sprains and other soft tissue injuries. Also used to treat post-operative pain, headache, migraine, menstrual and dental pain, and fever and pain in children.
Side-effects: heartburn, indigestion.

Imipramine (tricyclic antidepressant)

Less sedating than some other antidepressants, it is used for long-term treatment of depression and also for nocturnal enuresis (bedwetting) in children.
Side-effects: drowsiness, sweating, dry mouth, blurred vision, dizziness, fainting, palpitations, gastrointestinal upset.

Indinavir (antiretroviral – protease inhibitor)

Used to treat HIV infection in combination with other antiretroviral drugs.
Side-effects: gastrointestinal upset, anorexia, hepatic dysfunction, pancreatitis, blood disorders, sleep disturbances, fatigue, headache, dizziness, paraesthesia, myalgia, myositis, taste disturbance, rash, itching, anaphylaxis.

Insulin (peptide hormone)

Lowers blood sugar and is given by injection to control type I and sometimes type II diabetes mellitus.
Side-effects: injection site irritation, weakness, sweating, hypoglycaemia, weight gain.

Interferon (antiviral and anticancer)

Group of proteins produced by the body in response to viral infection that stimulate the immune response:

Interferon alfa – used for certain lymphomas and tumours (e.g. leukaemia) and chronic active hepatitis B and C.

Side-effects: anorexia, nausea, influenza-like symptoms, lethargy.

Interferon beta – used for relapses of multiple sclerosis.

Side-effects: irritation at injection site, influenza-like symptoms.

Interferon gamma – used in conjunction with antibiotics to treat chronic granulomatous disease.

Side-effects: fever, headache, chills, myalgia, fatigue, nausea, vomiting, arthralgia, rashes and injection-site reactions.

Ipratropium (antimuscarinic)

Bronchodilator that is used to treat reversible airways obstruction, particularly in chronic obstructive pulmonary disease.
Side-effects: dry mouth and throat.

Isoprenaline (inotropic sympathomimetic)

Increases heart rate and cardiac contractility. Used to treat heart block and severe bradycardia.
Side-effects: tachycardia, arrhythmias, hypotension, sweating, tremor, headache.

Isosorbide mononitrate (organic nitrate)

A coronary and peripheral vasodilator. Used as prophylaxis in angina and as an adjunct in congestive heart failure.
Side-effects: headaches, dizziness, flushing, postural hypotension, tachycardias.

Ketamine (intravenous anaesthetic)

Used to induce and maintain anaesthesia during surgery.
Side-effects: hallucinations and other transient psychotic sequelae, increased blood pressure, tachycardia, increased muscle tone, apnoea, hypotension.

Lactulose (osmotic laxative)

Used to relieve constipation. Also used to treat hepatic encephalopathy.
Side-effects: flatulence, belching, stomach cramps, diarrhoea.

Lansoprazole (proton-pump inhibitor)

Reduces the amount of acid produced by the stomach and is used to treat stomach and duodenal ulcers as well as gastro-oesophageal reflux and oesophagitis.

Side-effects: headache, gastrointestinal upset, dizziness.

Levodopa/L-dopa (dopamine precursor)

Used to treat idiopathic Parkinson's disease by replacing the depleted dopamine in the brain. It is combined with an inhibitor such as carbidopa (to form co-caraldopa) or benserazide (to form co-beneldopa) which prolongs and enhances its action. It becomes less effective with continued use.
Side-effects: nausea, vomiting, abdominal pain, anorexia, postural hypotension, dysrhythmias, dizziness, discoloration of urine and other bodily fluids, abnormal involuntary movements, nervousness, agitation.

Levothyroxine (thyroid hormone)

Used in the treatment of hypothyroidism.
Side-effects: usually at excessive dosage. Include cardiac arrhythmias, tachycardia, anxiety, weight loss, muscular weakness and cramps, sweating, diarrhoea.

Lidocaine/lignocaine (local anaesthetic, class I anti-arrhythmic agent)

Used as a local anaesthetic and for ventricular dysrhythmias, especially following myocardial infarction.
Side-effects: nausea, vomiting, drowsiness, dizziness.

Lisinopril (ACE inhibitor)

Vasodilator that is used to treat hypertension, congestive heart failure and following myocardial infarction.
Side-effects: nausea, vomiting, dry cough, altered sense of taste, hypotension.

Lithium (antimanic)

Used to prevent and treat mania, bipolar disorders and recurrent depression. Its effects (including toxicity) are increased if it is combined with a thiazide diuretic.
Side-effects: weight gain, nausea, vomiting, diarrhoea, fine tremor.

Loperamide (antimotility)

Inhibits peristalsis and prevents the loss of water and electrolytes. Used to treat diarrhoea.
Side-effects: none.

Losartan (angiotensin-II receptor antagonist)

Shares similar properties to ACE inhibitors and is used to treat hypertension, heart failure and diabetic neuropathy. Does not cause a persistent dry cough, which commonly complicates ACE inhibitor therapy.
Side-effects: dizziness.

Mannitol (osmotic diuretic)

Reduces cerebral oedema and therefore intracranial pressure. Used preoperatively to reduce intraocular pressure in glaucoma.
Side-effects: chills, fever, fluid/electrolyte imbalance.

Meloxicam (NSAID)

Used to relieve the symptoms of rheumatoid arthritis, ankylosing spondylitis and acute episodes of osteoarthritis. Has a relatively selective action on the inflammatory response compared to other NSAIDs, causing less gastrointestinal disturbances. However, it is also associated with a greater risk of cardiovascular adverse effects.
Side-effects: gastrointestinal upset, headache, dizziness, vertigo, rash.

Metformin (biguanide)

Used to treat type II diabetes mellitus by decreasing glucose production, increasing peripheral glucose utilization and reducing glucose absorption in the digestive tract.
Side-effects: anorexia, nausea, vomiting, diarrhoea.

Methotrexate (cytotoxic and immunosuppressive)

Inhibits DNA, RNA and protein synthesis leading to cell death. Used to treat leukaemia, lymphoma and a number of solid tumours. Also used for rheumatoid arthritis and psoriatic arthritis.
Side-effects: bone marrow suppression, anorexia, diarrhoea, nausea, vomiting, hepatotoxicity, dry cough, mouth and gum ulcers and inflammation.

Methyldopa (antihypertensive)

Used to treat high blood pressure, especially in pregnancy.
Side-effects: drowsiness, headache, postural hypotension, depression, impotence.

Metoclopramide (dopamine antagonist)

Used to treat nausea and vomiting caused by radiotherapy, anti-cancer drug and opioid treatment, migraines, and following surgery. Also used to reduce symptoms of gastro-oesophageal reflux.

Side-effects: acute dystonic reactions, especially in children and young adults.

Midazolam (benzodiazepine)

Water-soluble and short-acting, it is given by injection or infusion to relieve anxiety and to provide sedation with amnesia. Used during small procedures under local anaesthetic and in ITU units for those on ventilatory support.

Side-effects: apnoea, hypotension, drowsiness, light-headedness, confusion, ataxia, amnesia, dependence, muscle weakness.

Milrinone (phosphodiesterase inhibitor)

A positive inotrope with vasodilating properties, it increases cardiac contractility and reduces vascular resistance. Used to treat severe congestive heart failure and myocardial dysfunction.

Side-effects: hypotension, cardiac arrhythmias, tachycardia, headache, insomnia, nausea, vomiting, diarrhoea.

Morphine (opioid analgesic)

Used to relieve severe pain and suppress cough in palliative care. Also effective in the relief of acute left ventricular failure.

Side-effects: drowsiness, nausea, vomiting, constipation, dizziness, dry mouth and respiratory depression.

Naloxone (antagonist for central and respiratory depression)

Used to reverse respiratory depression caused by opioid analgesics, mainly in overdose.

Side-effects: nausea, vomiting, tachycardia, fibrillation.

Naproxen (NSAID)

Used to relieve the symptoms of adult and juvenile rheumatoid arthritis, acute musculoskeletal disorders, acute gout and menstrual cramps.

Side-effects: gastrointestinal disturbances.

Nelfinavir (antiretroviral – protease inhibitor)

Used to treat HIV infection in combination with other antiretroviral drugs.
Side-effects: gastrointestinal upset, anorexia, hepatic dysfunction, pancreatitis, blood disorders, sleep disturbances, fatigue, headache, dizziness, paraesthesia, myalgia, myositis, taste disturbance, rash, itching, anaphylaxis.

Nevirapine (antiretroviral – NNRTI)

Used to treat HIV infection, specifically HIV type 1 (HIV-1) in combination with other antiretroviral drugs. Not effective for HIV-2.
Side-effects: gastrointestinal upset, rash, itching, anxiety, depression, sleep disturbances, dizziness, headache, impaired concentration, toxic epidermal necrolysis, hepatitis.

Nicorandil (potassium-channel activator)

Used for the prevention and treatment of angina. Acts on both the coronary arteries and veins to cause dilation, thus improving blood flow.
Side-effects: headache, flushing, nausea.

Nifedipine (calcium channel blocker)

Used to treat hypertension, angina and Raynaud's disease.
Side-effects: headache, flushing, ankle swelling, dizziness, fatigue, hypotension.

Nimodipine (calcium channel blocker)

Relaxes vascular smooth muscle, acting preferentially on the cerebral arteries. Used to treat cerebral vasospasm associated with subarachnoid haemorrhage.
Side-effects: hypotension, ECG abnormalities, headache, gastrointestinal disorders, nausea, sweating.

Nitrous oxide (inhalational agent)

Used for maintenance of anaesthesia and, in smaller doses, for analgesia without loss of consciousness, especially in labour.
Side-effects are rare.

Noradrenaline/norepinephrine (sympathomimetic agent)

Administered intravenously to constrict peripheral vessels to raise blood pressure in patients with acute hypotension.
Side-effects: hypertension, headache, bradycardia, arrhythmias, peripheral ischaemia.

Omeprazole (proton-pump inhibitor)

Reduces the amount of acid produced by the stomach and is used to treat stomach and duodenal ulcers as well as gastro-oesophageal reflux and oesophagitis.
Side-effects: headache, gastrointestinal upset, dizziness.

Ondansetron (serotonin antagonist)

Used to treat nausea and vomiting associated with anti-cancer drug therapy, radiotherapy and following surgery.
Side-effects: headache, constipation.

Orphenadrine (antimuscarinic)

Blocks the action of the neurotransmitter acetylcholine and is used to reduce rigidity and tremor in younger patients with parkinsonism. Not useful for bradykinesia.
Side-effects: dry mouth/skin, constipation, blurred vision, retention of urine.

Oxybutinin (antimuscarinic)

Reduces unstable contractions of the bladder, thereby increasing its capacity. Used to treat urinary frequency, urgency and incontinence, nocturnal enuresis and neurogenic bladder instability.
Side-effects: dry mouth and eyes, gastrointestinal upset, difficulty in micturition, skin reactions, blurred vision.

Oxytetracycline (tetracycline antibiotic)

See antibiotics in 'Drug classes'.

Pancuronium (muscle relaxant)

Long-acting, it is used as a muscle relaxant during surgical procedures and to facilitate tracheal intubation. Also used on patients receiving long-term mechanical ventilation.
Side-effects: tachycardia, hypertension, skin flushing, hypotension, bronchospasm.

Paracetamol (non-opioid analgesic)

Used to treat mild pain and reduce fever. Does not irritate the gastric mucosa and so can be used by those who have peptic ulcers or can be used in place of aspirin for those who are aspirin-intolerant.

Side-effects are rare but overdose is dangerous, causing liver failure.

Paroxetine (selective serotonin re-uptake inhibitor)

Increases serotonin levels and is used in depression, obsessive-compulsive disorder, panic disorder, social phobia, post-traumatic stress disorder and generalized anxiety disorder.

Side-effects: as for amitriptyline and, in addition, yawning. Extrapyramidal reactions (e.g. parkinsonian symptoms) and withdrawal syndrome appear to be more common than with other selective serotonin re-uptake inhibitors (SSRIs).

Pethidine (opioid analgesic)

Used to treat moderate to severe pain, especially during labour.

Side-effects: dizziness, nausea, vomiting, drowsiness, confusion, constipation.

Phenytoin (anticonvulsant)

Used to treat all forms of epilepsy (except absence seizures) as well as trigeminal neuralgia.

Side-effects: dizziness, headache, confusion, nausea, vomiting, insomnia, acne, increased body hair.

Piroxicam (NSAID)

Has a long duration of action and is used to relieve the symptoms of adult and juvenile rheumatoid arthritis, acute gout, osteoarthritis and acute musculoskeletal disorders.

Side-effects: gastrointestinal upset.

Pizotifen (antimigraine)

Inhibits the action of histamine and serotonin on blood vessels in the brain and is used in the prevention of vascular headache including classical and common migraines and cluster headache.

Side-effects: increased appetite, weight gain, drowsiness.

Pravastatin (statin)

Lowers LDL cholesterol and is prescribed for those who have not responded to diet and lifestyle modification to protect them from cardiovascular disease.
Side-effects: mild: gastrointestinal upset, headache, fatigue, rarely myositis.

Prednisolone (corticosteroid)

In high doses it is used to suppress inflammatory and allergic disorders, e.g. asthma, eczema, inflammatory bowel disease, rheumatoid arthritis. Also used as an immunosuppressant following organ transplant and to treat leukaemia. It is used in lower doses for replacement therapy in adrenal deficiency, though cortisol (hydrocortisone) is preferred.
Side-effects: indigestion, acne, increased body hair, moon-face, hypertension, weight gain/oedema, impaired glucose tolerance, cataract, glaucoma, osteoporosis, peptic ulcer, candida, adrenal suppression.

Propofol (IV anaesthetic)

Used to induce and maintain anaesthesia. Also used as a sedative on ITU and during investigative procedures.
Side-effects: hypotension, tremor.

Propranolol (β-blocker)

Used to treat hypertension, angina, arrhythmias, hyperthyroidism, migraine, anxiety and for prophylaxis after myocardial infarction.
Side-effects: fatigue, cold peripheries, bronchoconstriction, bradycardia, heart failure, hypotension, gastrointestinal upset, sleep disturbances.

Quinine (antimalarial)

Used for the treatment of malaria. Also used to prevent nocturnal leg cramps.
Side-effects: tinnitus, headache, blurred vision, confusion, gastrointestinal upset, rash, blood disorders.

Raloxifene (selective oestrogen receptor modulator (SERM))

Used to prevent vertebral fractures in postmenopausal women at increased risk of osteoporosis.

Side-effects: hot flushes, leg cramps, peripheral oedema, venous thromboembolism, thrombophlebitis.

Ramipril (ACE inhibitor)

As a vasodilator it is used to treat hypertension and congestive heart failure. Also used following myocardial infarction.
Side-effects: nausea, dizziness, headache, cough, dry mouth, taste disturbance.

Repaglinide (meglitinide)

Oral, short-acting, antidiabetic drug that lowers blood glucose levels after eating. Used to treat type II diabetes mellitus.
Side-effects: gastrointestinal upset.

Rifampicin (antituberculous agent)

Antibacterial used to treat tuberculosis, leprosy and other serious infections such as Legionnaires' disease and osteomyelitis. Used as a prophylactic against meningococcal meningitis and *Haemophilus influenzae* (type b) infection.
Side-effects: red-orange-coloured tears and urine.

Riluzole (no classification)

Used to extend life or delay mechanical ventilation in patients with motor neurone disease.
Side-effects: gastrointestinal upset, headache, dizziness, weakness.

Risperidone (antipsychotic)

Used for acute psychiatric disorders and long-term psychotic illness such as schizophrenia.
Side-effects: insomnia, agitation, anxiety, headache, weight gain, postural hypotension, mild extrapyramidal symptoms (e.g. parkinsonian symptoms).

Rivastigmine (anticholinesterase)

Inhibits the breakdown of acetylcholine. Used to improve cognitive function in mild to moderate dementia due to Alzheimer's disease, although the underlying disease process is not altered.
Side-effects: weakness, weight loss, dizziness, gastrointestinal upset, drowsiness, tremor, confusion, depression.

Salbutamol (β_2 agonist)

A bronchodilator, it is used to relieve asthma, chronic bronchitis and emphysema. It is also used in premature labour to relax uterine muscle.
Side-effects: tremor, tachycardia, anxiety, nervous tension, restlessness.

Salmeterol (β_2 agonist)

A bronchodilator that is used to treat asthma and bronchospasms. It is longer-acting than salbutamol and so is useful in preventing nocturnal asthma. It should not be used to relieve acute asthma attacks as it has a slow onset of effect.
Side-effects: fine tremors, especially in the hands.

Saquinavir (antiretroviral – protease inhibitor)

Used to treat HIV infection in combination with other antiretroviral drugs.
Side-effects: gastrointestinal upset, anorexia, hepatic dysfunction, pancreatitis, blood disorders, sleep disturbances, fatigue, headache, dizziness, paraesthesia, myalgia, myositis, taste disturbance, rash, itching, anaphylaxis, peripheral neuropathy and mouth ulcers.

Senna (stimulant laxative)

Used to treat constipation by increasing the response of the colon to normal stimuli.
Side-effects: abdominal cramps, diarrhoea.

Simvastatin (statin)

Lowers LDL cholesterol and is prescribed for those who have not responded to diet and lifestyle modification to protect them from cardiovascular disease.
Side-effects: mild: gastrointestinal upset, headache, fatigue, rarely myositis.

Sodium aurothiomalate (gold salt)

Used in the treatment of active progressive rheumatoid arthritis and juvenile arthritis with the aim of suppressing the disease process.
Side-effects: mouth ulcers, proteinuria, skin reactions, blood disorders.

Sodium cromoglicate (mast cell inhibitor)

Used to prevent the onset of asthma and other allergic conditions. It has a slow onset of action and so is not useful in treating acute asthma. It is also used to prevent allergic conjunctivitis, allergic rhinitis and for food allergies.
Side-effects: cough, hoarseness, throat irritation, bronchospasm.

Sodium valproate (antiepileptic)

Used to treat all types of epilepsy.
Side-effects: nausea, vomiting, weight gain.

Streptokinase (fibrinolytic agent)

An enzyme that dissolves blood clots by acting on the fibrin contained within it. Due to its fast-acting nature it is useful in treating acute myocardial infarction. Also used to treat a number of thromboembolic events such as pulmonary embolism and thrombosed arteriovenous shunts.
Side-effects: excessive bleeding, hypotension, nausea, vomiting, allergic reactions.

Sulfasalazine (aminosalicylate)

Used as an anti-inflammatory to treat ulcerative colitis and active Crohn's disease. Also found to help in the treatment of rheumatoid arthritis.
Side-effects: nausea, vomiting, loss of appetite, headache, joint pain, abdominal discomfort, anorexia.

Sumatriptan ($5HT_1$ (serotonin) agonist)

Used to treat severe acute migraine and cluster headaches (subcutaneous injection only).
Side-effects: feeling of tingling/heat, flushing, feeling of heaviness/weakness, lethargy.

Tamoxifen (anti-oestrogen)

Used in the treatment of breast cancer (when the tumour is oestrogen-receptor positive) to slow the growth of a tumour and to prevent the recurrence of the cancer following surgical removal. Also used in the treatment of infertility due to failure of ovulation.
Side-effects: gastrointestinal upset, hot flushes, vaginal bleeding.

Tamsulosin (α-blocker)

Used to treat urinary retention due to benign prostatic hypertrophy by causing the urethral smooth muscle to relax.
Side-effects: dizziness, postural hypotension, headache, abnormal ejaculation, drowsiness, palpitations.

Temazepam (benzodiazepine)

Used as a short-term treatment for insomnia and as a premedication before surgery.
Side-effects: daytime drowsiness, dependence.

Terbutaline (β_2 agonist)

Acts as a bronchodilator and is used to treat and prevent bronchospasm associated with asthma, chronic bronchitis and emphysema.
Side-effects: nausea, vomiting, fine tremor, restlessness, anxiety.

Tetracycline (tetracycline antibiotic)

See antibiotics in 'Drug classes'.

Theophylline (methylxanthine)

Acts as a bronchodilator and is used to treat asthma, bronchitis and emphysema.
Side-effects: headache, nausea, vomiting, palpitations.

Thiopental (barbiturate)

Used to induce general anaesthesia, as well as reducing intracranial pressure in patients whose ventilation is controlled.
Side-effects: cardiovascular and respiratory depression.

Tibolone (hormone replacement therapy)

A synthetic steroid used as a short-term treatment for symptoms of menopause, especially hot flushes. Has both oestrogenic and progestogenic activity. Also used as a second-line preventative treatment for postmenopausal osteoporosis.
Side-effects: weight changes, dizziness, headache, dermatitis, gastrointestinal upset, increased facial hair, vaginal bleeding.

Timolol (β-blocker)

Used to treat hypertension, angina and for prophylaxis following myocardial infarction. Also commonly administered

as eye drops for glaucoma and occasionally given for the prevention of migraine.
Side-effects: see propranolol.

Tizandine (α_2-adrenoceptor agonist)

Acts centrally to reduce muscle spasticity associated with multiple sclerosis or spinal cord injury or disease.
Side-effects: drowsiness, fatigue, dizziness, dry mouth, gastrointestinal upset, hypotension.

Tolterodine (antimuscarinic)

Reduces unstable contractions of the bladder, thereby increasing its capacity. Used to treat urinary frequency, urgency and incontinence.
Side-effects: dry mouth and eyes, gastrointestinal upset, headache, drowsiness.

Tramadol (opioid analgesic)

Used to treat moderate to severe pain.
Side-effects: nausea, vomiting, dry mouth, tiredness, drowsiness, dependence.

Trazodone (antidepressant)

Used to treat depression and anxiety, particularly where sedation is required. Has fewer cardiovascular effects than tricyclic antidepressants and therefore commonly prescribed to the elderly.
Side-effects: drowsiness.

Trihexyphenidyl/benzhexol (antimuscarinic)

Blocks the action of the neurotransmitter acetylcholine and is used to reduce rigidity and tremor in younger patients with parkinsonism. Not useful for bradykinesia.
Side-effects: dry mouth/skin, constipation, blurred vision, retention of urine.

Vancomycin (glycopeptide antibiotic)

Administered intravenously for the treatment of serious infections caused by Gram-positive bacteria or in situations where patients are allergic to, or have failed to respond to other less toxic antibiotics such as penicillins or cephalosporins. Commonly used for MRSA infections and

endocarditis. Given orally exclusively for the treatment of gastrointestinal infections, notably pseudomembranous colitis caused by the *Clostridium difficile* organism.
Side-effects: nephrotoxicity, ototoxicity (damage to the auditory nerve), blood disorders.

Vecuronium (muscle relaxant)

Used as a muscle relaxant during surgical procedures and to facilitate tracheal intubation, it has an intermediate duration of action.
Side-effects: skin flushing, hypotension, bronchospasm are rare.

Verapamil (calcium channel blocker)

Used in the treatment of hypertension, angina of effort and supraventricular dysrhythmias.
Side-effects: constipation, headache, ankle swelling, nausea, vomiting.

Warfarin (oral anticoagulant)

Prevention and treatment of pulmonary embolism and deep vein thrombosis. Decreases the risk of transient ischaemic attacks as well as thromboembolism in people with atrial fibrillation and following artificial heart valve surgery.
Side-effects: haemorrhage, bruising.

Zalcitabine (antiretroviral – NRTI)

Prevents the replication of HIV and therefore the progression of AIDS by blocking the action of the reverse transcriptase enzyme. Usually used in combination with other antiretroviral drugs.
Side-effects: pancreatitis, peripheral neuropathy, headache, insomnia, gastrointestinal upset, fatigue, breathlessness, cough, blood disorders, rash, liver damage, oral and oesophageal ulcers.

Zidovudine (antiretroviral – NRTI)

Action, uses and side-effects similar to zalcitabine. Also used to prevent maternal–fetal HIV transmission.
Other side-effects: anaemia, myopathy, paraesthesia, taste disturbance, chest pain, impaired concentration, urinary frequency, itching, influenza-like symptoms.

Prescription abbreviations

Abbreviation	Latin	English
a.c.	ante cibum	before food
b.d.	bis die	twice a day
o.d.	omni die	daily
o.m.	omni mane	in the mornings
o.n.	omni nocte	at night
p.c.	post cibum	after food
p.r.n.	pro re nata	when required
q.d.s.	quater die sumendum	four times a day
q.q.h.	quaque quarta hora	every 4 hours
stat.	statim	immediately
t.d.s.	ter die sumendum	three times a day
t.i.d.	ter in die	three times a day

Further reading

BMA/RPSGB 2007 British National Formulary, 54th edn. British Medical Association and Royal Pharmaceutical Society of Great Britain, London

Bennett P N, Brown M J 2003 Clinical pharmacology, 9th edn. Churchill Livingstone, Edinburgh

Chatu S, Milson A, Tofield C 2000 Hands-on guide to clinical pharmacology. Blackwell Science, Oxford

Greenstein B, Gould D 2004 Trounce's Clinical pharmacology for nurses, 17th edn. Churchill Livingstone, Edinburgh

Henry J A 2007 BMA new guide to medicine and drugs, 7th edn. British Medical Association, London

MacConnachie A M, Hay J, Harris J, Nimmo S 2002 Drugs in nursing practice: an A–Z guide, 6th edn. Churchill Livingstone, Edinburgh

Rang H P, Dale M M, Ritter J M, Flower R 2007 Rang and Dale's pharmacology, 6th edn. Churchill Livingstone, Edinburgh

Volans G, Wiseman H 2006 Drugs handbook 2006, 27th edn. Palgrave Macmillan, Basingstoke

Appendices

Maitland symbols **318**

Grades of mobilization/manipulation **319**

Abbreviations **319**

Prefixes and suffixes **331**

Adult basic life support **336**

Paediatric basic life support **337**

Conversions and units **338**

Laboratory values **339**

Physiotherapy management of the spontaneously breathing, acutely breathless patient **342**

SECTION 7

Maitland symbols (Hengeveld & Banks 2005, with permission)

Peripheral joints

F	Flexion
E	Extension
Ab	Abduction
Ad	Adduction
↷	Medial rotation
↶	Lateral rotation
HF	Horizontal flexion
HE	Horizontal extension
HBB	Hand behind back
Inv	Inversion
Ev	Eversion
DF	Dorsiflexion
PF	Plantarflexion
Sup	Supination
P	Pronation
El	Elevation
De	Depression
Protr	Protraction
Retr	Retraction
Med	Medial
Lat	Lateral
OP	Overpressure
PPIVM	Passive physiological intervertebral movements
PAIVM	Passive accessory intervertebral movements
ULNT	Upper limb neural tests
LLNT	Lower limb neural tests
Q	Quadrant
Lock	Locking position
F/Ab	Flexion abduction
F/Ad	Flexion adduction
E/Ab	Extension abduction
E/Ad	Extension adduction
Distr	Distraction
↓	Posteroranterior movement
↑	Anteroposterior movement
→	Transverse movement in the direction indicated
↕	Gliding adjacent joint surfaces
⟼⟻	Compression
	Longitudinal movement:
Ceph	Cephalad
Caud	Caudad

Spine

	↓	Central posteroanterior (PAs) ↙with a Ⓛ inclination
	↑	Central anteroposterior pressures (Aps)
	↱	Unilateral PAs on Ⓛ < with a medial inclination
	↰	Unilateral APs on the Ⓛ
	←	Transverse pressure towards Ⓛ
	↺	Rotation of head, thorax or pelvis towards Ⓛ
	↷	Lateral flexion towards Ⓛ
	↔	Longitudinal movement (state cephalad or caudad)
	↴	Unilateral PAs at angle of Ⓡ 2nd rib
	↴	Further laterally on Ⓡ on 2nd rib
	↗	Unilateral APs on Ⓡ
CT	↑	Cervical traction in flexion
CT	↑	Cervical traction in neutral
IVCT	↗	Sitting
IVCT	↗	Lying
IVCT 10 3/0 15		Intermittent variable cervical traction in some degree of neck flexion, the strength of pull being 10 kg with a 3-second hold period, no rest period, for a treatment time lasting 15 minutes
LT		Lumbar traction
LT 30/15		Lumbar traction, the strength of pull being 30 kg for a treatment time of 15 minutes
LT crk 15/5		Lumbar traction with hips and knees flexed: 15 kg for 5 minutes
IVLT 50 0/0 10		Intermittent variable lumbar traction, the strength of pull being 50 kg, with no hold period and no rest period, for a treatment time of 10 minutes

Figure A.1 Maitland symbols.

Grades of mobilization/manipulation (Hengeveld & Banks 2005, with permission)

Grade I – a small amplitude movement performed at the beginning of the available range. Usually performed as a slow smooth oscillatory movement.

Grade II – a large amplitude movement performed within a *resistance-free* part of the available range. If performed near the beginning of the available range, it will be classified as a grade II−, and if taken deep into the range, yet still not reaching resistance, it will be classified as a grade II+

Grade III – a large amplitude movement performed into resistance or up to the limit of the available range. If the movement is carried firmly to the limit of the available range it is expressed as a grade III+ but if it nudges gently into the resistance yet short of the limit of the available range, it is expressed as a grade III−.

Grade IV – a small amplitude movement performed into resistance or up to the limit of the available range. Can be expressed as 4+ or 4− in the same way as grade III.

Grade V – a small amplitude, high velocity general movement performed usually, but not always, at the end of the available range.

Grade loc V – a small amplitude high velocity thrust localized to a single joint movement usually, but not always, at the end of the available range.

Reference

Hengeveld E, Banks K 2005 Maitland's peripheral manipulation, 4th edn. Butterworth Heinemann, Edinburgh

Abbreviations

AAA	abdominal aortic aneurysm
Ab	antibody
ABGs	arterial blood gases
ABPA	allergic bronchopulmonary aspergillosis
ACBT	active cycle of breathing technique
ACE	angiotensin-converting enzyme

ACT	activated clotting time
ACTH	adrenocorticotrophic hormone
AD	autogenic drainage
ADH	anti-diuretic hormone
ADL	activities of daily living
ADR	adverse drug reaction
AE	air entry
AEA	above elbow amputation
AF	atrial fibrillation
AFB	acid-fast bacillus
AFO	ankle–foot orthosis
Ag	antigen
AGN	acute glomerulonephritis
AHRF	acute hypoxaemic respiratory failure
AI	aortic insufficiency
AIDS	acquired immune deficiency syndrome
AKA	above knee amputation
AL	acute leukaemia
ALD	alcoholic liver disease
ALI	acute lung injury
AML	acute myeloid leukaemia
AP	anteroposterior
APACHE	acute physiology and chronic health evaluation
ARDS	acute respiratory distress syndrome
ARF	acute renal failure
AROM	active range of movement
AS	ankylosing spondylitis
ASD	atrial septal defect
ATN	acute tubular necrosis
AVAS	absolute visual analogue scale
AVF	arteriovenous fistula
AVR	aortic valve replacement
AVSD	atrioventricular septal defect
AXR	abdominal X-ray
BE	bacterial endocarditis/barium enema/base excess
BEA	below elbow amputation
BiPAP	bilevel positive airway pressure
BIVAD	biventricular device
BKA	below knee amputation

BM	blood glucose monitoring
BMI	body mass index
BO	bowels open
BP	blood pressure
BPD	bronchopulmonary dysplasia
BPF	bronchopleural fistula
bpm	beats per minute
BS	bowel sounds/breath sounds
BSA	body surface area
BSO	bilateral salpingo-oophorectomy
BVHF	bi-ventricular heart failure
Ca	carcinoma
CABG	coronary artery bypass graft
CAD	coronary artery disease
CAH	chronic active hepatitis
CAL	chronic airflow limitation
CAO	chronic airways obstruction
CAPD	continuous ambulatory peritoneal dialysis
CAVG	coronary artery vein graft
CAVHF	continuous arterial venous haemofiltration
CBD	common bile duct
CBF	cerebral blood flow
CCF	congestive cardiac failure
CCU	coronary care unit
CDH	congenital dislocation of the hip
CF	cystic fibrosis
CFA	cryptogenic fibrosing alveolitis
CHD	coronary heart disease
CHF	chronic heart failure
CI	chest infection
CK	creatine kinase
CLD	chronic lung disease
CML	chronic myeloid leukaemia
CMV	controlled mandatory ventilation/cytomegalovirus
CNS	central nervous system
CO	cardiac output
C/O	complains of
COAD	chronic obstructive airways disease
COPD	chronic obstructive pulmonary disease

CP	cerebral palsy
CPAP	continuous positive airway pressure
CPM	continuous passive movements
CPN	community psychiatric nurse
CPP	cerebral perfusion pressure
CPR	cardiopulmonary resuscitation
CRF	chronic renal failure
CRP	C-reactive protein
CSF	cerebrospinal fluid
CT	computed tomography
CTEV	congenital talipes equinovarus
CV	closing volume
CVA	cerebrovascular accident
CVP	central venous pressure
CVS	cardiovascular system
CVVHF	continuous veno-venous haemofiltration
CXR	chest X-ray
D&C	dilation and curettage
D/C	discharge
D/W	discussed with
DBE	deep breathing exercises
DDH	developmental dysplasia of the hips
DH	drug history
DHS	dynamic hip screw
DIB	difficulty in breathing
DIC	disseminated intravascular coagulopathy
DIOS	distal intestinal obstruction syndrome
DLCO	diffusing capacity for carbon monoxide
DM	diabetes mellitus
DMD	Duchenne muscular dystrophy
DN	district nurse
DNA	deoxyribonucleic acid/did not attend
DSA	digital subtraction angiography
DU	duodenal ulcer
DVT	deep vein thrombosis
DXT	deep X-ray therapy
EBV	Epstein–Barr virus
ECG	electrocardiogram
EEG	electroencephalogram

EIA	exercise-induced asthma
EMG	electromyography
ENT	ear, nose and throat
EOR	end of range
Ep	epilepsy
EPAP	expiratory positive airway pressure
EPP	equal pressure points
ERCP	endoscopic retrograde cholangiopancreatography
ERV	expiratory reserve volume
ESR	erythrocyte sedimentation rate
ESRF	end-stage renal failure
$ETCO_2$	end-tidal carbon dioxide
ETT	endotracheal tube
EUA	examination under anaesthetic
FB	foreign body
FBC	full blood count
FDP	fibrin degradation product
FET	forced expiration technique
FEV_1	forced expiratory volume in 1 second
FFD	fixed flexion deformity
FG	French gauge
FGF	fibroblast growth factor
FH	family history
FHF	fulminant hepatic failure
FiO_2	fractional inspired oxygen concentration
FRC	functional residual capacity
FROM	full range of movement
FVC	forced vital capacity
FWB	full weight-bearing
GA	general anaesthetic
GBS	Guillain–Barré syndrome
GCS	Glasgow Coma Scale
GH	general health
GIT	gastrointestinal tract
GOR	gastro-oesophageal reflux
GPB	glossopharyngeal breathing
GTN	glyceryl trinitrate
GU	gastric ulcer/genitourinary
H^+	hydrogen ion

[H^+]	hydrogen ion concentration
HASO	hip abduction spinal orthosis
Hb	haemoglobin
HC	head circumference
Hct	haematocrit
HD	haemodialysis
HDU	high dependency unit
HF	heart failure
HFCWO	high-frequency chest wall oscillation
HFJV	high-frequency jet ventilation
HFO	high-frequency oscillation
HFOV	high-frequency oscillatory ventilation
HFPPV	high-frequency positive pressure ventilation
HH	hiatus hernia/home help
HI	head injury
HIV	human immunodeficiency virus
HLA	human leukocyte antigen
HLT	heart–lung transplantation
HME	heat and moisture exchanger
HPC	history of presenting condition
HPOA	hypertrophic pulmonary osteoarthropathy
HR	heart rate
HRR	heart rate reserve
HT	hypertension
IABP	intra-aortic balloon pump
ICC	intercostal catheter
ICD	intercostal drain
ICP	intracranial pressure
ICU	intensive care unit
IDC	indwelling catheter
IDDM	insulin-dependent diabetes mellitus
Ig	immunoglobulin
IHD	ischaemic heart disease
ILD	interstitial lung disease
IM	intramedullary
IM/i.m.	intramuscular
IMA	internal mammary artery
IMV	intermittent mandatory ventilation
INR	international normalized ratio

IPAP	inspiratory positive airway pressure
IPPB	intermittent positive pressure breathing
IPPV	intermittent positive pressure ventilation
IPS	inspiratory pressure support
IRV	inspiratory reserve volume
IS	incentive spirometry
ITU	intensive therapy unit
IV/i.v.	intravenous
IVB	intervertebral block
IVC	inferior vena cava
IVH	intraventricular haemorrhage
IVI	intravenous infusion
IVOX	intravenacaval oxygenation
IVUS	intravascular ultrasound
JVP	jugular venous pressure
KAFO	knee–ankle–foot orthosis
KO	knee orthosis
LA	local anaesthetic
LAP	left atrial pressure
LBBB	left bundle branch block
LBP	low back pain
LED	light-emitting diode
LFT	liver function test/lung function test
LL	lower limb/lower lobe
LOC	level of consciousness
LP	lumbar puncture
LRTD	lower respiratory tract disease
LSCS	lower segment caesarean section
LTOT	long-term oxygen therapy
LVAD	left ventricular assist device
LVEF	left ventricular ejection fraction
LVF	left ventricular failure
LVRS	lung volume reduction surgery
MAP	mean airway pressure/mean arterial pressure
MAS	minimal access surgery
MCH	mean corpuscular haemoglobin
MC&S	microbiology, culture and sensitivity
MCV	mean corpuscular volume
MDI	metered dose inhaler

ME	metabolic equivalents/myalgic encephalomyelitis
MI	myocardial infarction
ML	middle lobe
MM	muscle
MMAD	mass median aerodynamic diameter
MND	motor neurone disease
MOW	meals on wheels
MRI	magnetic resonance imaging
MRSA	meticillin-resistant *Staphylococcus aureus*
MS	mitral stenosis/multiple sclerosis
MSU	midstream urine
MUA	manipulation under anaesthetic
MVO_2	myocardial oxygen consumption
MVR	mitral valve replacement
MVV	maximum voluntary ventilation
NAD	nothing abnormal detected
NAI	non-accidental injury
NBI	no bony injury
NBL	non-directed bronchial lavage
NBM	nil by mouth
NCPAP	nasal continuous positive airway pressure
NEPV	negative extrathoracic pressure ventilation
NFR	not for resuscitation
NG	nasogastric
NH	nursing home
NIDDM	non-insulin-dependent diabetes mellitus
NIPPV	non-invasive intermittent positive pressure ventilation
NITU	neonatal intensive care unit
NIV	non-invasive ventilation
NOF	neck of femur
NOH	neck of humerus
NP	nasopharyngeal
NPA	nasopharyngeal airway
NPV	negative pressure ventilation
NR	nodal rhythm
NREM	non-rapid eye movement
N/S	nursing staff
NSAID	non-steroidal anti-inflammatory drug

NSR	normal sinus rhythm
NWB	non-weight-bearing
OA	oral airway/osteoarthritis
OB	obliterative bronchiolitis
OD	overdose
O/E	on examination
OGD	oesophagogastroduodenoscopy
OHFO	oral high-frequency oscillation
OI	oxygen index
OLT	orthotopic liver transplantation
OPD	outpatient department
ORIF	open reduction and internal fixation
OT	occupational therapist
PA	pernicious anaemia/posteroanterior/pulmonary artery
P_ACO_2	partial pressure of carbon dioxide in alveolar gas
$PaCO_2$	partial pressure of carbon dioxide in arterial blood
PADL	personal activities of daily living
P_AO_2	partial pressure of oxygen in alveolar gas
PaO_2	partial pressure of oxygen in arterial blood
PAP	pulmonary artery pressure
PAWP	pulmonary artery wedge pressure
PBC	primary biliary cirrhosis
PC	presenting condition/pressure control
PCA	patient-controlled analgesia
PCD	primary ciliary dyskinesia
PCIRV	pressure-controlled inverse ratio ventilation
PCP	*Pneumocystis carinii* pneumonia
PCPAP	periodic continuous positive airway pressure
PCV	packed cell volume
PCWP	pulmonary capillary wedge pressure
PD	Parkinson's disease/peritoneal dialysis/postural drainage
PDA	patent ductus arteriosus
PE	pulmonary embolus
PEEP	positive end-expiratory pressure
PEF	peak expiratory flow
PEFR	peak expiratory flow rate
PEG	percutaneous endoscopic gastrostomy

PeMax	peak expiratory mouth pressure
PEP	positive expiratory pressure
PFC	persistent fetal circulation
PFO	persistent foramen ovale
PHC	pulmonary hypertension crisis
PID	pelvic inflammatory disease
PIE	pulmonary interstitial emphysema
PIF	peak inspiratory flow
PIFR	peak inspiratory flow rate
PiMax	peak inspiratory mouth pressure
PIP	peak inspiratory pressure
PMH	previous medical history
PMR	percutaneous myocardial revascularization
PN	percussion note
PND	paroxysmal nocturnal dyspnoea
POMR	problem-oriented medical record
POP	plaster of paris
PROM	passive range of movement
PS	pressure support/pulmonary stenosis
PTB	pulmonary tuberculosis
PTCA	percutaneous transluminal coronary angioplasty
PTFE	polytetrafluoroethylene
PTT	partial thromboplastin time
PVC	polyvinyl chloride
PVD	peripheral vascular disease
PVH	periventricular haemorrhage
PVL	periventricular leucomalacia
PVR	pulmonary vascular resistance
PWB	partial weight-bearing
QOL	quality of life
RA	rheumatoid arthritis/room air
RAP	right atrial pressure
RBBB	right bundle branch block
RBC	red blood cell
RDS	respiratory distress syndrome
REM	rapid eye movement
RFT	respiratory function test
RH	residential home
RhF	rheumatic fever

RIP	rest in peace
RMT	respiratory muscle training
R/O	removal of
ROM	range of movement
ROP	retinopathy of prematurity
RPE	rating of perceived exertion
RPP	rate pressure product
RR	respiratory rate
RS	respiratory system
RSV	respiratory syncytial virus
RTA	road traffic accident
RV	residual volume
RVF	right ventricular failure
SA	sinoatrial
SAH	subarachnoid haemorrhage
SALT	speech and language therapist
SaO_2	arterial oxygen saturation
SB	sinus bradycardia
SBE	subacute bacterial endocarditis
SCI	spinal cord injury
SDH	subdural haematoma
SG_{AW}	specific airway conductance
SH	social history
SHO	senior house officer
SIMV	synchronized intermittent mandatory ventilation
SLAP	superior labrum, anterior and posterior
SLE	systemic lupus erythematosus
SMA	spinal muscle atrophy
SN	Swedish nose
SOA	swelling of ankles
SOB	shortness of breath
SOBAR	short of breath at rest
SOBOE	short of breath on exertion
SOOB	sit out of bed
SpO_2	pulse oximetry arterial oxygen saturation
SpR	special registrar
SPS	single point stick
SR	sinus rhythm
SS	social services

ST	sinus tachycardia
SV	self-ventilating
SVC	superior vena cava
SVD	spontaneous vaginal delivery
SVG	saphenous vein graft
SVO_2	mixed venous oxygen saturation
SVR	systemic vascular resistance
SVT	supraventricular tachycardia
SW	social worker
T21	trisomy 21 (Down's syndrome)
TAA	thoracic aortic aneurysm
TAH	total abdominal hysterectomy
TAVR	tissue atrial valve repair
TB	tuberculosis
TBI	traumatic brain injury
$TcCO_2$	transcutaneous carbon dioxide
TcO_2	transcutaneous oxygen
TED	thromboembolic deterrent
TEE	thoracic expansion exercises
TENS	transcutaneous electrical nerve stimulation
TFA	transfemoral arteriogram
TGA	transposition of the great arteries
THR	total hip replacement
TIA	transient ischaemic attack
TKA	through knee amputation
TKR	total knee replacement
TLC	total lung capacity
TLCO	transfer factor in lung of carbon monoxide
TLSO	thoracolumbar spinal orthosis
TM	tracheostomy mask
TMR	transmyocardial revascularization
TMVR	tissue mitral valve repair
TOP	termination of pregnancy
TPN	total parenteral nutrition
TPR	temperature, pulse and respiration
TURBT	transurethral resection of bladder tumour
TURP	transurethral resection of prostate
TV	tidal volume
TWB	touch weight-bearing

Tx	transplant
U&E	urea and electrolytes
UAO	upper airway obstruction
UAS	upper abdominal surgery
UL	upper limb/upper lobe
URTI	upper respiratory tract infection
USS	ultrasound scan
UTI	urinary tract infection
V	ventilation
V_A	alveolar ventilation/alveolar volume
VAD	ventricular assist device
VAS	visual analogue scale
VATS	video-assisted thoracoscopy surgery
VBG	venous blood gas
VC	vital capacity/volume control
V_E	minute ventilation
VE	ventricular ectopics
VEGF	vascular endothelial growth factor
VER	visual evoked response
VF	ventricular fibrillation/vocal fremitus
V/P shunt	ventricular peritoneal shunt
V/Q	ventilation/perfusion ratio
VR	vocal resonance
VRE	vancomycin-resistant enterococcus
VSD	ventricular septal defect
V_T	tidal volume
VT	ventricular tachycardia
WBC	white blood count
WCC	white cell count
WOB	work of breathing
W/R	ward round

Prefixes and suffixes

Prefix/suffix	Definition	Example
adeno-	gland	adenoma
-aemia	blood	hyperglycaemia

Prefix/suffix	Definition	Example
-algia	pain	neuralgia
angio-	vessel	angiogram
ante-	before	antenatal
arteri-	artery	arteriosclerosis
arthro-	joint	arthroscopy
-asis	condition	homeostasis
atel-	imperfect	atelectasis
athero-	fatty	atherosclerosis
auto-	self	autoimmunity
baro-	pressure	barotrauma
bi-	two, twice or double	bilateral, biconcave
bili-	bile	bilirubin
-blast	cell	osteoblast
brachi-	arm	brachial artery
brady-	slow	bradycardia
carcin-	cancer	carcinogen
cardio-	heart	cardiology
carpo-	wrist	carpal tunnel
-centesis	to puncture	amniocentesis
cephal-	head	cephalad
cerebro-	brain	cerebrospinal fluid
cervic-	neck	cervical fracture
chol-	bile	cholestasis
chondro-	cartilage	chondromalacia
contra-	against	contraindicated
costo-	rib	costochondral junction
cranio-	skull	craniotomy
cryo-	cold	cryotherapy
cut-	skin	cutaneous
cyano-	blue	cyanosis
cysto-	bladder	cystoscopy

Prefix/suffix	Definition	Example
cyto-	cell	cytoplasm
dactyl-	finger	dactylomegaly
derm-	skin	dermatome
diplo-	double	diplopia
dors-	back	dorsum
dys-	difficult	dyspnoea
-ectasis	dilatation	bronchiectasis
ecto-	outside	ectoplasm
-ectomy	excision	appendectomy
encephalo-	brain	encephalitis
endo-	within	endochondral
entero-	intestine	enterotomy
erythro-	red	erythrocyte
extra-	outside	extrapyramidal
ferro-	iron	ferrous sulphate
gastro-	stomach	gastroenteritis
-genic	producing	iatrogenic
haem-	blood	haematoma
hepato-	liver	hepatectomy
hetero-	dissimilar	heterosexual
homo-	same	homosexual
hydro-	water	hydrotherapy
hyper-	excessive	hyperactive
hypo-	deficiency	hypoxaemia
iatro-	medicine, doctors	iatrogenic
idio-	one's own	idiopathic
infra-	beneath	infrapatellar
inter-	among	interrater
intra-	inside	intrarater
iso-	equal	isotonic
-itis	inflammation	tendinitis
laparo-	loins, abdomen	laparotomy

Prefix/suffix	Definition	Example
lipo-	fat	liposuction
-lysis	breakdown	autolysis
macro-	large	macrodactyly
mal-	bad, abnormal	malignant
-malacia	softening	osteomalacia
mammo-	breast	mammogram
mast-	breast	mastectomy
-megalo	enlarged	cardiomegaly
mening-	membranes	meninges
-morph	form or shape	ectomorph
myel-	spinal cord, marrow	myelitis
myo-	muscle	myotonic
naso-	nose	nasopharyngeal
necro-	death	necrosis
nephr-	kidney	nephritis
oculo-	eyes	monocular
-oid	resembling	marfanoid
oligo-	deficiency	oliguria
-oma	tumour	lymphoma
oophoro-	ovaries	oophorectomy
-opsy	examine	biopsy
-osis	state, condition	nephrosis
osseo-	bone	osseous
osteo-	bone	osteolysis
-ostomy	to form an opening	colostomy
oto-	ear	otalgia
-otomy	to make a cut	osteotomy
para-	beside	paraspinal
-penia	deficiency	thrombocytopenia
peri-	around	periosteum
phago-	eat, destroy	phagocytosis

Prefix/suffix	Definition	Example
pharyngo-	throat	pharyngoscope
-philia	love of	hydrophilia
phleb-	vein	phlebitis
-phobia	fear of	hydrophobia
-plasia	formation	hyperplasia
-plasty	moulding	rhinoplasty
-plegia	paralysis	hemiplegia
pneum-	breath, air	pneumothorax
-pnoea	breathing	dyspnoea
poly-	many	polymyositis
pseud-	false	pseudoplegia
pyelo-	kidney	pyeloplasty
reno-	kidneys	renography
retro-	behind	retrograde
rhino-	nose	rhinitis
-rrhagia	abnormal flow	haemorrhage
salping-	fallopian tube	salpingostomy
sarco-	flesh	sarcoma
sclero-	hardening	scleroderma
-scopy	examination	endoscopy
somat-	body	somatic
spondyl-	vertebrae	spondylosis
-stasis	stagnation	haemostasis
steno-	narrow	stenosis
-stomy	surgical opening	colostomy
supra-	above	suprapubic
syn-	united with	syndesmosis
tachy-	swift	tachycardia
thoraco-	chest	thoracotomy
thrombo-	clot	thrombolytic
-tomy	incision	gastrostomy
trans-	across	transection
-trophy	growth	hypertrophy

Prefix/suffix	Definition	Example
uro-	urine	urology
vaso-	vessel	vasospasm
veno-	vein	venography

Adult basic life support

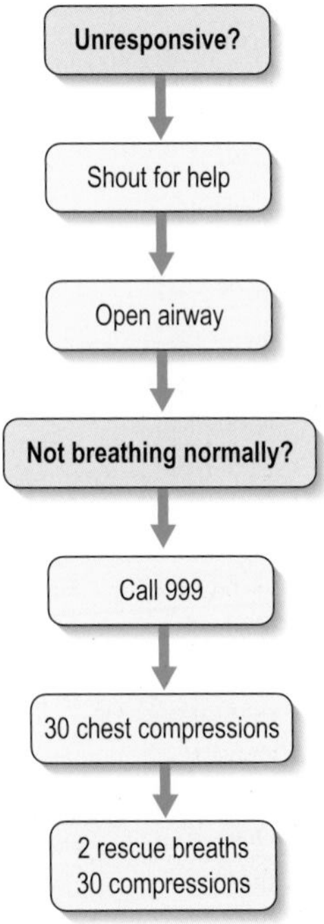
Unresponsive?
Shout for help
Open airway
Not breathing normally?
Call 999
30 chest compressions
2 rescue breaths
30 compressions

Figure A.2 Adult basic life support. (From the 2005 Resuscitation Guidelines, with permission of the Resuscitation Council UK; www.resus.org.uk.)

Paediatric basic life support

(Healthcare professionals with a duty to respond.)

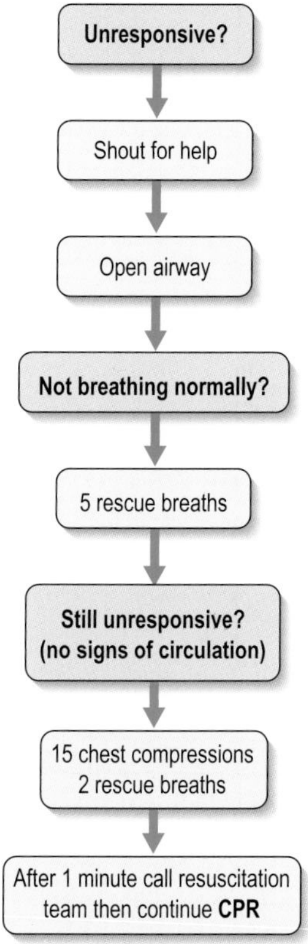
Unresponsive?
Shout for help
Open airway
Not breathing normally?
5 rescue breaths
Still unresponsive?
(no signs of circulation)
15 chest compressions
2 rescue breaths
After 1 minute call resuscitation
team then continue CPR

Figure A.3 Paediatric basic life support. (From the 2005 Resuscitation Guidelines, with permission of the Resuscitation Council UK.)

Conversions and units

Pounds/kg

lb	kg
1	0.45
2	0.91
3	1.36
4	1.81
5	2.27
6	2.72
7	3.18
8	3.63
9	4.08
10	4.54
11	4.99
12	5.44
13	5.90
14	6.35

Stones/kg

Stones	kg
1	6.35
2	12.70
3	19.05
4	25.40
5	31.75
6	38.10
7	44.45
8	50.80
9	57.15
10	63.50
11	69.85
12	76.20

Stones	kg
13	82.55
14	88.90
15	95.25
16	101.60
17	107.95
18	114.30

Mass

1 kilogram (kg)	= 2.205 pounds (lb)
1 pound (lb)	= 454 milligrams (mg)
	= 16 ounces (oz)
1oz	= 28.35 grams (g)

Length

1 inch (in)	= 2.54 centimetres (cm)
1 metre (m)	= 3.281 feet (ft)
	= 39.37 in
1 foot (ft)	= 30.48 cm
	= 12 in

Volume

1 litre (L)	= 1000 millilitres (mL)
1 pint	≈ 568 mL

Pressure

1 millimetre of mercury (mmHg)	= 0.133 kilopascal (kPa)
1 kilopascal (kPa)	= 7.5 mmHg

Laboratory values

Biochemistry

Alanine aminotransferase (ALT)	10–40 U/L
Albumin	36–47 g/L
Alkaline phosphatase	40–125 U/L
Amylase	90–300 U/L

Aspartate aminotransferase (AST)	10–35 U/L
Bicarbonate (arterial)	22–28 mmol/L
Bilirubin (total)	2–17 mmol/L
Caeruloplasmin	150–600 mg/L
Calcium	2.1–2.6 mmol/L
Chloride	95–105 mmol/L
Cholesterol (total)	Desirable level <5.2 mmol/L
Cholesterol (HDL)	
Men	0.5–1.6 mmol/L
Women	0.6–1.9 mmol/L
Copper	13–24 mmol/L
Creatine kinase (total)	
Men	30–200 U/L
Women	30–150 U/L
Creatinine	55–150 mmol/L
Globulins	24–37 g/L
Glucose	3.6–5.8 mmol/L
Iron	
Men	14–32 mmol/L
Women	10–28 mmol/L
Lactate (arterial)	0.3–1.4 mmol/L
Lactate dehydrogenase (total)	230–460 U/L
Magnesium	0.7–1.0 mmol/L
Osmolality	275–290 mmol/kg
Phosphate (fasting)	0.8–1.4 mmol/L
Potassium (serum)	3.6–5.0 mmol/L
Protein (total)	60–80 g/L
Sodium	136–145 mmol/L
Transferrin	2–4 g/L
Urea	2.5–6.5 mmol/L
Vitamin A	0.7–3.5 mmol/L
Vitamin C	23–57 mmol/L
Zinc	11–22 mmol/L

Haematology

Activated partial thromboplastin time (APTT)	30–40 s
Bleeding time (Ivy)	2–8 min

Erythrocyte sedimentation rate (ESR)	
Adult men	1–10 mm/h
Adult women	3–15 mm/h
Fibrinogen	1.5–4.0 g/L
Folate (serum)	4–18 mg/L
Haemoglobin	
Men	130–180 g/L (13–18 g/dL)
Women	115–165 g/L (11.5–16.5 g/dL)
International normalized ratio (INR)	0.89–1.10
Mean cell haemoglobin (MCH)	27–32 pg
Mean cell haemoglobin concentration (MCHC)	30–35 g/dL
Mean cell volume (MCV)	78–95 fL
Packed cell volume (PCV or haematocrit)	
Men	0.40–0.54 (40–54%)
Women	0.35–0.47 (35–47%)
Platelets (thrombocytes)	$150–400 \times 10^9$/L
Prothrombin time (PT)	12–16 s
Red cells	
Men	$4.5–6.5 \times 10^{12}$/L
Women	$3.85–5.30 \times 10^{12}$/L
White cell count (leukocytes)	$4.0–11.0 \times 10^9$/L

Values vary from laboratory to laboratory, depending on testing methods used. These reference ranges should be used as a guide only. All reference ranges apply to adults only; they may differ in children.

Physiotherapy management of the spontaneously breathing, acutely breathless patient

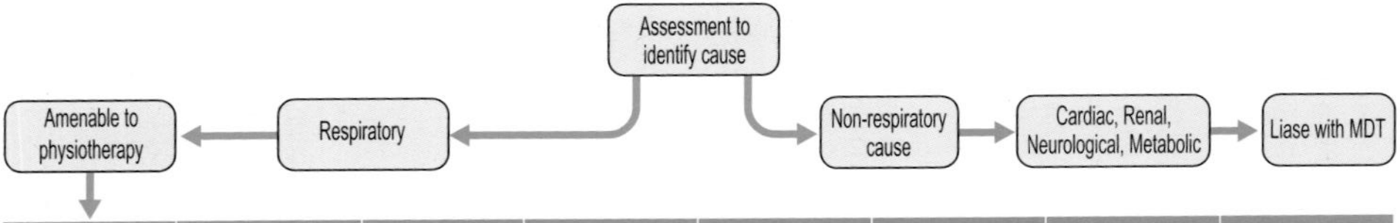
Assessment to identify cause
Respiratory
Amenable to physiotherapy
Non-respiratory cause
Cardiac, Renal, Neurological, Metabolic
Liase with MDT

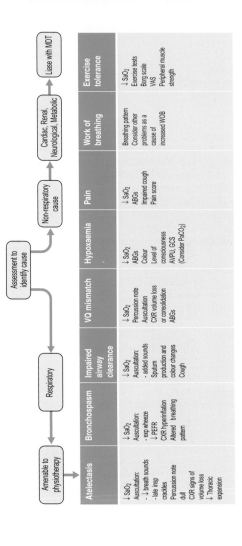

Atelectasis	Bronchospasm	Impaired airway clearance	VQ mismatch	Hypoxaemia	Pain	Work of breathing	Exercise tolerance
↓ SaO_2 Auscultation: - ↓ breath sounds - late insp crackles Percussion note dull CXR signs of volume loss ↓ Thoracic expansion	↓ SaO_2 Auscultation: - exp wheeze ↓ PEFR CXR hyperinflation Altered breathing pattern	↓ SaO_2 Auscultation: - added sounds Sputum production and colour changes Cough	↓ SaO_2 Percussion note Auscultation CXR volume loss or consolidation ABGs	↓ SaO_2 ABGs Colour Level of consciousness AVPU, GCS (Consider $PaCO_2$)	↓ SaO_2 ABGs Impaired cough Pain score	Breathing pattern Consider other problems as a cause of increased WOB	↓ SaO_2 Exercise tests Borg scale VAS Peripheral muscle strength

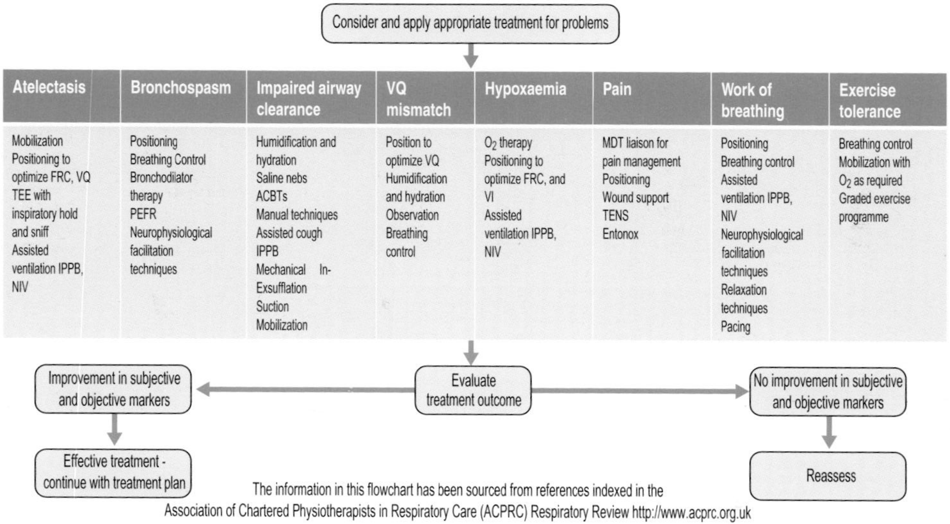

Consider and apply appropriate treatment for problems
Atelectasis
Mobilization
Positioning to optimize FRC, VQ
TEE with inspiratory hold and sniff
Assisted ventilation IPPB, NIV
Bronchospasm
Positioning
Breathing Control
Bronchodilator therapy
PEFR
Neurophysiological facilitation techniques
Impaired airway clearance
Humidification and hydration
Saline nebs
ACBTs
Manual techniques
Assisted cough
IPPB
Mechanical In-Exsufflation
Suction
Mobilization
VQ mismatch
Position to optimize VQ
Humidification and hydration
Observation
Breathing control
Hypoxaemia
O_2 therapy
Positioning to optimize FRC, and VI
Assisted ventilation IPPB, NIV
Pain
MDT liaison for pain management
Positioning
Wound support
TENS
Entonox
Work of breathing
Positioning
Breathing control
Assisted ventilation IPPB, NIV
Neurophysiological facilitation techniques
Relaxation techniques
Pacing
Exercise tolerance
Breathing control
Mobilization with O_2 as required
Graded exercise programme
Evaluate treatment outcome
Improvement in subjective and objective markers
Effective treatment - continue with treatment plan
No improvement in subjective and objective markers
Reassess
The information in this flowchart has been sourced from references indexed in the Association of Chartered Physiotherapists in Respiratory Care (ACPRC) Respiratory Review http://www.acprc.org.uk

Figure A.4 Physiotherapy management of the spontaneously breathing, acutely breathless patient. (Used with kind permission of the Association of Chartered Physiotherapists in Respiratory Care.)

Index

A

Abbreviations, 319–331
prescriptions, 316
Abducens nerve, 181
Abduction tests *see* Valgus stress tests
Abductor digiti minimi (foot), 57
Abductor digiti minimi (hand), 57
Abductor hallucis, 57
Abductor pollicis brevis, 58
Abductor pollicis longus, 58
Abscess, lung, 260
Acalculia, 187
Accessory nerve, 182
ACE (angiotensin-converting enzyme) inhibitors, 286, 293–294, 298, 303, 310
Acetylcysteine, 289–290
Aciclovir, 290
Acid-base disorders, 208–210
Acidosis, 208–209
Acquired immune deficiency syndrome (AIDS), 246–247
see also Antiretrovirals
Activated partial thromboplastin time, 231, 340
Active compression test, shoulder, 115
Active cycle of breathing technique, 235
Acute breathlessness, physiotherapy management, 342–343
Acute respiratory distress syndrome (ARDS), 246
Adduction tests *see* Varus stress tests
Adductor brevis, 58
trigger point, 94
Adductor hallucis, 58
Adductor longus, 58
Adductor magnus, 58–59
trigger point, 94
Adductor pollicis, 59
Adenosine, 290
Adhesive capsulitis, 246
Adrenaline, 290
Adson's manoeuvre, 129–130
Afterload, heart, 218
Agnosia, 187
Agraphia, 187
AIDS *see* Acquired immune deficiency syndrome
Airway
impaired clearance, 342, 343
suction, 235–236
Akinesia, 187
Alanine aminotransferase, 339
Albumin, 225, 339
Alendronate, 290
Alexia, 187
Alfentanil, 290–291
Alkaline phosphatase, 339
Alkalosis, 208–209, 210

Allopurinol, 291
α_2-adrenoceptor agonists, 295, 314
Alzheimer's disease, 247
  donepezil, 297
Aminoglycosides, 286
Aminophylline, 291
Amiodarone, 291
Amitriptyline, 291
Amlodipine, 291
Amnesia, 187
Amoxicillin, 286
Ampicillin, 286
Amusia, 187
Amylase, 339
Amyotrophic lateral sclerosis, 262
Anaesthesia
  intravenous, 302, 309
  local, 303
Analgesics, 286
Anatomical planes and directions, 2
Anconeus, 59
Angiotensin-II receptor antagonists, 304
Angiotensin-converting enzyme inhibitors, 286, 293–294, 298, 303, 310
Ankle joint, 26
  close packed positions and capsular patterns, 102
  fractures, Weber's classification, 113–114
  muscles listed by function, 56–57
  musculoskeletal tests, 129
  ranges of movement, 98
Ankylosing spondylitis, 247
Anomia, 187
Anosmia, 187
Anosognosia, 187
Anterior cerebral artery
  anatomy, 172
  lesions, 172–173
  territory, 169
Anterior drawer tests
  ankle, 129
  knee, 126
  shoulder, 115
Anterior slide test, shoulder, 115–116
Anteroposterior chest X-rays, 204
Anti-arrhythmics, 303
  amiodarone, 291
Antibiotics, 286
  ciprofloxacin, 295
  vancomycin, 314–315
Anticancer drugs, 301–302, 304
Anticholinergics, bronchodilators, 288
Anticholinesterases, 310
  donepezil, 297
Anticoagulants, 300, 315
Antidepressants
  fluoxetine, 299
  trazodone, 314
  tricyclic antidepressants, 291, 297, 301
Antidiuretic hormone, 254
Antiemetics, 286, 305
Antiepileptics (anticonvulsants), 287, 294, 299–300, 308, 312
Antimuscarinics, 292, 301, 302, 307, 314
Antipsychotics, 294, 300, 310
Antiretrovirals, 287, 296, 298, 301, 306, 311, 315
Antivirals
  aciclovir, 290

interferons, 301
Aphasia, 187
Apley scarf test, 117
Apley's test, knee, 126–127
Apprehension tests
knee (Fairbank's), 127
shoulder, 116
Arterial blood gases, 208–210
Arterial blood pressure, 215
Ascending tracts, spinal cord, 170
Ashworth scale, muscle tone, 192
Aspartate aminotransferase, 340
Aspirin, 292
Assist/control ventilation (ACV), 212
Astereognosis, 187
Asthma, 248
Ataxia, 187
Atelectasis, 342, 343
Atenolol, 292
Athetosis, 187
Atlanto-axial joint, 19
Atlanto-occipital joint, 19
Atorvastatin, 292
Atracurium, 292
Atrial fibrillation, 222–223
Atropine, 292
Auditory cortex
lesions, 177
primary, 168
Auscultation, lungs, 206–208
Axillary nerve, 31, 140, 144
Azathioprine, 292

B

Babinski reflex, 42, 190
Back
muscles, 5–7
pain, 154–160
Baclofen, 293
Baker's cyst, 248
Bamboo spine, 247
Barton's fracture, 111
Base excess, base deficit, 208, 210
Basic life support
adults, 336
paediatric, 337
Basilar artery, lesions, 174–175
Basophils, blood counts, 229
Beclometasone, 293
Beighton hypermobility score, 108–110
Bell's palsy, 248
Bendrofluazide, 293
Bendroflumethiazide, 293
Bennett's fracture, 112
Benserazide, 303
Benzhexol (trihexyphenidyl), 314
Benzodiazepines, 287–288, 296, 305
Benzylpenicillin, 286
β-blockers, 287, 292, 309, 313–314
Bicarbonate *see* HCO_3^-
Biceps brachii, 59
Biceps femoris, 59
see also Hamstring muscles
Biceps load tests, shoulder, 116
Biguanides, 304
Bilevel positive airway pressure (BiPAP), 214
Bilirubin, 225, 340
Biochemistry, serum, 225–228, 339–340
Bisphosphonates, 290, 298–299
Bleeding time, 340

Blood *see* Haematology
Blood gases, 208–210
Blood pressure, arterial, 215
  mean, 217
Blue bloaters, 250
Bones
  foot, 28
  hand, 27
  mineral density, DEXA, 283
Boutonnière deformity, 248
Brachial plexus, 29, 139
Brachialis, 60
Brachioradialis, 60
Bradycardia
  ECG, 221
  rates, 216
Bradykinesia, 187
Bradypnoea, respiratory rate, 218
Brain, 166–169
Breath sounds, 206
  reduced, 206
Breathlessness, physiotherapy management, 342–343
Brittle bone disease, 264
Broca's dysphasia, 171, 248–249
Bronchi
  anatomy, 199
  chest X-rays, 205
Bronchial breath sounds, 206
Bronchiectasis, 249
Bronchiolitis, 249
Bronchitis, 249–250
Bronchodilators, 288
Bronchospasm, 342, 343
  chest auscultation, 207
Brown-Séquard syndrome, 250
Brush test, 127
Budesonide, 293
Bulbar palsy, 250
  progressive, 262
  see also Pseudobulbar palsy
Bursitis, 250

C

C-reactive protein, 225
Caeruloplasmin, 340
Cafaclor, 286
Calcaneal branch of medial plantar nerve, 36
Calcitonin, 293
Calcium, 226, 340
Calcium channel blockers, 288, 291, 297, 306, 315
Calf, muscles, 16–18
Capsular patterns of joints, 101–102
Capsulitis, glenohumeral joint, 246
Captopril, 293–294
Carbamazepine, 294
Carbidopa, 303
Carbon dioxide, arterial tension *see* $PaCO_2$
Carbonic anhydrase inhibitors, 288, 289
Cardiac glycosides, 289, 296
Cardiac index, 215
Cardiac output, 215
Cardiophrenic angle, 206
Carpal tunnel syndrome, 250
Cauda equina syndrome, 155
Causalgia, 252
Cefaclor, 286
Cefotaxime, 286
Cefuroxime, 286
Celecoxib, 294
Central venous pressure, 216
Cephalosporins, 286
Cerebellum

function tests, 189, 191
lesions, 179
Cerebral arteries
lesions, 171–174
territories, 169
Cerebral hemispheres, 166–169
lesions, 175–177
Cerebral palsy, 250–251
Cerebral perfusion pressure, 216
Cerebrovascular lesions, 171–175
see also Strokes
Cervical spine
close packed position and capsular pattern, 101
injury, functional implications, 184–186
musculoskeletal tests, 115
Charcot–Marie–Tooth disease, 251
Chest
examination, 206–208
muscles, 8–9
physiotherapy, 232–237
X-rays, 203–206
Chloride, 340
Chlorpromazine, 294
Cholesterol, 340
Chondromalacia patellae, 251
McConnell test, 128
Chorea, 187
Choreoathetosis, 251
Chronic bronchitis, 249–250
Chronic fatigue syndrome, 251
Chronic obstructive pulmonary disease (COPD), 251–252
Ciclosporin, 294–295
Cimetidine, 295
Ciprofloxacin, 295
Claw toe, 252
Clomipramine, 295
Clonidine, 295
Clonus, 41, 42, 187
Close packed positions of joints, 101–102
Clotting, tests, 230–231
Club foot, 278
Clunk test, shoulder, 116
Coccydynia, 252
Codeine phosphate, 295
Colles' fracture, 111
Common peroneal nerve, 35, 36, 151, 153
Compartment syndrome, 252
Compensation issues, back pain, 157
Complex regional pain syndrome, 252–253
Compression tests
active, shoulder, 115
pelvis, 123
Computed tomography, 281–282
Conduction system, heart, 218–219
Conduction velocity, nerves, 284
Continuous positive airway pressure (CPAP), ventilation, 213–214
Contractility, heart, 218
Controlled mechanical ventilation (CMV), 212
Conversion disorder, 253
Conversions between metric and imperial units, 338–339
Copper, 340
Coracobrachialis, 60
Corticosteroids, 288, 293, 295–296, 300, 309
Costophrenic angle, 206

Coxa vara, 253
Crackles, chest auscultation, 207
Cranial nerves, 179–182
Crank test, shoulder, 116–117
Creatine kinase, 226, 340
Creatinine, 226, 340
Cromoglicate (of sodium), 312
Crossed-arm adduction test, 117
Cubital tunnel syndrome, 253
Cuffs, tracheostomy tubes, 238–239
Cutaneous distribution, nerves
  dermatomes, 39
  foot, 38
  lower limb, 38
  upper limb, 37
Cystic fibrosis, 253–254

D

De Quervain's tenosynovitis, 121, 278
Deep peroneal nerve, 35, 152, 153
Deep vein thrombophlebitis, Homan's test, 130
Deltoid, 60
Dermatomes, 39
Dermatomyositis, 269
Descending tracts, spinal cord, 170
Developmental dysplasia of hip, 254
Dexamethasone, 295–296
DF118 (dihydrocodeine), 296–297
Diabetes insipidus, 254
Diabetes mellitus, 254
Diaphragm, 60–61
  chest X-ray, 206
  surface markings, 199
Diazepam, 296
Diclofenac, 296
Didanosine, 296
Diffuse idiopathic skeletal hyperostosis (DISH), 255
Digoxin, 289, 296
Dihydrocodeine, 296–297
Diltiazem, 297
Diplopia, 187
Disability, back pain and, 159–160
Distraction test
  cervical spine, 115
  see also Gapping test
Diuretics, 288–289, 304
  loop diuretics, 288, 289, 299
  thiazide diuretics, 288, 289, 293
Dobutamine, 289, 297
Donepezil, 297
Dopamine, 289, 297
Dopamine antagonists, 305
Dopamine precursor, 303
Dornase alfa, 297
Dorsal interossei (foot and hand), 61
Dosulepin (dothiepin), 297
Double lumen tubes, tracheostomy, 239
Doxapram, 298
Drop test, shoulder, 117
Drug history, 161
Dual energy X-ray absorptiometry (DEXA), 283
Duchenne muscular dystrophy, 263

Dull percussion, chest, 208
Dupuytren's contracture, 255
Dysaesthesia, 187
Dysarthria, 188
Dysdiadochokinesia, 188, 191
Dysmetria, 188
Dysphagia, 188
Dysphasia, 171, 188
  Broca's, 171, 248–249
  Wernicke's, 171, 280
Dysphonia, 188
Dyspnoea, physiotherapy management, 342–343
Dyspraxia, 188
Dyssynergia, 188
Dystonia, 188

E

ECGs (electrocardiography), 218
Ectopics, ventricular, 223
Efavirenz, 298
Ehlers–Danlos syndrome (EDS), 255
Elbow joint, 21
  close packed position and capsular pattern, 101
  muscles listed by function, 55
  musculoskeletal tests, 120–121
  ranges of movement, 97
Electrocardiography (ECG), 218
Electroencephalography (EEG), 283
Electromyography, 284
Emotional factors, back pain, 157–158
Emphysema, 255–256
Emphysema (surgical), 204
Empty can test, 119
Empyema, 256
Enalapril, 298
Endotracheal tube, correct position, 205
Enteropathic arthritis, 256
Eosinophils, blood counts, 229
Epicondylitis
  lateral, 120, 278
  medial, 120, 257
Epinephrine (adrenaline), 290
Equinovarus deformity, 278
Erector spinae, 61
Erythrocyte sedimentation rate, 231, 341
Erythromycin, 286
Estradiol, 298
Etidronate, 298–299
Evoked potentials, 284
Examination (physical), 161–162
  chest, 206–208
  neurological, 189–192, 193–195
    cranial nerves, 180–181
  see also Subjective examination
Exercise, breathlessness and tolerance, 342, 343
Expansion exercises, thoracic, 235
Expiratory reserve volume (ERV), 201
Exposure, chest X-rays, 204
Extensor(s), forearm, 12
  trigger points, 91
Extensor carpi radialis brevis, 61
  trigger point, 91

Extensor carpi radialis longus, 61
trigger point, 91
Extensor carpi ulnaris, 62
trigger point, 91
Extensor digiti minimi, 62
Extensor digitorum, 62
Extensor digitorum brevis, 62
Extensor digitorum longus, 62
trigger point, 95
Extensor hallucis longus, 62–63
Extensor indicis, 63
trigger point, 91
Extensor pollicis brevis, 63
Extensor pollicis longus, 63
External oblique muscle, 63
External rotation lag sign, shoulder, 117
External rotation recurvatum test, 127
Exudates, pleural effusion, 267
Eye, cranial nerve tests, 180, 181

F

Faber's test, 124
Facial nerve, 181
Bell's palsy, 248
Fairbank's apprehension test, 127
Family history, 161
Femoral nerve, 35, 149, 154
Femoral shear test, 123
Femur, neck fractures, Garden classification, 112–113
Fenestrated tracheostomy tubes, 239
Fentanyl, 299
Ferrous sulphate, 299
Fibrinogen, 341
Fibrinolytic agents, 312
Fibromyalgia, 256
Finger–nose test, 189
Fingers
muscles listed by function, 55
musculoskeletal tests, 121–122
Finkelstein test, 121
FiO_2 (fractional inspired oxygen concentration), 211
First metacarpophalangeal joint, close packed position and capsular pattern, 102
Flat-back posture, 105, 107
Flexor(s), forearm, 11
Flexor carpi radialis, 63
Flexor carpi ulnaris, 64
Flexor digiti minimi brevis (foot and hand), 64
Flexor digitorum accessorius, 64
Flexor digitorum brevis, 64
Flexor digitorum longus, 65
trigger point, 96
Flexor digitorum profundus, 65
Flexor digitorum superficialis, 65
Flexor hallucis brevis, 65
Flexor hallucis longus, 65–66
trigger point, 96
Flexor pollicis brevis, 66
Flexor pollicis longus, 66
Fluoxetine, 299
Folate, 341
Foot
bones, 28
joints, close packed

positions and capsular patterns, 102
musculoskeletal tests, 129
nerves, cutaneous distribution, 38
Forced expiration technique, 235
Forearm, muscles, 11–12
trigger points, 91
Forestier's disease, 255
Fowler's sign, 119
Fractional inspired oxygen concentration (FiO_2), 211
Fractures, classifications, 110–114
Freiberg's disease, 256
Fremitus, vocal, 208
Froment's sign, 121
Frontal lobe, 166
lesions, 175–176
Frusemide (furosemide), 299
Functional residual capacity (FRC), 202
Furosemide, 299

G

Gabapentin, 299–300
Gag reflex, 181
Gait, examination headings, 195
Galeazzi fracture-dislocation, 111
Ganglion, 257
Gapping test, pelvis, 123
Garden classification, fractures of neck of femur, 112–113
Gastrocnemius, 66
trigger points, 96
Gemellus inferior, 66
Gemellus superior, 66
Gentamicin, 286
Gillet's test, 123
Glenohumeral joint, 20
adhesive capsulitis, 246
close packed position and capsular pattern, 101
see also Shoulder
Glicazide, 300
Globulins, 340
Glossopharyngeal nerve, 181
Glucose, 226, 340
Gluteal nerves, 36
Gluteus maximus, 67
Gluteus medius, 67
trigger points, 93, 94
Gluteus minimus, 67
Glyceryl trinitrate (GTN), 300
Glycopeptides, 286
Gold salts, 311
Golfer's elbow (medial epicondylitis), 120, 257
Gout, 257
allopurinol, 291
Gower's sign, 263
Gracilis, 67
Graphanaesthesia, 188
GTN (glyceryl trinitrate), 300
Guillain–Barré syndrome (GBS), 257

H

Haematocrit (packed cell volume), 230, 341
Haematology, 229–231, 340–341
Haemoglobin, 341
blood levels, 230
Haemoptysis, 212
Haemothorax, 257

Hallux valgus, 258
Haloperidol, 300
Hammer toe, 258
Hamstring muscles, trigger points, 95
Hand
bones, 27
joints, 22
muscles, 11–12
musculoskeletal tests, 121–123
Hawkins–Kennedy impingement test, 117
HCO_3^- (bicarbonate), 208, 209, 340
respiratory failure, 210
Head and neck, muscles listed by function, 54
Head-down position, 233–234
Hearing, testing, 181
Heart
chest X-ray, 205
conduction system, 218–219
monitoring, 215
Heart rate, 216
Heel–shin test, 189
Hemianopia, 188
Hemiballismus, 188
Hemiparesis, 188
Hemiplegia, 188
Heparin, 300
Herbert classification, scaphoid fractures, 112
Hereditary motor sensory neuropathy (HMSN), 251
Herpes zoster, 273
High dependency care units, charts, 240
High-frequency ventilation, 213
Hila (lungs), 205
Hip joint, 24
close packed position and capsular pattern, 101
developmental dysplasia, 254
muscles listed by function, 56
musculoskeletal tests, 124–125
ranges of movement, 97
History-taking, 160–161
HIV infection *see* Acquired immune deficiency syndrome
Hoffman reflex, 42, 189
Homan's test, 130
Homonymous (term), 188
Hormone replacement therapy, 298, 313
Hornblower's sign, 117
Horner's syndrome, 258
Hotchkiss modification of Mason's classification, radial head fractures, 111
Hughston plica test, 127
Humeroulnar joint, close packed position and capsular pattern, 101
Humerus, proximal fractures, Neer's classification, 110
Huntington's disease, 258
Hydrocortisone, 300
Hyoscine, 301
Hyper-resonant percussion, chest, 208
Hyperacusis, 188
Hypercalcaemia, 226
Hyperinflation, manual, 236
Hyperkalaemia, 228

Hypermobility, 260
Beighton score, 108–110
Ehlers–Danlos syndrome, 255
Hypernatraemia, 228
Hyperparathyroidism, 258
Hyperreflexia, 188
Hypertension, blood pressure level, 215
Hyperthyroidism, 259
Hypertonia, 188
Hypertrophy, 188
Hyperventilation syndrome, 259
Hypocalcaemia, 226
Hypoglossal nerve, 182
Hypokalaemia, 228
Hyponatraemia, 228
Hypotension, blood pressure level, 215
Hypothyroidism, 259
Hypoxaemia, 342, 343
Hypoxaemic respiratory failure, 210

I

Ibuprofen, 301
Iliacus, 67–68
Iliocostalis cervicis, 68
Iliocostalis lumborum, 68
Iliocostalis thoracis, 68
Iliopsoas trigger points, 92
Imaging, diagnostic, 281–283
Imipramine, 301
Immunosuppressants, 292, 294–295, 304
Imperial units, conversions to metric, 338–339
Impingement tests, shoulder, 117, 118
Indinavir, 301
Inferior gluteal nerve, 36
Inferior oblique muscle, 68
Inflammatory bowel disease, enteropathic arthritis, 256
Inflammatory disorders, spine, 156
Infraspinatus, 68
trigger points, 89
Inotropes, 289, 297, 302, 305
Inspiration, for chest X-rays, 204
Inspiratory capacity (IC), 202
Inspiratory reserve volume (IRV), 201
Insulin, 301
Intensive care units, charts, 240
Intention tremor, 189
Intercostal spaces, 205
Intercostales externi, 69
Intercostales interni, 69
Interferons, 301–302
Intermediate cutaneous nerve of the thigh, 35
Intermittent mandatory ventilation (IMV), 212
Intermittent positive pressure breathing (IPPB), 237
Internal oblique muscle, 69
International normalized ratio (clotting time measure), 231, 341
Interossei
dorsal (foot and hand), 61
palmar, 73
plantar, 74
Interspinales (muscles), 69
Interstitial lung disease, 259
Intertransversarii, 69
Intracranial pressure, 216–217

Intracranial pressure (*continued*)
raised, chest physiotherapy in, 236
Ipratropium bromide, 288, 302
Iron (serum), 340
Iron salts, 299
Isoprenaline, 302
Isosorbide mononitrate, 302

J

Jendrassik's manoeuvre, 41
Jerk test, shoulder, 117
Jet ventilation, high-frequency, 213
Joints
capsular patterns, 101–102
close packed positions, 101–102
position sense, 190
ranges of movement, 97–98
see also Hypermobility
Jones fracture, 260

K

Kaposi's sarcoma, 247
Kartagener's syndrome, 270
Ketamine, 302
Kinaesthesia, 188
Knee joint, 25
anterior drawer tests, 126
close packed position and capsular pattern, 101
muscles listed by function, 56
musculoskeletal tests, 126–129
range of movement, 98
slump knee bend, 137
Köhler's disease, 260
Kyphosis–lordosis posture, 105, 106

L

L-dopa, 303
Laboratory values, normal ranges, 339–441
Lachman's test, 127
Lactate, 340
Lactate dehydrogenase, 227, 340
Lactulose, 302
Lansoprazole, 302
Lateral collateral ligament, 25
Lateral cutaneous nerve of the calf, 35
Lateral cutaneous nerve of the thigh, 35
Lateral epicondylitis, 120, 278
Lateral plantar nerve, 36
Latissimus dorsi, 70
trigger points, 88
Laxatives, 302, 311
Leg, muscles, 15–18
Leg length test, 124
Length, units, conversions, 339
Levator scapulae, 70
trigger point, 86
Levodopa, 303
Levothyroxine, 303
Lidocaine, 303
Life support
adults, 336
paediatric, 337
Lift-off test, shoulder, 117–118
Ligamentous instability test, fingers, 121

Ligaments, grading of sprains, 114
Lignocaine (lidocaine), 303
Limbic lobe, 166
lesions, 177
Linburg's sign, 121–122
Lisinopril, 303
Lithium, 303
Load and shift test, shoulder, 118
Locked-in syndrome, 260
Long sitting test, 124
Longissimus capitis, 70
Longissimus cervicis, 70
Longissimus thoracis, 70
Longus capitis, 71
Longus colli, 71
Loop diuretics, 288, 289, 299
Loperamide, 303
Losartan, 304
Lower limb
muscles, 13–18
nerve root levels, 52–53
nerves
cutaneous distribution, 38
pathways, 35–36, 146–154
Lower motor neurone lesions, 183
reflexes, 41
Lumbar spine injury, functional implications, 185–186
Lumbosacral plexus, 30, 147
Lumbricals (foot and hand), 71
Lungs
abscesses, 260
bronchopulmonary segments, 200
capacities (function tests), 202
interstitial disease, 259
physiotherapy techniques, 232–237
pneumonia, 267–268
surface markings, 198–199
volumes (function tests), 201–202
see also Chest
Lunotriquetral ballottement, 122
Lymphocytes, blood counts, 229

M

Macrolides, 286
Magnesium, 227, 340
Magnetic resonance imaging, 282
Maitland symbols, 318
Mallet toe/finger, 261
Manipulation, grades, 319
Mannitol, 304
Manual chest clearance techniques, 234
Manual hyperinflation, 236
March fracture, 261
Marfan syndrome, 261
Mason's classification, radial head fractures, 111
Mass, units, conversions, 339
McConnell test, 128
McMurray test, 128
Mean arterial pressure, 217
Mean cell haemoglobin, 341
Mean cell haemoglobin concentration, 341
Mean cell volume, 341
Medial cutaneous nerve of the arm, 33
Medial cutaneous nerve of the forearm, 33

Medial cutaneous nerve of the thigh, 35
Medial epicondylitis, 120, 257
Medial plantar nerve, calcaneal branch, 36
Median nerve, 32, 141, 142, 145
  carpal tunnel syndrome, 250
Median nerve bias, neurodynamic test, 132
Mediastinum, shift on X-ray, 205
Medical Research Council, muscle power scale, 84
Meloxicam, 304
Meningitis, 261
Meningocele, 274
Metabolic acidosis, 209, 210
Metabolic alkalosis, 209, 210
Metacarpals, thumb, fractures, 112
Metformin, 304
Methotrexate, 304
Methyldopa, 304
Metoclopramide, 305
Metric units, conversions to imperial, 338–339
Mid-tarsal joint, close packed position and capsular pattern, 102
Midazolam, 305
Middle cerebral artery, 171
  lesions, 171–172
  territory, 169
Migraine
  pizotifen for, 308
  sumatriptan for, 312
Milrinone, 289, 305
Mini tracheostomy, 239
Minimal volume (lungs), 202
Miosis, 188
Mobile machines, chest X-rays taken with, 204
Mobilization, grades, 319
Monitoring, cardiorespiratory, 215
Monocytes, blood counts, 229
Monophonic wheeze, 207
Monteggia fracture-dislocation, 111
Morphine, 305
Morton's metatarsalgia, 261–262
Motor cortical areas, 168, 169
  lesions, 175, 176
Motor neurone disease, 262
Mucolytics, 289, 297
Multifidus, 71–72
Multiple sclerosis, 262–263
Muscle relaxants, 292, 293, 307, 315
Muscles
  anatomy, 3–18
  innervation *see* Myotomes
  listed alphabetically, 57–83
  listed by function, 54–57
  nerve root levels, 49–53
  posture, 103–107
  power scale, 84
  sprains, grading, 114
  tone
    Ashworth scale, 192
    examination headings, 194
Muscular dystrophy, 263
Musculocutaneous nerve, 34, 141, 144
Musculoskeletal tests, 114–130
Myalgic encephalomyelitis, 251
Myasthenia gravis, 263
Myelomeningocele, 275

Myositis ossificans, 263
Myotomes, 40, 49–53
see also Muscles, nerve root levels

N

Naloxone, 305
Naproxen, 305–306
Nasal cannula, FiO_2 levels, 211
Neck
muscles, 3–4
listed by function, 54
passive flexion (test), 136–137
see also Cervical spine
Neck of femur, fractures, Garden classification, 112–113
Neer impingement test, shoulder, 118
Neer's classification, proximal fractures of humerus, 110
Nelfinavir, 306
Nerve(s) *see* Peripheral nerves
Nerve conduction studies, 284
Nerve root levels, muscles, 49–53
Nerve root pain, 155
Neuroanatomy, 166–170
Neurodynamic tests, 130–137
precautions, 138
Neurology, 165–195
assessment, 192–195
examination, 189–192, 193–195
cranial nerves, 180–181
glossary, 187–189
Neutrophils, blood counts, 229
Nevirapine, 306
Nicorandil, 306
Nifedipine, 306
Nimodipine, 306
Nitrates, organic
glyceryl trinitrate (GTN), 300
isosorbide mononitrate, 302
Nitrous oxide, 306
Non-invasive ventilation (NIV), 214–215
Non-nucleoside reverse transcriptase inhibitors, 287, 298, 306
Non-steroidal anti-inflammatory drugs (NSAIDs), 289, 292, 294, 296, 301, 304, 305–306, 308
Noradrenaline, 307
Normal ranges, laboratory values, 339–441
Nucleoside reverse transcriptase inhibitors, 287, 296, 315
Nystagmus, 188

O

Ober's sign, 124
O'Brien test, 115
Obstructive sleep apnoea, 274
Obturator externus, 72
Obturator internus, 72
Obturator nerve, 35, 150, 153–154
Occipital lobe, 166
lesions, 177
Occupation, back pain and, 158–160

Oculomotor nerve, 180
Oestrogens, 298
Olfactory cortex, 168, 169
Olfactory nerve, 180
Omeprazole, 307
Ondansetron, 307
Opioids, 286, 290–291, 295, 296–297, 299, 305, 308, 314
Opponens digiti minimi, 72
Opponens pollicis, 72
Optic nerve, 180
Orphenadrine, 307
Oscillation ventilation, 213
Osgood–Schlatter disease, 264
Osmolality, serum, 340
Osmotic diuretics, 288, 289, 304
Osteoarthritis, 264
Osteochondritis, 264
Osteochondritis dissecans, 264
Osteogenesis imperfecta, 264
Osteomalacia, 265
Osteomyelitis, 265
Osteopenia, DEXA, 283
Osteoporosis, 265
  DEXA, 283
Oxybutynin, 307
Oxygen
  arterial tension (PaO_2), 208
  fractional inspired concentration (FiO_2), 211
  saturation (SpO_2), 217
  therapy, FiO_2 levels, 211
Oxytetracycline, 286

P

P wave (of ECG), 219
Packed cell volume, 230, 341
$PaCO_2$ (arterial carbon dioxide tension), 208, 209
  respiratory failure, 210
Paediatric basic life support, 337
Paget's disease, 265
Pain
  back, 154–160
  breathlessness with, 342, 343
Palmar interossei, 73
Palmaris longus, 73
Pancuronium, 307
PaO_2 (arterial oxygen tension), 208
Paracetamol, 308
Paraesthesia, 189
Paraphasia, 189
Paraplegia, 189
Parathyroid hormone, 258
Paresis, 189
Parietal lobe, 166
  lesions, 176
Parkinson's disease, 265–266
  levodopa for, 303
Paroxetine, 308
Passive neck flexion (test), 136–137
Past medical history, 161
Past pointing, finger–nose test, 189
Patrick's test, 124
Patte's test, 118
Pectineus, 73
Pectoralis major, 73
  trigger points, 87
Pectoralis minor, 73
  trigger point, 88
Pellegrini–Stieda syndrome, 266
Pelvis
  fractures, Tile classification, 112

musculoskeletal tests, 123–124
Penicillins, 286
Percussion
chest clearance, 234
chest examination, 208
Peripheral nerves
cutaneous distribution
foot, 38
lower limb, 38
upper limb, 37
see also Dermatomes
pathways, 139–154
lower limb, 35–36, 146–154
upper limb, 31–34, 139–146
Peritendinitis, 278
Peroneus brevis, 73–74
trigger point, 95
Peroneus longus, 74
trigger point, 95
Peroneus tertius, 74
Perthes' disease, 266
Pethidine, 308
PH of blood, 208–209
respiratory failure, 210
Phenytoin, 308
Phosphate, 227, 340
Phosphodiesterase inhibitors, 289, 305
Photophobia, 189
Physical examination, 161–162
Physiotherapy, techniques, 232–237
Piedallu's sign, 123
Pin prick test, 190
Pinch grip test, 120
Pink puffers, 256
Piriformis, 74
trigger points, 94
Piriformis syndrome, 266
Piriformis test, 125
Piroxicam, 308
Pizotifen, 308
Planes, cardinal, 2
Plantar fasciitis, 266–267
Plantar interossei, 74
Plantar nerves, 36
Plantar reflex, 42, 190
Plantaris, 74–75
Plateau fractures of tibia, Schatzker classification, 113
Platelet counts, 230, 341
Pleural effusion, 267
Pleural rub, 207
Pleurisy, 267
Pneumonia, 267–268
Pneumothorax, 268
Poliomyelitis, 268–269
post polio syndrome, 269–270
Polyarteritis nodosa, 269
Polymyalgia rheumatica, 269
Polymyositis, 269
Polyphonic wheeze, 207
Pons, lesions, 178
Popliteal bursa, Baker's cyst, 248
Popliteus, 75
'Portable' chest X-rays, 204
Position sense, joints, 190
Positioning of patient
lung physiotherapy, 232–234
raised intracranial pressure, 217
Positive-pressure ventilation, high-frequency, 213
Post polio syndrome, 269–270
Posterior cerebral artery, 173
lesions, 173–174
territory, 169

Posterior cutaneous nerve of the thigh, 36
Posterior drawer tests
knee, 128
shoulder, 118
Posterior interosseous nerve, 146
Posterior sag sign, 128
Posteroanterior chest X-rays, 204
Postural drainage, 232–234
Postures, 103–107
faulty alignment, 105–107
nursing for raised intracranial pressure, 217
see also Positioning of patient
Potassium, 228, 340
Potassium-sparing diuretics, 288
Power scale, muscles, 84
PR interval (of ECG), 220
Pravastatin, 309
Prednisolone, 309
Prefixes and suffixes, 331–336
Preload, heart, 218
Premature ventricular contractions, 223
Prescriptions, abbreviations, 316
Pressure, units, conversions, 339
Pressure-cycled SIMV, 213
Pressure support (PS), ventilation, 213
Primary ciliary dyskinesia, 270
Progressive bulbar palsy, 262
Progressive muscle atrophy, 262
Pronator quadratus, 75
Pronator teres, 75
trigger point, 92
Propofol, 309
Propranolol, 309
Proprioception, testing, 190
Prosopagnosia, 189
Protease inhibitors, 287, 301, 306, 311
Protein, total serum, 340
Prothrombin time, 230, 341
Proton-pump inhibitors, 302, 307
Provocation elevation test, 130
Prozac (fluoxetine), 299
Pseudobulbar palsy, 270
Psoas major, 75
Psoas minor, 75
Psoriatic arthritis, 270
Psychosocial yellow flags, back pain, 156–160
Ptosis, 189
Pulmonary artery pressure, 217
Pulmonary artery wedge pressure, 217–218
Pulmonary embolus, 270–271
Pulmonary oedema, 271
Pulses
heart rate, 216
locations, 43–44
Putamen, lesions, 178

Q

QRS complex (of ECG), 220
QT interval (of ECG), 220
Quadrant test, 125
Quadrantanopia, 189
Quadratus femoris, 76
Quadratus lumborum, 76

trigger points, 93
Quadriplegia, 189
Quinine, 309

R

Radial nerve, 31, 140, 143, 145–146
Radial nerve bias, neurodynamic test, 133
Radiocarpal joint, close packed position and capsular pattern, 101
Radiography *see* X-rays
Radionuclide scanning, 282–283
Radius, fractures, 111
Raloxifene, 309–310
Ramipril, 310
Ranges of movement
joints, 97–98
segmental, 99–100
Raynaud's phenomenon, 271
Reactive arthritis, 271
Reagan's test, 122
Rebreathing bag, manual hyperinflation, 236
Rectus abdominis, 76
Rectus capitis anterior, 76
Rectus capitis lateralis, 76
Rectus capitis posterior major, 76
Rectus capitis posterior minor, 77
Rectus femoris, 77
contracture test, 125
Red blood cell counts, 229, 341
Red flags, spine, 155–156
Reflex sympathetic dystrophy, 252–253
Reflexes, 40–42, 194
see also named reflexes
Reinforcement manoeuvres, reflexes, 40–41
Reiter's syndrome *see* Reactive arthritis; Seronegative spondyloarthropathies
Relocation test, shoulder, 119
Repaglinide, 310
Residual volume (RV), 201
Resonance, vocal, chest auscultation, 207
Resonant percussion, chest, 208
Respiratory acidosis, 209
Respiratory alkalosis, 209
Respiratory depression, naloxone for, 305
Respiratory distress syndrome, acute (ARDS), 246
Respiratory failure, 210
Respiratory rate, 218
Respiratory stimulants, doxapram, 298
Respiratory tract, 197–243
assessment, 240–242
Resuscitation *see* Basic life support
Retrolisthesis, 276
Reverse Phalen's test, 122
Reverse transcriptase inhibitors, 287, 296, 298, 306, 315
Rheumatoid arthritis, 271–272
Rhomboid major, 77
Rhomboid minor, 77
Rhomboideus, trigger points, 91
Rifampicin, 310
Riluzole, 310
Risperidone, 310
Rivastigmine, 310

Rolando's fracture, 112
Romberg's test, 191
Rotatores, 77

S

Sacral injury, functional implications, 186
Sacroiliac joint, 23
Salbutamol, 288, 311
Salcatonin, 293
Salmeterol, 311
Saphenous nerve, 35
Saquinavir, 311
Sarcoidosis, 272
Sartorius, 77
Scaleni, 78
  trigger points, 87
Scaphoid fractures, Herbert classification, 112
Scaphoid shift test, 122–123
Scapula, muscles, 10
  listed by function, 54
  see also named muscles
Schatzker classification, tibial plateau fractures, 113
Scheuermann's disease, 272
Sciatic nerve, 36, 146, 148
Scleroderma, 277
Segmental movement, ranges, 99–100
Segments, lungs, 200
Selective oestrogen receptor modulators, raloxifene, 309–310
Selective serotonin reuptake inhibitors, 299, 308
Semimembranosus, 78
  see also Hamstring muscles
Semispinalis capitis, 78
  trigger point, 85
Semispinalis cervicis, 78–79
  trigger points, 85
Semispinalis thoracis, 79
Semitendinosus, 79
  see also Hamstring muscles
Senna, 311
Sensory cortical areas, 168, 169
Sensory function, examination headings, 194
Septic arthritis, 272
Seronegative spondyloarthropathies, 272–273
Serratus anterior, 79
  trigger point, 88
Sever's disease, 273
Shaking, for chest clearance, 234
Shingles, 273
Shoulder
  adhesive capsulitis, 246
  muscles listed by function, 54–55
  musculoskeletal tests, 115–119
  ranges of movement, 97
  see also Glenohumeral joint
Sinding–Larsen–Johansson disease, 273
Single lumen tubes, tracheostomy, 239
Sinus rhythm, 221–222
Sitting flexion, 123
Situs inversus, 270
Sjögren's syndrome, 273–274
Sleep apnoea, 274
Slocum tests, 128, 129
Slump knee bend, 137
Slump test, 135–136
Smith's fracture, 111
Social history, 161
Sodium, 228, 340

Sodium aurothiomalate, 311
Sodium cromoglicate, 312
Sodium valproate, 312
Soleus, 79
trigger points, 96
Spasmodic torticollis, 279
Speed's test, 119
Spina bifida, 274–275
Spinal cord
injury, functional implications, 184–186
tracts, 170
Spinal muscular atrophies (SMA), 275
Spinal stenosis, 275
Spinalis, 79
Spine
ankylosing spondylitis, 247
nerve root pain, 155
ranges of segmental movement, 99–100
red flags, 155–156
Splenius capitis, 80
trigger point, 86
Splenius cervicis, 80
trigger point, 86
Spondyloarthropathies, seronegative, 272–273
Spondylolisthesis, 275–276
Spondylolysis, 276
Spondylosis, 276
Sprains, grading, 114
Spurling's test, 115
Sputum, 211–212
ST segment (of ECG), 220
Standing flexion (test), 124
Statins, 292, 309
Stereognosis, 189
Sternocleidomastoid, 80
cranial nerve test, 182
trigger points, 85
Straight leg raise (test), 136
Strains, muscles, grading, 114
Streptokinase, 312
Stroke volume, 218
Strokes, 276–277
Subjective examination, 160–161
neurological, 193
respiratory assessment, 240
Suboccipital trigger point, 85
Subscapularis, 80
trigger points, 90
Subtalar joint, close packed position and capsular pattern, 102
Suction, airway, 235–236
Sudeck's atrophy, 252–253
Suffixes and prefixes, 331–336
Sulcus sign, 119
Sulfasalazine, 312
Sulphonylureas, 300
Sumatriptan, 312
Superficial peroneal nerve, 152, 153
Superior gluteal nerve, 36
Superior oblique muscle, 80
Supinator, 81
trigger points, 92
Supine to sit test, 124
Supraspinatus, 81
Supraspinatus tendon tests, 117, 118, 119
Sural nerve, 36
Surface markings, lungs, 198–199
Surgical emphysema, 204
Swan–Ganz catheters, 217
Swan neck deformity, 277
Sway-back posture, 105, 106
Sweater finger sign, 122
Sympathomimetics, 302, 307
adrenaline, 290
bronchodilators, 288

Symptoms, subjective examination, 160–161
Synchronized intermittent mandatory ventilation (SIMV), 213
Systemic lupus erythematosus, 277
Systemic sclerosis, 277
Systemic vascular resistance, 218

T

T-scores, bone mineral density, 283
T wave (of ECG), 220
Tachycardia
  ECG, 222
  heart rate, 216
Tachypnoea, respiratory rate, 218
Talar tilt (test), 129
Talipes calcaneovalgus, 277
Talipes equinovarus, 278
Talocrural joint, close packed positions and capsular patterns, 102
Tamoxifen, 312
Tamsulosin, 313
Tarsal tunnel syndrome, 278
Temazepam, 313
Temperature sensation, testing, 191
Temporal lobe, 166
  lesions, 177
Temporomandibular joint, close packed position and capsular pattern, 101
Tendon reflexes, deep, 41
Tennis elbow (lateral epicondylitis), 120, 278
Tenosynovitis, 278
  de Quervain's, 121, 278
Tenovaginitis, 278
Tension pneumothorax, 268
Tensor fasciae latae, 81
  trigger points, 94
Terbutaline, 313
Teres major, 81
  trigger point, 90
Teres minor, 81
  trigger point, 90
Tetracyclines, 286
Tetraplegia, 189
TFCC load test, 122
Thalamic syndrome, 174
Thalamus, lesions, 178
Theophylline, 313
Thiazide diuretics, 288, 289, 293
Thigh, muscles, 13–14
Thiopental, 313
Thomas test, 125
Thompson's test, 129
Thoracic expansion exercises, 235
Thoracic outlet syndrome, 129–130, 278–279
Thoracic spine injury, functional implications, 185
THREAD (mnemonic), 161
Thumb
  metacarpal fractures, 112
  muscles listed by function, 56
Thyroid gland, disorders, 259
Thyroxine (levothyroxine), 303
Tibia, Schatzker classification of plateau fractures, 113

Tibial nerve, 36, 146–153, 151
Tibialis anterior, 81–82
  trigger point, 95
Tibialis posterior, 82
  trigger point, 96
Tibolone, 313
Tidal volume (V_T), 201
Tile classification, pelvis fractures, 112
Timolol, 313–314
Tinel's sign
  elbow, 120
  wrist, 122
Tizanidine, 314
Toes, muscles listed by function, 57
Tolterodine, 314
Tone, muscles
  Ashworth scale, 192
  examination headings, 194
Torticollis, 279
Total lung capacity (TLC), 202
Touch (light), test, 190
Trachea
  bifurcation, surface markings, 199
  X-ray, 205
Tracheostomies, 237–240
Tramadol, 314
Transferrin, 340
Transient ischaemic attacks, 277
Transudates, pleural effusion, 267
Transverse myelitis, 279–280
Transversus abdominis, 82
Trapezius, 82–83
  trigger points, 85, 86
Trazodone, 314
Trendelenburg's sign, 125
Triangular fibrocartilage complex load test, 122
Triceps brachii, 83
Tricyclic antidepressants, 291, 297, 301
Trigeminal nerve, 180
Trigeminal neuralgia, 280
Trigger finger, 278
Trigger points, sites, 85–96
Trihexyphenidyl, 314
Trochlear nerve, 180
Trunk muscles, 6–7
  listed by function, 54
Tuberculosis, 280
Two-point discrimination, 191

U

Ulna, fractures, 111
Ulnar nerve, 33, 141, 142, 144–145
  cubital tunnel syndrome, 253
Ulnar nerve bias, upper limb neurodynamic test, 134
Ultrasound, 283
Units, 338–339
Upper cutaneous nerve of the arm, 31
Upper limb
  muscles, 8–12
    nerve root levels, 49–51
  nerves
    cutaneous distribution, 37
    pathways, 31–34, 139–146
  neurodynamic tests, 130–135
Upper motor neurone lesions, 183, 189, 190
  reflexes, 41
Urea, 228, 340

V

Vagus nerve, 181
Valgus stress tests
  elbow, 121
  knee, 126
Valproate (of sodium), 312
Vancomycin, 286, 314–315
Varus stress tests
  elbow, 121
  knee, 126
Vascular resistance, systemic, 218
Vascular tests, 129–130
Vastus intermedius, 83
Vastus lateralis, 83
Vastus medialis, 83
Vecuronium, 315
Ventilation, mechanical, 212–215
Ventilatory failure, 210
Ventricular ectopics, 223
Ventricular fibrillation, 224
Ventricular tachycardia, 223–224
Verapamil, 315
Vertebral arteries, 174–175
Vestibulocochlear nerve, 181
Vibration sense, testing, 192
Vibrations for chest clearance, 234
Visual cortical areas, 168, 169
  lesions, 177
Vitamin A, 340
Vitamin C, 340
Voice sounds, chest auscultation, 207–208
Volkmann's ischaemic contracture, 252
Volume, units, conversions, 339
Volume-cycled SIMV, 213
VQ mismatch, breathlessness, 342, 343

W

Warfarin, 315
Watson test, 122–123
Weber–Barstow manoeuvre, 125
Weber's classification, ankle joint fractures, 113–114
Weber's syndrome, 174
Weight, units, conversions, 338–339
Werdnig–Hoffman disease, 275
Wernicke's dysphasia, 171, 280
Wheeze, chest auscultation, 207
White blood cell counts, 229, 341
Wohlfart–Kugelberg–Welander disease, 275
Wrist joint, 22
  close packed position and capsular pattern, 101
  muscles listed by function, 55
  musculoskeletal tests, 121, 122–123
  ranges of movement, 97

X

X-rays, 281
  chest, 203–206
  see also Dual energy X-ray absorptiometry

Y

Yellow flags, psychosocial, back pain, 156–160
Yergason's test, 119

Z

Zalcitabine, 315
Zidovudine, 315
Zinc, 340